Teaching
in the
Hospital

Books in the ACP Teaching Medicine Series

Theory and Practice of Teaching Medicine
Jack Ende, MD, MACP
Editor

Methods for Teaching Medicine
Kelley M. Skeff, MD, PhD, MACP
Georgette A. Stratos, PhD
Editors

Teaching in Your Office, A Guide to Instructing Medical Students and Residents, Second Edition
Patrick C. Alguire, MD, FACP
Dawn E. DeWitt, MD, MSc, FACP
Linda E. Pinsky, MD, FACP
Gary S. Ferenchick, MD, FACP
Editors

Teaching in the Hospital
Jeff Wiese, MD, FACP
Editor

Mentoring in Academic Medicine
Holly J. Humphrey, MD, MACP
Editor

Leadership Careers in Medical Education
Louis Pangaro, MD, MACP
Editor

Teaching Medicine Series

Jack Ende, MD, MACP
Series Editor

Teaching in the Hospital

Jeff Wiese, MD, FACP
Editor

ACP Press
American College of Physicians • Philadelphia, Pennsylvania

Director, Publishing Operations: Linda Drumheller
Developmental Editor: Marla Sussman
Production Editor: Suzanne Meyers
Publishing Coordinator: Angela Gabella
Cover Design: Kate Nichols
Index: Kathleen Patterson

Printed in the United States of America
Printing/Binding by Versa Press
Composition by ACP Graphic Services

Library of Congress Cataloging-in-Publication Data

Wiese, Jeff.
  Teaching in the hospital / Jeff Wiese.
      p. ; cm. -- (ACP teaching medicine series)
  Includes bibliographical references.
  ISBN 978-1-934465-44-8
  1. Hospitals--Medical staff--Study and teaching. 2. Medicine--Study and
teaching. I. American College of Physicians. II. Title. III. Series: ACP teaching
medicine series.
  [DNLM: 1. Medical Staff, Hospital. 2. Teaching--methods. 3. Education,
Medical--methods. WX 18 W651t 2010]
  RA975.T43.W54 2010
  362.11068'3--dc22
                                        2009053110

10 11 12 13 14 / 10 9 8 7 6 5 4 3 2

Contributors

Lorenzo DiFrancesco, MD
Associate Professor Medicine
Senior Associate Program Director
Emory University School of Medicine
Atlanta, Georgia

Jeffrey J. Glasheen, MD
Associate Professor
University of Colorado, Denver
Director, Hospital Medicine Program
University of Colorado Hospital
Denver, Colorado

Jeannette Guerrasio, MD
Assistant Professor of Medicine
University of Colorado Hospital
Denver, Colorado

Richard Kopelman, MD, FACP
Endicott Professor of Medicine
Tufts University School of Medicine
Vice Chairman of Medicine
Tufts Medical Center
Boston, Massachusetts

Kevin J. O'Leary, MD
Associate Program Director
Internal Medicine Residency and Unit
    Director
Associate Chief, Division of Hospital
    Medicine
Northwestern University Feinberg School
    of Medicine
Chicago, Illinois

Joseph Rencic, MD, FACP
Assistant Professor of Medicine
Tufts University School of Medicine
Associate Program Director, Internal
    Medicine
Tufts Medical Center
Boston, Massachusetts

Marianne Tschoe, MD
Assistant Professor
Northwestern University Feinberg School
    of Medicine
Chicago, Illinois

Jeff Wiese, MD, FACP
Professor of Medicine
Associate Dean of Graduate Medical
    Education
Tulane University Health Sciences Center
New Orleans, Louisiana

Neil Winawer, MD, FHM
Associate Professor of Medicine
Emory University School of Medicine
Atlanta, Georgia

To all hospitalists, who have devoted their careers and lives to the advancement of patient safety and quality and to the education of their residents and students.

Acknowledgments

The editor would like to acknowledge the Tulane University residents and hospitalists, whose dedication to the underserved inspires him to advance high-quality health care that is safe, effective, and equitable for all people.

The authors would like to acknowledge the support and contributions of their families. They also thank the staffs of the Society of Hospital Medicine, the Association of Program Directors in Internal Medicine, and the American College of Physicians for their dedication to quality, patient safety, and education in the practice of internal medicine.

Contents

Visit www.acponline.org/acp_press/teaching
for additional information.

About the *Teaching Medicine* Series

This book series, *Teaching Medicine*, represents a major initiative from the American College of Physicians. It is intended for College members but also for the profession as a whole. Internists, family physicians, subspecialists, surgical colleagues, nurse practitioners, and physician assistants—indeed, anyone involved with medical education—should find this book series useful as they pursue one of the greatest privileges of the profession: the opportunity to teach and make a difference in the lives of learners and their patients. The series is composed of six books:

- *Theory and Practice of Teaching Medicine*, edited by me, considers how medical learners learn (how to be doctors), how medical teachers teach, and how they (the teachers) might learn to teach better.

- *Methods for Teaching Medicine*, edited by Kelley M. Skeff and Georgette A. Stratos, builds on this foundation but focuses on the actual methods that medical teachers use. This book explores the full range of techniques that encourage learning within groups. The authors present a conceptual framework and guiding perspectives for understanding teaching; the factors that support choices for particular teaching methods (such as lecturing vs. small group discussion); and practical advice for preceptors, attendings, lecturers, discussion leaders, workshop leaders, and, finally, course directors charged with running programs for continuing medical education.

- *Teaching in Your Office*, edited by Patrick C. Alguire, Dawn E. DeWitt, Linda E. Pinsky, and Gary S. Ferenchick, will be familiar to many teaching internists. It has been reissued as part of this series. This book remains the office-based preceptor's single most useful resource for preparing to receive medical students and residents into an ambulatory practice setting or, among those already engaged in office-based teaching, for learning how to do it even better.

- *Teaching in the Hospital* is edited by Jeff Wiese and considers the challenges and rewards of teaching in that particular setting. Hospitalists as well as more traditional internists who attend on the inpatient service will be interested in the insightful advice that this book provides. This advice focuses not only on how to conduct rounds and encourage learning among students and house officers but also on how to frame and orient the content of rounds for some of the more frequently encountered inpatient conditions.

- *Mentoring in Academic Medicine,* edited by Holly J. Humphrey, considers professional development across the continuum of medical education, from issues pertaining to students to residents to faculty themselves, as well as issues pertaining to professional development of special populations. Here is where the important contributions of mentors and role models are explored in detail.

- *Leadership Careers in Medical Education* concludes this series. Edited by Louis Pangaro, this book is written for members of the medical faculty who are pursuing—or who are considering—careers as clerkship directors, residency program directors, or educational leaders of departments or medical schools, careers that require not only leadership skill but also a deep understanding of the organization and administration of internal medicine's educational enterprise. This book explores the theory and practice of educational leadership, including curricular design and evaluation; and offers insightful profiles of many of internal medicine's most prominent leaders.

Jack Ende, MD, MACP
Philadelphia, 2010

Introduction: The Uniqueness of Hospital Medicine

Teaching in the hospital setting is unique. The complexity and variability of patients require the hospital medicine educator (the attending physician) to adapt to the circumstances and be prepared to teach a wide range of clinical topics, while serving as a role model for an expanded patient care team. The attending is routinely required to interact with various components of the hospital system: the emergency department, the intensive care unit, the laboratory, the pharmacy, and the social work department, in addition to the variable ecosystems on each hospital ward. Furthermore, the attending must interact with multiple services, many of which are not internal medicine–based: surgery, neurology, and obstetrics, for example, in addition to subspecialty services.

On top of all of this is the pressure to ensure timely patient throughput and adherence to billing, coding, and documentation standards. Through each patient's course, the attending has the responsibility of ensuring patient safety and quality, while addressing systems issues that might impair either. And at the end of each patient's course is the responsibility of ensuring a safe and effective transition of care from the inpatient system to the ambulatory system. A whole other series of challenges for the attending arise from the hospital medicine system and the responsibilities of teaching students and residents. Traditional ward teams are distinctly heterogeneous, both in level of training and career interest. Experienced senior residents and novice third-year medical students on the same team are the rule, making it challenging to find content that is suitable for all learners.

Even with the new work hours regulations, the team is also likely to be fatigued, and the unpredictability of a ward service often leads to meals that do not come at planned times. The attending's audience, the students and residents, will more often than not arrive tired, hungry, and distracted by the stress of the rapidly changing patient care environment. Work hours regulations have increased the intensity of the work day (there is more to be done in a shorter amount of time) and have increased the fragmentation of care (for example, shift work, day call, night float). The attending may be faced with a dynamically changing team composition, depending on the residency program's system of shift-based coverage, clinic scheduling, and required days off. The team that was present on Monday is unlikely to be the team that is present on Tuesday.

The attending physician is faced with the challenge of assuring the balance of patient safety and sufficient resident-physician autonomy, a critical component to active and sustained learning. The balance of trust and supervision varies for each resident, even at the same level of training; it requires that the attending physician quickly analyze and assess the resident's performance and determine the latitude that she will allow for that resident to make decisions him- or herself.

The attending physician is accountable to the educational and hospital systems, ensuring simultaneous compliance with accrediting bodies such as the Joint Commission, the accrediting body for hospitals; the Accreditation Council for Graduate Medical Education (ACGME), the accrediting body for graduate medical education; and the Liaison Committee on Medical Education, the accrediting body for medical schools.

The attending is tasked with all of these responsibilities, working within a system that does not have defined units of time (like clinic visits), with time requirements changing from day to day. And at the end of the day, the attending physician is simultaneously charged with the tasks of reviewing the previous day's work in the form of the residents' and students' notes, recording a note herself, and preparing for the day that will follow. It is little wonder that great education is often lost in this environment, defaulting to just getting the work done and hoping for a better day tomorrow.

But despite its challenges, I wouldn't do anything else. Indeed, it is because of its challenges that I chose medical education in hospital medicine as a career. For with great challenges come great opportunities, and nowhere is that more true than on the inpatient medical wards. The rapid pace of the wards and the complexity and diversity of each day can be daunting, but both provide the opportunity to see students and residents at their best. Almost every aspect of medical care can be taught, and at a magnification that allows for precise assessment of learners' skills, deficits, and needs. If medical education were a stress test, the hospital medicine environment is a 5-MET stress, allowing for the easy diagnosis of learners' abilities and requirements.

Because of the fast-paced and diverse environment, I have the opportunity to role-model skills and behaviors in a manner not available to teachers in other settings. Professionalism, communication, interpersonal skills, patient advocacy, systems change, and "equanimitas" are but a few of the opportunities. The diversity of patient care experiences adds to this, while allowing me the opportunity to teach about a broad range of topics. And finally, the wards offer an opportunity to be a part of a team. If only for a month or so at a time, the intensity of the experience creates the perception of having walked that common road for much longer. The fulfillment that comes with the team interaction is immeasurable.

Hospital medicine, however, is not a venue where education can be left to chance. The demands are too severe and the pace is too fast. To be successful in meeting these responsibilities while ensuring effective clinical education requires planning, and not in the form of simply assembling PowerPoint lectures.

This book is designed to empower hospital medical educators with the tools and skills necessary to be successful during their time on the wards, as well as enable them to extract the greatest fulfillment from this experience. Chapter 1 ("Teaching to Improve Performance: The Clinical Coach") outlines the essential attributes of making the transition from phase 1, 2, and 3 teaching (phases in which the teacher is mostly concerned with himself) to phase 4 teaching (in which the teacher focuses on the learner's performance). This chapter provides practical strategies for making this transition from "the teacher" to "the coach." It also outlines simple strategies to establish and maintain the "glue" that holds the ward team together, thereby improving each learner's performance.

Establishing expectations is the cornerstone of ensuring that a ward month operates efficiently and effectively. Furthermore, it is central to establishing the culture on the wards (ideally, a culture of accountability without "blame," wherein learners feel free to express concerns about issues related to patient safety, and to admit errors so that they can be corrected. Chapter 2 ("The First Day On Service: The Attending's Role in Setting Expectations") provides techniques for establishing and communicating expectations for each member of the ward team. A sizable proportion of an attending physician's expectations will be unique to him or her. This is the artistry of attending on the wards, which is to be embraced. Some proportion of these expectations, however, are relatively universal, and this chapter outlines elements to be considered in delivering expectations, along with strategies for making the expectations explicit.

Inpatient attending physicians must use their time effectively, avoiding wasted or duplicated efforts. They must multitask, such as documenting clinical care while teaching how to write progress notes. They must enter the hospital each day with a general idea of the direction in which the patient care needs will take the team, and have an idea of how they will meld educational opportunities during that journey. Chapter 3 ("Strategies for Succeeding as an Inpatient Attending Physician") provides suggestions for time management and discusses two of the more challenging issues for hospital medicine attendings: dealing with heterogeneity in the team and establishing the appropriate level of autonomy for each learner. The chapter provides strategies for conducting rounds to optimize education without sacrificing patient care. Chapter 3 also addresses strategies for the practical aspect of attending on the wards: billing, coding, and ensuring safe and effective transitions of care as the patients leave the hospital.

A large part of the attending's role is to teach and evaluate clinical reasoning. The attending physician should anticipate that most learners will be somewhere to the left or middle on the reporter-interpreter-manager-educator spectrum (1). Chapter 4 ("Teaching Clinical Reasoning on the Inpatient Service") provides strategies for assessing each learner's clinical reasoning abilities and strategies to move learners farther along the spectrum toward the educator physician. An important goal of hospital medicine is patient safety and quality, and this chapter also discusses methods for teaching these skills in the context of diagnosing and correcting medical errors.

The ACGME's Six Core Competencies shifted the paradigm of graduate medical education, moving the focus away from "knowledge-only" and toward a paradigm of overall competence. Chapter 5 ("Teaching the Important Nonclinical Skills on the Inpatient Service") provides strategies for improving the learners' performance in the components that will be lifelong requisites for their success in medicine: time management, data organization, interpersonal skills, independent study, and communication skills.

To truly assume the role of "coach" in augmenting performance, attending physicians must be astute in evaluation, reading small clues about each team member's needs and abilities. They must be prepared to integrate that information into decisions on to how much autonomy they will allow for each team member. At least twice during a rotation (mid-rotation and end of rotation), the attending should consolidate the day-to-day formative feedback into summative feedback, ensuring that each learner precisely knows the magnitude of his or her abilities, and where improvement is needed. Without a proper method, feedback and evaluation can be uncomfortable, usually translating into feedback and evaluation that are ineffective. Chapter 6 ("Feedback, Evaluation, and Remediation on the Inpatient Service") provides strategies and methods for delivering feedback and enabling continued improvement if the attending is not there.

Section II of this book is unique. It presents actual examples of the dialogues, referred to as teaching scripts, between an inpatient teacher and his team, focused on the clinical content of 15 common internal medicine problems. Ten are presented in this book; the remaining five appear in the Web-based version of this series, available at www.acponline.org/acp_press/teaching. The scripts here unfold in Socratic fashion, emphasizing that learners understand the methods of approaching diagnostic conundrums rather than merely memorizing protocols. Each dialogue, or script, is a product of the author's approach, which should not be construed as the best or only approach. Each attending will develop his or her own teaching scripts over time, and this too should be embraced as part of the artistry of hospital medicine education. Section II seeks merely to provide examples and, where no teaching script exists in the reader's repertoire, to provide a starting point from which the reader's own personalized teaching script will emerge. The purpose here is to have inpatient attendings consider not only how they will teach a given topic but also the clinical approach they will encourage their learners to learn. Thus, this section is both pedagogic and clinical.

In total, this book will, it is hoped, provide attending physician with the skills, strategies, and knowledge necessary to appreciate the fulfillment that is found in hospital medicine education like nowhere else: The fulfillment of watching students and residents develop into competent and compassionate physicians.

The dialogues that appear throughout this book rely on a cast of characters of a typical ward team, consisting of Dr. Phaedrus, the attending physician; Moni, the resident physician; Stef, the intern physician; and Paul, the medical student.

Jeff Wiese, MD, FACP
New Orleans, Louisiana, 2010

Section I

Core Competencies of Hospital Teaching

1

Teaching to Improve Performance: The Clinical Coach

Jeff Wiese, MD, FACP

Many physicians mistakenly see teaching merely as the dissemination of knowledge. Yet while knowledge is necessary, it is not sufficient. It is of little consequence that students have vast knowledge if they cannot enact it for the benefit of the patient. The translation of knowledge to practice, or *performance*, is what matters, and changing the paradigm from being a great "teacher" to being a great "coach" (ensuring performance) is the first step to educational excellence in the hospital setting.

There are four critical components to becoming a effective clinical coach: *motivation, visualization, anticipation,* and selecting *content* that has *utility*. The attending must recognize that even the most motivated learners will not be so each day. This chapter identifies strategies to motivate learners to want to learn the knowledge and skills the attending has to impart. Providing a vision of how learners will use the skill (visualization), the attending can increase learner interest and help learners see the practical application of the skill rather than just knowledge acquisition. By anticipating where learners will make mistakes as they attempt to apply the skill, the attending can prevent these areas of error or confusion. This can be done even as the initial content is taught. Choosing content that has utility refers to identifying topic areas that are most likely to be useful to the learners' future career. The attending has to remain flexible: What has utility for one learner may

KEY POINTS

- Inpatient attendings should consider a new paradigm for teaching in which the attending functions as a coach.
- Four measures that enhance inpatient teaching effectiveness are motivation, visualization, anticipation, and selection of content focused upon utility.
- Inpatient attendings may progress through four phases of development as inpatient teachers: phase 1: the teacher needs to establish credibility; phase 2: the teacher begins to receive positive comments; phase 3: teachers are focused on gaining recognition, such as teaching awards; and phase 4: teachers are focused less on their own success and more on the success and skill of their students.
- Inpatient teachers can motivate students in several ways, including addressing them by name, using physical touch, tapping into the students' own motivation for learning; using visualization; emphasizing methods rather than content; and taking steps to ensure that not only the quality but also the quantity of teaching is appropriate.
- Several techniques are available to promote learners' memory and retention, including use of advanced organizers (such as illustrations and pneumonics) and ensuring that what is taught follows an orderly sequence, starting from a foundation and building upward.
- Inpatient teachers should take care to use questions appropriately: Socratic questions move students to higher levels of understanding, while non-Socratic questions can be used to assess students' levels of understanding and learning and, therefore, as a check on the coach's success in enabling learning.

not have utility for others. This chapter addresses strategies for defining utility for different learners; chapter 3 discusses strategies for dealing with the heterogeneity of the ward team (that is, different definitions of utility for different team members).

Mastery of each of these four central tenets of "clinical coaching" enables successful evolution through the four phases of the educator's development until phase 4 is reached—the point at which ensuring learners' optimal performance is the goal.

❖ The Phases of a Teacher's Development

Phase 1: "It's All About Me"

The phase 1 teacher is focused on himself. After years of not knowing acid-base, he finally has his arms around it. To prove this competency to himself (and to impress his students), he sets out to teach it. Perhaps you remember the days, sitting in the back of a dark lecture hall in medical school, listening to a lecturer drone on about the details of acid-base—right down to the chloride channels, and how ammonia does this and aldosterone does that. All the while, you ask yourself, "Wow, this looks like a lot of work. I'm not sure the juice is worth the squeeze on this one … maybe I'll just take the hit on the exam and learn it later." And after successive iterations of the same internal dialogue over the next few year, you finally learn it. To prove it, witnesses will be required—students who will see a barrage of details littering a white board, right down to the difference between the Bartter and the Gitelman syndromes. And while the teacher feels proud of all that he can recall, a student sits in the back of the conference room saying to herself, "Wow, this looks like a lot of work. I'm not sure the juice is worth the squeeze on this one … maybe I'll just take the hit on the exam and learn it later." Phase 1 teaching is about teachers showing how much they know, but it has little effect on the student's performance.

Phase 2: "It's About How It Makes Me Feel"

Despite its inefficacy in improving performance, eventually an approbation will evolve—some student will say, "Wow, thank you for teaching us. That was really great." This is roughly equivalent to saying, "Thank you for acknowledging my presence." It is a sad commentary on the paucity of teaching on the clinical wards as the pace and time pressures have increased over the years. But the approbation feels good, and it becomes its own motivation for subsequent teaching. And that's fine—at least teaching occurs. Still, it is all about the teacher: The motivation is what makes her feel good, with little regard for the performance of the student.

Phase 3: "Going for the Prize"

After enough approbations, some student group nominates the teacher for an award. Given the paucity of grants and research, the attending exalts, "This could be a way for me to get promoted!" The award feels good, further motivating the teacher to teach. There is nothing wrong with this, except that the motivation for the teaching continues to be all about the teacher— what feels good … what is good … for *the teacher*, with little regard for the student's performance. It is fine to classify phases 2 and 3 together as an ego-motivated exercise driven by public opinion. Yet as any great artist will say, once artists pander to public opinion, they have given away their art. Imperceptibly, the teacher begins to teach what students want to hear, but not necessarily what they need to hear. Put another way, no coach gained great favor by making his players run wind sprints, but that is exactly what they needed to be ready to perform come game time.

Phase 4: "It's About the Student's Performance"
And then there is phase 4, the nirvana of clinical coaching. Phase 4 is defined by its image, and the image is important—for the more this image rests in the back of the attending physician's mind, the more it will drive her practice of clinical education, and the better the result will be. The image is this: Someday, you will turn the corner on some lonely hospital ward, and at the end of the hallway, you will see a former student doing right by a patient because of something you have enabled him to do. There will be no applause at that moment, and there will be no awards. In fact, no one else will know about it all—but you will. For you will know that the performance you have enabled in that student has benefited a patient. Enabling performance distant from the time of contact with the student is at the heart of phase 4, and it is what sets clinical education in the hospital setting apart from classroom instruction. To achieve phase 4 requires a paradigm switch away from the mere dissemination of knowledge and toward a focus on performance: in a word, coaching.

❖ Motivation Techniques

One of the unique aspects of education in the hospital setting is the nature of those being coached. The wards are a flurry of activity, with someone always wanting something for a patient: the nurses needing orders to be written; the social workers needing forms and discharge instructions to be completed; the pharmacist needing detailed patient data to release the appropriate pharmaceuticals; and the hospital administration pressing for discharge by 11 a.m., patients from the intensive care unit to be transferred immediately, and emergency department consults within the hour. The residents and students are working just shy of 80 hours per week—tired and hungry, their meals coming at odd hours, they struggle to satisfy everyone, all the while wondering what will become of their careers (*"Will I pass the boards? Who will write my letters? Did I get my applications in on time?"*). And after all of this, the student or resident has very little emotional voltage remaining to *learn*. This monstrous challenge before the teaching moment even begins is what makes teaching on the hospital wards challenging and unique, but it is also what makes motivation a critical component in ensuring performance.

The first step in motivating your learners is to acknowledge and deal with the sentiment that will hold you back if it is not consciously addressed: "Should I *have* to motivate students and residents to learn clinical medicine? I mean, seriously, it's only something as *trivial* as a patient's life!" Here's an analogy to answer that question. Should an NFL football coach have to motivate a prima donna wide receiver to catch the ball—even after he's been paid 5 billion dollars to do so? No. But if he doesn't, then the receiver doesn't catch the ball and the team loses. Should the attending physician have to motivate students to learn medicine? No. But if the coach does not motivate, the student's performance falls short and patient care suffers. So, *should* you have to motivate students to learn? The short answer: No. *Must* we motivate students to learn in order to be effective? Yes.

Using Names

There is one word that will ensure your motivational effectiveness. To any given person, in any society, in any time in history, the most magical, motivating word is … her name.

And using people's names cannot be done enough. Take this example extracted from the wards:

> *"Paul, you had a patient with a hemoglobin of 9, Paul … and you diagnosed anemia, Paul. Fantastic. And Paul, the way you ordered a ferritin, Paul, well it was … inspirational! And Paul, the way you did the rectal exam, Paul, to exclude GI bleeding, Paul … I mean, what more can I say, Paul? Fantastic, Paul."*

The remainder of the team might be thinking, "Who is this freak?"; but not Paul. He's thinking, "This guy is great—I'm going to nominate him for a teaching award!" And that's the simple trick to winning awards (if you are only interested in phase 3). Just walk around the hospital or medical school calling people by their names for a year; you'll win an award.

Why is using people's names so powerful? It communicates that you care about the person as a person—as a unique person; not just a moon that orbits your planet. With this one word, it establishes the relationship requisite for the coach–player relationship. It says, "I see you as a person who is valuable to me; and I care enough about you as a unique person to know your name."

The hospital wards can be a lonely place, with most students and residents feeling lost and over their head. Sum this up in one sentiment:

People are not going to care what you know until they know that you care. The best way to achieve that critical first step is simply to use people's names.

And if you are thinking, "That's fine and all ... but I'm just not very good with names." Well, here is the inside-the-actor's-studio tip number two: You don't have to be good with names. All you have to remember is one person's name. Begin with this student or resident each day, using the name as often as possible, and then end that segment of rounds by saying, *"Paul, I've picked on you enough. Choose someone else on the team, but call him by name."* Paul will give you the next person's name. See? Easy. Just offload the responsibility of remembering names onto someone else.

Physicality

The second step in motivation is to use *physicality*. Recognize that the students we coach have grown up with a very different perspective of entertainment. As opposed to previous generations, for whom entertainment was "live" (the symphony had in-person artists playing, the play or musical had in-person performers, sports events were intimate enough that the players appeared in person), this generation has grown up in front of a glass screen. DVD players, TVs, movies, computers ... these have been the source of this generation's entertainment. If at any time the entertainment went south or became uncomfortable, they simply changed the channel, left the room, or engaged in another activity (such as answering a cell phone). Students will carry this psychological perception of entertainers "behind glass screens" with them onto the wards, seeing their attending (that is, the entertainer) as being behind a protective glass screen. It is the reason that a hospital ward team is spatially defined by an attending, surrounded by a 3-foot force field with all team members in orbit at a safe distance. Do not be perplexed when a student answers his cell phone during rounds or begins to surf the Web on his BlackBerry. He is simply changing the channel, and feels comfortable enough to do so because of the psychological glass screen.

After mastery of names, the next step in motivation is to *break the glass screen*. If you find yourself in a small conference room on the wards doing a quick talk, immediately move away from the whiteboard or chalkboard. As you circulate about the room, you'll see the progress notes go back into the pockets and the phones back into their holsters. The energy of the room will rise, and this energy is what you need to fuel the motivation for the session. If you are on the wards conducting rounds, simply step across the semi-circle that surrounds you and assume a new position on the ward team. Even though the 3-foot force field will reset, it will temporarily bring down the glass screen and generate some much-needed energy.

Use the *power of physical touch*. A simple handshake for a job well done or a touch on the shoulder for encouragement sends the sentiment you long for: "I see you as a person. I am not a hologram, I am your coach." The power of touch is motivating, especially when well timed; it acknowledges great performance in a way that words cannot achieve and supports the player during difficult times (the pat on the shoulder) when things don't go well. And while shaking hands is a filthy custom, it is ours—so embrace it. It will remind you to wash your hands and ensure that your students do the same. Finally, despite the power of touch, it is worth noting that there are safe touch zones and unsafe touch zones. Further explanation is not needed.

Given enough time on the wards as a clinical coach, you will encounter those special students who have lost all pluripotency—there is no longer flexibility in the career decision, and the student has differentiated into, say, orthopedics (or some other career not remotely close to your own). Sadly, many of these students will arrive with the mental stance that they "don't need to know internal medicine to do orthopedics." So the question becomes, "What do I do with this student? Should I simply sequester him in the back, and teach to the students who might want to do medicine? After all, it's his problem, not mine. Right?" Wrong. This student, more than any other, needs a healthy dose of internal medicine—it may be his last trip through formal instruction in internal medicine, and the truth is that the more internal medicine he knows, the better an orthopedic surgeon he will become. But how do you motivate the student who doesn't want to learn internal medicine?

The Hook
The answer is the *hook*. Every student has one: some reason that she will want to know what it is you have to teach. As an example, take this excerpt from the clinical wards:

> *"So Stef, you told me that you are going to do orthopedic surgery. Is that correct?"*

> *"That's right." Stef's face momentarily lights up, though the arms remain crossed.*

> *"Okay, well listen, let me paint a mental image for you.... It's 3 years from now, 5 p.m. on Friday. You've had a busy day on the orthopedics service, doing some really exciting cases. And you're*

super excited because you have dinner plans with your family, and you're ready to leave the hospital. Can you see yourself there?"

"Yes." Stef's grin begins to show the twinge of nervousness at the thought of being the resident.

"All right, well imagine that just as you start to leave the hospital, the pager goes off. The 62-year-old woman for whom you put in an artificial hip is now in atrial fibrillation with a rapid ventricular rate. Wow ... what to do? So here will be your two options, Stef. Option 1, you can call me when that day arrives. As the med consult, I'll come see her, but it might take awhile. I have a lot of consults on Friday afternoon, for whatever reason, and it will probably mean that you are going to have to call your family and cancel that dinner .... Or option 2, I can teach you in the next 5 minutes all that you need to know about rate control and clot control, and when that day comes, you can fix the problem yourself and be home in time for dinner. So which option do you want?"

"Hey, sounds good to me. Tell me what I need to know." Stef's apprehension is turning to genuine excitement.

The unique feature of hospital medicine teams is the great heterogeneity of the team members. Some students will be interested in internal medicine as a career; others will have other careers in mind. Even among the residents there will be diverse career trajectories: some in general medicine, some in subspecialties, and some in careers that are not internal medicine (such as the preliminary interns). Each of these members will have a hook, and couching the instruction in utility—how the student will eventually use the information—generates the motivation that you need to ensure performance down the line.

But how do you deal with this heterogeneity? Doesn't couching the content in the orthopedic student's future career alienate the other team members? The answer is no. Despite our evolution, people have retained their *herd mentality*. When the lion stares down one antelope, the whole herd feels the same emotion. So it is with hooks on the wards—as the content is couched in utility for one team member, the other team members will begin to envision their own future and feel the same utility. The effect of motivation will be felt by all.

But how do you teach content that has no obvious utility? What if, say, a faculty member wonders, "I want to teach prion disease, and I just can't see how any of my students are going to use that. What do I do?" The answer is, "Well ... don't teach that." The truth is that in the grand scheme, the teacher's time with a ward team is short—it is impossible to teach all of internal medicine in this time frame, and something will have to be sacrificed. You might as well sacrifice according to utility: Teach what people will use, and this will establish the motivation necessary for overcoming the monstrous time and energy challenges that oppose you.

❖ Using Visualization to Empower Interest and Promote Retention

As noted in the preceding section, one of the most powerful hooks is the ability to create a vision for how the student will use the skill or knowledge. That hook is important because it generates motivation for learning the skill and keeps the content of the coaching session focused on topics that have utility. When you consider that the mind has a difficult time distinguishing between what was imagined and what actually happened, the principle of visualization takes on even greater importance. The coach who can create a palpable vision of performing the skill effectively gives the student one "repetition" of doing that skill without ever having done it. It is the reason that great coaches in whatever venue—performing arts, music, athletics—have the same mantra: "See it before you do it." It is the same reason that you'll find actors backstage and athletes in the locker room, all with eyes closed, rocking back and forth, seeing themselves doing the dance steps, or hitting the ball, or whatever task is immediately before them as they prepare to perform.

Teaching procedures on the internal medicine wards, though not as involved as on a surgical service, is the most tangible example of this coaching strategy. The time for the teacher to get the residents to visualize each step of the procedure is before they begin the procedure, as the "hard stop" is proceeding with the nursing and ancillary staff. The art lies in asking the questions that drive the vision:

"Can you see yourself prepping and draping the patient? Don't do it yet ... just visualize it. Can you see it? Yes, good. Where will your procedure tray be? What will it look like? Is there anything not on that tray that you need? Now would be the time to get it.

"Can you see yourself finding the landmarks? Will you do that before or after your drape the neck? Can you see yourself putting the iodine on? Okay, now, can you see yourself loading the anesthesia syringe? Where will you inject? What will you do with the needle after you are finished with it? Where will you position your body as you insert the finder needle? Can you reach everything on your tray? It would suck to have found the vein, but have to change body positions to reach the inserting needle, huh?

"Can you hear the pager going off? Who will answer it? Yeah, maybe it's best to hand off the pager now before you begin....

"Now the inserting needle is in. Can you see the blood return in the syringe? It's dark red, isn't it? That's good, because that means you're in the vein. Now, how is the guidewire positioned? Can you see the little 'J' at the end? Probably good to insert the wire such that the 'J' is pointing toward the heart. That will make sure that the wire, and eventually the catheter, heads down toward the heart and not up to the head.... Okay. The guidewire is in. See yourself holding it as you remove the needle. Don't let go."

But visualization is not exclusive to procedure training. The more that teaching topics can be pursued with a vision of how students will use it, with as much detail created in their minds as possible, the better the retention of that topic will be. And retention is requisite for phase 4 performance. It will matter little if the student masters the topic in the moment but cannot recall it at a later date. Long-term performance suffers without proper visualization. Later in this chapter, examples of creating a vision are discussed, although there are an infinite number of degrees of freedom: Visualization is the art of the attending physician.

It is important that all visions be positive. Positive visualization leads to positive results; negative visions lead to negative results. Students and residents, on average, are terrified of failure, and it is the prospect of failure or mistakes that dominates their thoughts. This is of great risk to their performance. The analogy is the golfer who hits the golf ball into the water and then immediately proclaims, "I knew I was going to do that." And he's absolutely right. If failure is on your mind (hitting the ball in the water), the body will accommodate accordingly. The coach's job is to ensure that the vision is positive—it is appropriate to get the student to visualize the pitfalls and potential mistakes inherent in a clinical task, but it is vital that the vision is created such that the residents can see themselves avoiding the pitfall or overcoming the obstacle.

You may wonder, "But do I have time to create these visions?" If you stay with the paradigm of teaching as much knowledge as you have (phase 1), the answer is no. But if performance is the goal, then the paradigm shift to being a coach liberates you from the compulsion to teach all details, enabling the time to create the vision. Therein lies retention, and eventually performance.

❖ Anticipating Learner Pitfalls: The Power of Methods

The goal in hospital medicine is to establish a culture where everyone feels free to admit and learn from mistakes because this atmosphere advances patient safety and quality. A central tenet of this "no-blame culture" is that mistakes will be made and are an inherent part of practicing medicine, especially in a training environment. Building this culture begins with acknowledgment that medical errors can and do occur, and the focus will be on strategies to address and hopefully prevent them.

The art of the coach is to anticipate where mistakes will be made and to address these potential pitfalls even as the topic or skill is being taught. Regardless of an attending's self-esteem as to how much she does or does not know, this is her area of expertise—all physicians have been down the road that the students and residents are just now embarking upon. We have made the mistakes and are familiar with these pitfalls; this is an area of expertise that, unlike details of medical content, cannot be easily obtained from textbooks.

A great sports coach would not merely teach the team the playbook and then call it a day. No, she would teach the offensive plays (the playbook) but would then alert the players about what the opposing team (the defense) will try to do to prevent the team from succeeding. The analogy in clinical coaching is teaching students where the common errors lurk and preparing them accordingly while the topic is being taught.

The important maxim of anticipation is that people do not rise to some super-human level of understanding in the setting of crisis; instead, they fall to their lowest level of incompetence. A cluster of residents can sit through an hour-long lecture on hypotension on a Friday afternoon, and at the conclusion of that lecture can readily recite the causes of hypotension. In the traditional model, this recitation (an examination score) would mark success. But the experienced clinician knows that it is a very different task to recite those same causes of hypotension at 2 a.m. after being awoken from sleep in a hospital call room. Rushing to the patient's bedside, the resident can only say, "Call 911" and, to his dismay, is reminded that he *is* 911. The coach must anticipate the drop-off in performance under periods of crisis and plan accordingly to temper the resident's fall in competence. The two best measures to prevent the sudden decline in performance during duress are *to teach methods instead of details* and *to create realistic visions of what the resident can expect* when the time comes.

❖ Techniques to Promote Retention

The presumption in medical education is that once knowledge is acquired, it is the student's to keep (dashed line 1 in Figure 1-1). The reality is that knowledge, like all things in the universe, decays. It is the reason that despite taking three semesters of French in high school, one might find that, years later, uttering the phrases, "I love you" and "Where is the bathroom?" in French might be all that remains.

The clinical coach must recognize the way in which medical students have been socialized to learn. The "bulimic" method of learning is characterized by doing without knowledge for a prolonged period (from, say, the beginning of a college semester or a medical school "block" until the week before midterm or block examination), gorging on knowledge (cramming), and vomiting the knowledge onto a Scantron examination, with subsequent removal of the knowledge from the system. The method of instruction (that is, in which content from one parcel of time is mutually exclusive from other parcels) and a focus on details have created an incentive for short-term memory strategies. While many colleges and medical schools are restructuring curricula to emphasize active learning, iterative learning, and long-term retention, the clinical coach should be prepared that many medical students will come to the wards with this bulimic mentality.

Any doubt about this mindset will be dispelled by laboratory coats laden with cards and textbooks and "quick fix" strategies (with titles such as "How to Survive on the Wards"). Failure to acknowledge and correct this mentality will limit the coach's success in teaching long-term strategies for retention and performance (methods of approach as opposed to

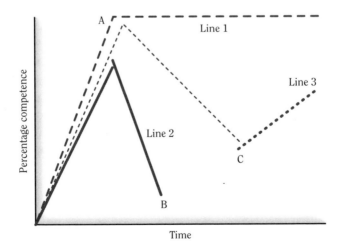

Figure 1-1 Skills decline graph.

details) because the student will resort to rote memorization of concrete facts in lieu of understanding the method. Even as coaching ensues, the student will frequently revert to the old strategy of trying to memorize content. The coach must recognize this behavior and redirect the student to the better strategy of learning methods and understanding as opposed to memorization.

If clinical education is focused on long-term performance, its goal should not be how high the "peak" rises (point A in Figure 1-1) but rather the slope of the decline in skill. In addition to visualization, there are three other methods for lessening the slope of the decline in skill: *teaching less by focusing on methods rather than details, using the Socratic method,* and *using advanced organizers.*

Teaching Less; Focusing on Methods Instead of Details

Sir William Osler (1) noted that, "The problem with medical students is that they try to learn too much; the problem with medical educators is that they try to teach too much. Teach them methods and the art of observation, and then give them patients to practice their skills." The clinical coach should be aware that medical students will come to the wards with the same mentality that was successful for them in the preclinical years: an obsessive focus on details and a belief that the knowledge base for clinical medicine can be "memorized" in lieu of understanding it. In the preclinical environment, there was a defined knowledge domain (for example, only renal disease in the renal block), and boundaries were clearly defined (students are accountable only for what was in the lecture or assigned readings). The distinguishing feature between an "A" grade and a "B" grade was the ability to recall details, and the two forces combined to create a mentality that everything about a topic *could* be learned (if only for a short time) and that it could be memorized. The clinical wards are different: No knowledge is out of bounds (that is, you can't say that it's unfair that a patient has a disease for which you have not been given a reading assignment), and all quarters of knowledge can be in play for any given patient (for example, the merging of the pulmonary, renal, and cardiac blocks). The result is that while some facts must be memorized, the "memorize it all strategy" is untenable. Even if that strategy is possible, memorized facts have a steep slope on the skills decline graph (solid line 2 in Figure 1-1), and the strategy is not effective in ensuring long-term performance (point B in Figure 1-1). This is especially important in hospital medicine, where multiorgan disease is the rule more than the exception, and the "typical" presenting pattern of a disease is changed to an "atypical" presentation that is not consistent with the student's memorized pattern recognition.

The role of the coach is to recognize that students will come with this mentality and to refocus them on learning strategies more conducive for long-term performance: methods of approach and understanding of disease. The first step is to teach less, jettisoning the details (as contained in phase 1 teaching) to free up more time for creating visualization, and for more in-depth time to ensure that students understand (as opposed to memorizing) the methods.

To balance this approach, the coach should be prepared to assign readings that will enable students to acquire the details on their own time. It is important to be realistic and honest in our abilities as educators: Even the greatest attending physicians cannot compete with a textbook or the Internet. Textbooks enable students to read and synthesize the content at their own pace, turning back the pages to re-review concepts that are not fully understood and referencing other information to help supplement the learning. A didactic lecture, at the teacher's pace (not the students'), has none of these luxuries (2). Details are best left for textbook reading; methods and approaches are the domain of the clinical coach. Chapter 5 outlines reading strategies that coaches can teach their students.

Asking Questions: The Socratic Method

It is important to begin with what the Socratic method is *not*. The Socratic method is not "pimping," the method of quizzing students about what they do and do not know. Pimping, otherwise known as the "traumatic Socratic," induces a high level of stress, redirecting students' mental energies away from the cerebral lobes and hippocampus (understanding and memory) and toward the amygdala (fight or flight). It is not effective for long-term performance, and it is usually a waste of time: If the student knows the answer to the question, there is no point in asking the question; if the student doesn't know the answer to the question, then the same time spent in asking the question could have been used to provide the answer. Proponents of the traumatic Socratic point to its utility as a motivating measure to ensure that residents are reading. This presupposes that the resident is reading *everything* in medicine (to prepare for every possible question), which is unrealistic. The reality is that the student cannot predict the questions that will be asked; thus, this approach does not accurately measure the student's reading. Further, the method induces anxiety, making reading uncomfortable, not motivating. The result is that residents read less, and the ward environment becomes a daunting exercise of day-to-day humiliation, which students learn to loathe.

The true Socratic method can be found in Plato's *Meno* (3). The method is not about ascertaining the student's knowledge but rather about moving the student's understanding from a baseline level of understanding to a higher level by asking questions that link concepts together. Consider the method as an exercise in "building neuron connections," with each neuron representing a concept, and each synapse representing the link between concepts. Each question in the Socratic method is meant to build a synapse. The questions are asked in a fashion that the answer is so intuitive (such as "But yes, of course" or "No, that wouldn't make sense") that the student's mental energy is devoted to the intuitive link between the two concepts, not on factual recall. Because the questions are intuitive, no mental energy is wasted on the amygdala (that is, the stress of fight or flight).

The power of the Socratic method is twofold. First, when knowledge has waned (see point C in Figure 1-1), students can re-create the knowledge by working through the line of questions on their own; this will raise the slope above the level of incompetence (dotted line 3 on Figure 1-1). Second, when an actual patient problem is not "typical" (for example, a patient with multiorgan dysfunctions or comorbid conditions that subsequently change the presenting pattern of the disease), the method allows the student to apply standard understanding of one problem (renal failure) to the complex patient, reasoning out the features unique to that patient.

The Socratic method in hospital-based medicine often follows the line of pathophysiology (see the teaching script for hyponatremia in section II of this book). The additional value is twofold: First, it draws on the student's past training in pathophysiology, linking scientific understanding to clinical medicine (as opposed to blind memorization of protocols); second, it allows transposing one topic to another (see the teaching scripts on acute renal failure and on hyponatremia in section II; the lines of questioning are very similar, although the answers are different).

Important to the Socratic method is that *wrong answers are not the fault of the student but rather of the coach*. The questions should be intuitive; wrong answers are usually due to questions that did not lead to an intuitive answer. In the neuron-building analogy, a wrong answer is the equivalent of a stroke. If a student answers incorrectly, the coach cannot merely correct the answer and move forward; this will require some rehab. The coach must back up three or four questions and repeat the line of questioning up to and through the missed question (with the student hopefully getting it right this time). The Socratic method works best one person at a time because this sets the expectation that the student (not someone else in the crowd) will be responsible for the next question in the sequence, thereby linking the concepts together. Do not worry; other learners on the team will follow along with the line of questioning by proxy, establishing the same linking of concepts. For instruction of topics that progressively build in their complexity, the earlier and easier parts of the Socratic method can be devoted to the least experienced learner. The line of questions can be of shifted to more experienced learners as the complex portion of the teaching ensues (see the teaching script on electrocardiograms in the online portion of this book, available at www.acponline.org/ acp_press/teaching/).

Advanced Organizers

Students will arrive on the wards with a belief that they can memorize clinical medicine. While memorization is effect for short-term recall, it is prone to a steep decline in competence over time. And yet if an alternative method of organizing content is not provided, students will resort to memorization. Central to Shulman's concept of pedagogic content knowledge, described in *Methods for Teaching Medicine*, another book in the *Teaching Medicine* series (2), advanced organizers, such as acronyms, pneumonics, algorithms, and diagrams, are mental constructions useful to organizing knowledge: They are "advanced" because they draw on previous experiences, and "organizers" because they are used to organize complex thoughts. Many of the teaching scripts in section II of this book illustrate this point. Advanced organizers are powerful because they enable students to organize their thoughts and methods and construct a differential diagnosis distant in time from the coaching session. There are no "right" advanced organizers; indeed, the way in which content is organized may be tailored to the students' interests and backgrounds. The artistry of clinical coaching is in discovering and developing your own advanced organizers. The teaching scripts in section II are meant to start this creative process.

❖ Blocking Coaching Sessions: Foundation Before Drywall

Like a house being constructed, a coaching session should be constructed in blocks. This is particularly important on the inpatient wards because time available for coaching often varies, with some days enabling longer coaching times and other days, far less time. By proactively thinking about the natural break points in a coaching session, the coach can do manageable components of a session, deferring subsequent components to future coaching sessions (see the teaching scripts on acid-base [in section II of this book] and electrocardiograms [at www.acponline.org/acp_press/ teaching]). This goes against the natural tendency of most teachers, however, wherein the predilection is to start and finish a lecture on a topic, including all of the details (phase 1 teaching), in one session. The reality is that the time to complete a topic from start to finish is rarely, if ever, present. The unpredictability of the inpatient wards makes it important to have considered the natural break points in a coaching session ahead of time because an unplanned interruption due to a change in a patient's condition can be accommodated by quickly finishing one block and then deferring subsequent blocks to later sessions.

To accomplish this task, however, the coach must think a priori of where the natural break points exist; otherwise the content is fragmented and disorganized. An important principle of learning is that *knowledge and skills are laid down in the student's mind in the way that they are delivered.* The transcription to the brain is like taking notes on a lecture with a pen and paper: As content is delivered, it is recorded. It is *not* like transcribing the lecture on a computer, where cutting and pasting can be used to easily reorganize the data. *Disorganized and random dissemination of knowledge on a topic leads to random and disordered thinking by the student.* Even when a lecture is well planned, students may try to take it to a higher level too early or to a lateral point in the content by asking the untimely question. The coach must have the discipline to maintain the linear nature of the lecture, delivering content in the way in which the coach would like to see the student recall the information later. This is particularly important in teaching methods and approaches, as illustrated in the teaching script on acid-base in section II of this book.

The a priori blocking of content into sessions that fit the rhythm of the inpatient service also has utility with respect to retention. At each break point between the blocks is the opportunity for the coach to assess the student's mastery to that point by asking questions or assigning tasks. Failure to demonstrate mastery of the "foundation" block necessitates that the coach and student return to the first block and not progress to the next "drywall" block.

When blocks are distributed over time, the first 2 minutes of each block should be devoted to a quick review of earlier blocks. This ensures that the content is being "laid down" in the student's mind in the correct order (see the teaching script for electrocardiograms at www.acponline.org/acp_press/teaching/).

❖ Checking on Learning

In this context, checking on learning relates not to the student's performance but rather to the *coach's* efficacy in ensuring the learner's performance. At each break point between blocks, the student's mastery of the preceding block should be ascertained before moving on to the next block.

There are numerous methods to ascertain competence, and it is part of the artistry of clinical coaches to design their own. Four of the most commonly used strategies for assuring yourself of the student's mastery of a block are 1) asking probing questions (non-Socratic) that establish the student's understanding of the content (see below), 2) asking the student to apply the content to a related but slightly different clinical task (see the teaching script on electrocardiograms in the online portion of this book, available at www.acponline.org/acp_press/teaching/), 3) asking the student to apply the material to new clinical data (see the teaching script on acid-base in section II), and 4) asking more experienced learners (residents) to teach the same content to less experienced learners (students).

Using Non-Socratic Questions to Assess a Learner's Competence

Questions asked outside of the Socratic method can help reduce the slope of skills decline, and when used, should have one of two primary purposes: 1) establishing the student's baseline understanding of the disease or concept and 2) evaluating the student's mastery of the topic as the coaching proceeds (evaluation of the coach's teaching by assessing the student's competence to that point). For both types of questioning, it is important that the questioning not induce excessive stress on the student; the fight-or-flight impulse will limit self-reflection, and the goal of discovering what the student knows may be obscured by the student's defensiveness.

To establish a baseline of understanding without inducing stress, ask questions with a broad latitude: "How have you seen this approached?" "After all that you have seen thus far, do you have a good method for approaching this problem?" Both examples have no "wrong" answer; whatever students have seen is what they have seen, even if it is incorrect. Broad-latitude questions encourage the student to engage in self-reflection before formulating an answer. In the second scenario, the questions should be designed to evaluate concepts taught in the preceding "block."

Importantly, when the teacher asks questions that require reasoning or introspection, the learner should be given protected time to think, formulate an answer, and then question. These questions should be directed to one learner at a time, and other team members who attempt to jump in on the designated learner's opportunity to answer the question should be restrained by the simple, *"Thanks, Stef, you're next. But let me give Paul a chance to answer this question."* Students and residents learn by experience; if the attending provides the answer to the question too quickly, or allows other learners to jump the question, they will either 1) guess at the answer in a hastened effort to get it in, which subverts the goal of analyzing the student's understanding of the concept, or 2) learn that it is futile to try to think about and answer subsequent questions because insufficient time will be provided to formulate an answer. The latter will be manifest as the quick "I don't know," and should be a sign to the attending that the answers are coming too quickly after the question was asked. *At least 5 seconds of protected time should be provided after each question to ensure appropriate introspection.*

Wrong answers can sometimes provide greater insight into a student's understanding of a concept than correct answers. The attending physician should avoid the temptation of brushing past a wrong answer by immediately correcting the response. Instead, see it as an autopsy moment: The bad event (the wrong answer) provides an opportunity to dissect and determine where the pathology rests. Great insight can be obtained by exploring why students came to the conclusions that they did (see the teaching script on antibiotics in section II). Once the systematic thought error is identified, it can be corrected.

Clinical medicine is about understanding disease; it is not about telepathy. Any question that begins with "This is a 'What am I thinking?' question" should not be asked. Just tell the student what you are thinking.

The Exponential Power of Teaching Others to Teach

Asking more experienced team members to teach less experienced team members is a powerful method to address several challenges of the hospital medicine ward team. Involving the more experienced members as the teachers and the less experienced ones as the learners addresses the challenge of dealing with the team's heterogeneity by actively involving all team members at once. Further, it allows teaching of the team when not all team members can be present. For example, when the students are in their clerkship classes or have the day off, the attending physician can teach the resident team members, with the directive that they will be teaching the students when they return. Even in the attending physician's absence, additional teaching can occur (the residents to the students), effectively doubling the attending physician's teaching efforts for the month. If the attending physician is present, it is an opportunity for him to sit in the back of the conference room and complete billing or coding cards while simultaneously listening to how the resident is teaching the material.

Observing a learner teach a block will clearly define, both to the coach and to the learner, her mastery of the topic. Areas of uncertainty or non-mastery will be painfully evident, serving as a powerful method of assessing the coach's teaching skills (that which she taught effectively and that which she did not) and the resident's mastery of the block prior. Further, this method allows the attending physician to teach topics that she believes the resident might not know, but also might find insulting if the attending physician tried to teach it. For example, a resident's ego may preclude an attending physician from teaching a "baby" topic such as anemia, even though the resident's competence may not be consistent with his ego. By couching the topic in the context of "I want you to teach this to the students," the attending physician is given the luxury of assuring that the resident has mastery over "baby" topics without insulting his ego.

❖ Conclusion

People are a product of their experience. Most students and residents will come to the hospital wards expecting to be taught in the same way in which they were taught in the classroom: The teacher talks, the students acquire knowledge. But as the Accreditation Council for Graduate Medical Education and Liaison Committee on Medical Education have defined, the practice of medicine is more than just medical knowledge (4). Proficiency is required in multiple skill domains: interpersonal skills/communication, using the practice to define areas of uncertainty (and the ability to shore up those areas of weakness), understanding the system in which the physician works, and demonstrating selflessness and empathy in caring for patients. In aggregate, each of the competencies contributes to the most important competency of them all: patient care. For learners to transition from students to fully competent physicians, they must be able to apply their knowledge for the benefit of their patients. Where *application* is the goal, *performance* is the measure of success in meeting that goal. The focus of the attending, then, is to ensure this performance by designing educational strategies (coaching) that motivate the learners to want to learn, anticipate where the learners are likely to go astray (and to prevent falling into those pitfalls), choosing content that has utility to the learners, and creating a vision for how the information or skill will be used.

REFERENCES

1. **Osler W.** Aequanimitas. Philadelphia: Blakiston; 1932.
2. **Skeff KM, Stratos GA, eds.** Methods for Teaching Medicine. Philadelphia: ACP Pr; 2010.
3. **Plato.** Meno. Jowett B, translator. Digireads.com Publishing; 2005.
4. **Accreditation Council for Graduate Medical Education.** Internal medicine program requirements. Accessed at www.acgme.org/acWebsite/RRC_140/140_prIndex.asp.

2

The First Day on Service: The Attending's Role in Setting Expectations

Kevin J. O'Leary, MD

Marianne Tschoe, MD

Jeff Wiese, MD, FACP

Despite the busyness of the hospital ward service, the first part of the first day should be devoted to a sit-down session with the team. One hour invested to clearly outline the goals and objectives for the rotation and the expectations for each team member will save 20 hours over the month that would have been otherwise wasted on miscommunication, absenteeism, and duplication of efforts. Further, it lays the groundwork for the midrotation and end-of-rotation evaluations, enabling honest and constructive feedback to each team member. *This first hour has to be prioritized above all other tasks, save the emergent code blue or rapid response.* The first day cannot end without this hour. Sitting the team down in a conference room or at a quiet location in the hospital is an important component of this first hour because it conveys the importance and primacy of this session and ensures that there will be time to ask questions and discuss any points of confusion in the initial game plan.

This chapter address the five core components of this initial orientation for the team: 1) setting goals and objectives, 2) discussing the organization of the team, 3) setting expectations of each team member, 4) describing the supervision-to-autonomy spectrum, and 5) ensuring communication. After a consideration of these five components of the initial orientation session, the chapter concludes with recommendations for promulgating a "no-blame" culture and establishing expectations for evaluation.

KEY POINTS

- The first day on service should include time set aside to establish goals and objectives for the teachers, interns, and residents, but also for the team as a whole.
- Issues pertaining to autonomy and supervision should be clarified, along with expectations for evaluation.
- This initial orientation is an opportunity for the inpatient teacher to help set the *tone* for the service, including the importance of facing one's mistakes, working within a "no-blame" system, and encouraging open lines of communication and feedback.

❖ Setting Team Goals and Objectives

Integrating Personal Objectives Into Institutional Objectives

The residency and the clerkship directors have probably already defined the goals and objectives for the rotation as it pertains to compliance with the Accreditation Council for Graduate Medical Education (ACGME) and Liaison Committee on Medical Education requirements. Before the rotation begins, the attending physician should review these goals and objectives. This is important not only to ensure compliance with accrediting bodies (the lifeblood of the residency and school) but also to establish consistency between rotations (that what was done on the last rotation for the residents is also done here). This improves understanding of the objectives and ensures that residents and students are not taught to "disrespect authority," which would be the unintended lesson if the attending did not respect the program's objectives. This last point is important because disrespect for authority becomes a habit that knows no specificity: It will eventually grow into disrespect for the attending physician's authority if the seed is planted early.

It is equally important that the attending establish his or her *personal goals for the team* and ensure that these are consistent with the program's goals. Given the wide spectrum of hospital medicine, it is unlikely that any attending will be an expert in all areas of clinical medicine. It is equally as likely, however, that attendings will possess greater expertise in some areas. While attending physicians cannot ignore areas in which they lack expertise (teaching should follow the patient's disease), they should also not be afraid of playing to their strengths in devoting time during the month to the areas where expertise lies. Admitting where you lack expertise and devoting time to finding the answers to these questions present an opportunity for role-modeling. Taking a personal inventory of strengths and weaknesses should precede each rotation.

Residency programs are required to integrate the ACGME competencies (1) into their curriculum (Table 2-1). The Clerkship Directors in Internal Medicine have similarly defined competencies for medical student (Box 2-1), and some medical schools have similarly defined competencies that they expect their students to demonstrate before graduation (2, 3). Because all medical students will eventually become residents, and because all specialties are held accountable to the six core competencies, these

---

Box 2-1. Clerkship Directors in Internal Medicine General Clinical Core Competencies

1. Diagnostic decision-making
2. Case presentation
3. History and physical examination
4. Communication and relationships with patients and colleagues
5. Interpretation of clinical information
6. Therapeutic decision-making
7. Bioethics of care
8. Self-directed learning
9. Prevention
10. Coordination of care and teamwork
11. Geriatric care
12. Basic procedures
13. Nutrition
14. Community health care
15. Continuous improvement in systems of medical care
16. Occupational and environmental health care
17. Advanced procedures

Data obtained from Alliance for Academic Internal Medicine. Clerkship Directors in Internal Medicine–Society for General Internal Medicine Core Medicine Clerkship Curriculum, 2009.

Table 2-1. Accreditation Council for Graduate Medical Education Competencies

Competency	Definition	Expectations: "I Expect You to:"
Patient care	Compassionate, appropriate, and effective treatment of health problems and the promotion of health	1. Demonstrate a caring and respectful behavior for your patients. 2. Gather essential and accurate information about your patients. 3. Make informed decisions about diagnostic and therapeutic interventions based on patient information and preferences, up-to-date scientific evidence, and clinical judgment. 4. Develop and enact patient management plans. 5. Counsel and educate your patients and their families. 6. Use information technology to support your patient care decisions. 7. Competently perform all procedures.
Medical knowledge	Knowledge about established and evolving biomedical, clinical, and cognate (e.g., epidemiologic and social-behavioral) sciences and the application of this knowlege to patient care	1. Demonstrate knowledge about established and evolving biomedical, clinical, and cognate (e.g., epidemiologic and social-behavioral) sciences and the application of this knowledge to patient care. 2. Demonstrate an investigatory and analytic thinking approach to knowledge to patient care clinical medicine. 3. Know and apply the basic sciences appropriate to their discipline.
Practice-based learning and improvement	Involves investigation and evaluation of physician's own patient care, appraisal and assimilation of scientific evidence, and improvements in patient care	1. Identify strengths, deficiencies, and limits in your knowledge and expertise. 2. Set learning and improvement goals. 3. Identify and perform appropriate learning activities. 4. Systematically analyze your practice using quality improvement methods, and implement changes with the goal of practice improvement. 5. Incorporate formative evaluation feedback into your daily practice.

		6. Locate, appraise, and assimilate evidence from scientific studies related to your patients' health problems.
		7. Use information technology to optimize your learning.
Interpersonal and communication skills	Communication practices that result in effective information exchange and teaming with patients, their families, and other health professionals	1. Communicate effectively with patients and families.
		2. Communicate effectively with physicians and other health professionals.
		3. Work effectively as a member or leader of the team.
		4. Act in a consultative role to other physicians and health professionals.
		5. Maintain comprehensive, timely, and legible medical records.
Professionalism	A commitment to carrying out professional responsibilities, adherence to ethical principles, and sensitivity to a diverse patient population	1. Demonstrate compassion, integrity, and respect for others.
		2. Demonstrate a responsiveness to patient needs that supersedes your self-interest.
		3. Demonstrate respect for patient privacy and autonomy.
		4. Demonstrate accountability to patients, society, and the profession.
		5. Demonstrate sensitivity and responsiveness to a diverse patient population, including diversity in sex, age, culture, race, religion, disabilities, and sexual orientation.
Systems-based practice	Manifested by actions that demonstrate an awareness of and responsiveness to the larger context and system of health care and the ability to effectively call on system resources to provide care that is of optimal value	1. Coordinate patient care within the health care system.
		2. Incorporate considerations of cost awareness and risk-benefit analysis in patient care.
		3. Advocate for quality patient care and optimal patient care systems.
		4. Work in interprofessional teams to enhance patient safety and improve patient care quality.
		5. Participate in identifying system errors and implementing potential systems solutions.

Data obtained from Accreditation Council for Graduate Medical Education Outcome Project. Accessed at www.acgme.org/outcome.

competencies serve as a useful paradigm for structuring the goals and objectives for all team members for the month. The added value to this paradigm is that it holds team members accountable for all aspects of their performance: The practice of medicine is analogous to a heptathlon (six events); exceptional performance in one event (medical knowledge) cannot compensate for dismal performance in other events (such as systems of care).

In addition, coaches should familiarize themselves with the tools that will be used to evaluate the learners. Evaluation is most effective when the goals and objectives for the rotation match the evaluation. Team members who do not perform well (see chapter 6) will attempt to dodge accountability for their poor performance on the basis of a communication error ("But I wasn't told that was expected of me"). This response prevents meaningful improvement from their evaluation. For example, even if it were reasonable to assume that seeing your patients every day is an *implied* expectation for an inpatient medicine ward, if this expectation is not explicitly stated students will have room to dodge the feedback instead of internalizing it. Reviewing the contents of this assessment tool before the rotation will help clarify how objectives are measured and prompt the attending to pay close attention for certain behaviors.

Learners' Goals

As noted in chapter 1, finding the "hook" for each team member is central to building motivation for the team. On the first day of the rotation, attending physicians should ask learners to define personal goals and objectives. Defining goals will be a new practice for many team members, and the attending physician should be prepared to help them make it a specific and achievable goal. For example, the initial response from a resident is likely to be "I want to learn a lot." The coach should help the resident better define this goal to make it more specific, and thus more tangible, by asking a direct question: *"Well, Stef, that's great. Much better than learning a little ... But if you had to choose, which two organ systems would you say you want to learn the most about?"* The student may say, *"I want to learn about taking care of patients."* This is too nebulous to be effective. The coach can help the student define the goal by asking, *"Well, Paul, you are in the right place. But let me ask you ... What career are you considering, and what parts of this rotation might be most useful to that career?"*

Analogous to planning a family vacation, each team member's goals should serve as a mental itinerary for the coach as he leads the team through the journey through the hospital wards: The combined goals of the attending and the team members are the destination, as well as the sites that need to be seen along the way. It is the coach's role to ensure that the goals are tangible; nebulous goals are not effective in defining the course. The coach should end this part of the session by defining and sharing his personal goals for the month in order to model this behavior.

❖ Organization of the Teaching Team

Setting the Schedule for the Month: Days Off and Teaching Schedules

The residency program usually determines the residents' call cycle and clinic schedules. The teaching attending may or may not be involved in determining which days the resident, interns, and students will be off-duty. However, the attending should consider how the call cycle and scheduled days off will affect team dynamics. The attending should ensure that days off have been scheduled for the month—once the month gets going, it is easy to miss ensuring that each team member has at least 1 day off in 7, averaged over the month. If it is in the attending's or the team's purview to schedule days off, the learners' personal needs should be considered in scheduling the days off for the month. This establishes the tone for the month that the clinical coach desires: Each team member is important as a *person*, not just as a position, and personal needs will be taken into account.

After personal considerations are taken into account, in general it is much more functional for the team if the resident's days off immediately precede on-call days, when the team's census of patients is likely to be lower. Moreover, the days when additional patients may be added to the service off of the call cycle (that is, days when overflow patients are distributed or short-call days) are less desirable as scheduled days off. Attention should be paid to the clinic requirements of the team to ensure that one team member does not have the day off while other team members are in clinic that afternoon. In either case, whether predetermined or assigned, the teaching attending needs to be aware of the days off scheduled for each team member, particularly the senior residents' days off, because the attending may have to be more available on those days.

Student Schedules

The teaching attending should also thoroughly understand students' schedules, including dates and times of required classroom experiences, and whether the student is expected to return to the wards after classes. Students will get the most out of their clinical rotations if they are an active part of patient care, and it should be emphasized that the more the students remain with the team, the greater the team will involve them in the management of their patients. Returning to the wards after classes should be expected.

Expectations for students will need to be adjusted according to the time of year and point of their rotation. For example, students in the first week of their third year of medical school would be expected to have a less advanced knowledge base than those at the end of the year. Similarly, students at the end of the rotation should be expected to perform at a higher level than during the first week of the rotation.

Setting Expectations for Each Team Member

The teaching attending should review his expectations for each learner. The single biggest error is failing to provide expectations at all. The second biggest error, however, is to provide nebulous expectations that have insufficient details to be meaningful (such as, "I expect all of you to work hard, and to be professional and conscientious"). The attending can improve the efficacy of the team by establishing expectations in the context of the anticipated day-to-day activities of the team. By providing expectations that are based on a sample day on the service, including rounding times and conference times, the attending can make these expectations more tangible and more meaningful. This method of expectations should be tailored for the three types of days on the service because expectations may change slightly depending on the type of day: 1) on-call days, 2) post-call days, and 3) other days.

Especially later in the year, students and residents are likely to bring preconceived expectations to the rotation on the basis of their experiences. Expectations that deviate from prior experiences are likely to be dismissed as "style" rather than "having a purpose." For this reason, it is important to *establish the rationale for each expectation*; once team members understand why the expectation exists, the probability for compliance with the expectation improves. It is fine to establish expectations that are based on personal preference. Clearly identifying these expectations as a style preference, in contrast to expectations that are critical because of their rationale, will highlight the importance of expectations that are based on some important reason (and not just style). The expectations should also be personal, with names used wherever possible, because this lends gravity to the expectation's importance by singling out the individual who is personally accountable for that expectation.

Following is a sample expectations talk (including statements that explain the rationale). The cast of characters includes Dr. Phaedrus (the attending), Moni (the resident), Stef (the intern), and Paul (the student). The dialogue is in italics to distinguish it from rationale and insights into teaching, which are in standard type. While a good deal of these expectations will already have been incorporated by residents and students as part of the program's "culture," it is important for the attending to assume ownership for how the service runs.

Before Rounds

> *"Okay, let's start with my expectations for what should happen before rounds. I'll start with the standard non-call, non–post-call day. For Paul and Stef, I'd like you to be here for prerounds early enough to collect all of the data that you will need to participate in the resident work rounds. You should be here as early as needed to accomplish this goal, but at any event, no later than 7 a.m. If you are not here early enough to collect these data, then you, and the team, cannot build a plan for your patients. You will have nothing to do during resident work rounds."*

Note how the attending conveys the expectation, and then provides the rationale for why the expectation exists.

> *"During prerounds, you should take a personal sign-out from the night-float intern. I do not want you taking sign-out over the phone, or just picking up the sign-out sheet. I want you to meet the intern in person and talk about what happened. I want you to see each patient as a very valuable baton ... extreme care needs to be given during each handoff, or things get dropped and patients get hurt."*

The attending anticipates the natural short cut that might occur when the intern or student gets pressed for time. He heads off this short cut by explicitly noting that it is not acceptable and providing the rationale.

> *"I want you to see each patient and talk with the patient to see how he or she did overnight, and how the symptoms have changed since yesterday. I'm going to tell your patients to be expecting you, so make sure you see them every day. Of all the data you collect, nothing replaces seeing the patient in person. Now, I realize that you do not have enough time to do a full physical examination on every patient, but I would like you to focus on the organ systems that are active for his or her admission."*

The attending keeps the expectation realistic by acknowledging the time limitations that will be present.

> *"We have to have that information to make decisions. If the patient is on telemetry, you should check with the telemetry clerk*

or the chart to see if there were any abnormal rhythms overnight. If a patient has had an arrhythmia, we need to know about it, as this could kill the patient if we do not fix the problem, and knowing about the arrhythmia was the whole point of having them on telemetry. If the nurse is available, and I realize sometimes that won't be the case, talk with the nurse who cared for the patient overnight. The nurses know the patients even better than you, and their insight is often lifesaving. I then would like you to check to see if any new laboratory results have come back, including culture results. Cultures sometimes take days to finally grow out, and we need to know if the culture turned positive overnight.

"Paul, I expect that you will talk with your intern before work rounds to get a sense of what the plan will be for the patient. For Paul and Stef, you should begin to think about what the plan will be for the patient, and be prepared to express that plan on work rounds. I do not expect that you will know all of the details, but I do expect that you will present a hypothesis as to the plan. If you do not learn to develop plans on your own, then you cannot advance to the next level of training. This is an important part of your development, and we need to see you practice doing this."

Resident Work Rounds

"For Paul and Stef, obviously you will want to present each patient's data to Moni, and you should end that concise presentation with your hypothesis as to the patient's plan. It is important that you are concise, since if you are not, there will not be enough time to see all of the patients on work rounds. Moni, I'd like you to be here early enough to round with the interns and students as a team, so that probably means 8 a.m. You should see the patients with the intern and students and not just card-flip. Once again, seeing a patient is worth all other data combined, and Paul and Stef do not have your level of experience in identifying which patients are really sick and need additional attention. I expect that the whole team will be on resident work rounds with you, and you will not split the team by rounding with one person at a time. This is important to ensure that we all learn from each other's patients, so that when one team member has the day off, another team member knows enough about his or her patients to help with the patient's care."

Again, the attending anticipates the "short cut" (splitting the team and not rounding as a team) and heads it off from the start, providing a rationale for why this can adversely affect patient care.

"The whole team should advance the patient's care plan during this time. If there are tests to be ordered, I want you to order them. If a patient looks to be ready for discharge, I want you to start the discharge process. We can always stop a discharge later in the morning if I disagree. I want you to be making these decisions, and allowing me the opportunity to evaluate your ability to make decisions that are safe and well-thought-out. To that end, I want you to show up for attending rounds prepared with a plan for each patient. If there are tests or medication orders that might harm the patient or that you do not feel comfortable doing, then please either call me first or hold those orders until attending rounds. The expectation I have for myself—and my promise to you—is that I will never be upset with you for calling me about a patient decision for which you are not comfortable."

The attending establishes the beginning of the "no-blame culture" by explicitly stating that he will not be angry with the team for doing the right thing (that is, calling about a patient decision about which the team is not comfortable).

"Finally, please end work rounds in time to attend morning report. If you find you need more time, then start earlier the next day so that you do have time for morning report."

Attending Rounds

"We should start attending rounds promptly at 10 a.m. Unless I tell Moni otherwise, we will meet on the 5-Center Ward. For attending rounds, as with work rounds, you should be prepared with a plan for each patient. If you have a plan prepared, I can better evaluate your decision-making and give you feedback that will make that decision-making even stronger. This will also free up time for more teaching on attending rounds if plans have already been established."

The attending anticipates that the predilection of most learners will be to remain in the comfort of the "reporter" role, merely reporting on data without having invested the intellectual courage required to make decisions. He notes why it is important that the team invest in making decisions by having a plan, and how this will help their development.

"I expect that all of us will show our respect for our patients by being neatly dressed and professional; that means no scrubs unless you are post-call and didn't have time to change into regular clothes. Remember, the more you assume the role of being the patient's physician, the more you are going to develop the skills necessary for your growth to the next level. Patients will recognize your scrubs as a sign that you are not 'the doctor in charge,' and they'll hold back on information; it will limit your patient rapport. Unsightly dress will make this even worse.

"Please no backpacks or purses on rounds; these are unnecessary pieces of baggage that serve to track MRSA and C. diff around the hospital. We'll find a secure place to store those if need be. This also means no drinks or food on rounds. Bringing food on the wards makes it look as if we are casually taking a walk; food is its own source of bacteria, and it is disrespectful to our patients who cannot eat. If, as a team, we are so tired as to need coffee, then we will sit at a conference table and talk about patients before seeing them."

Wearing scrubs may be acceptable at some institutions, and the attending should integrate dress code expectations according to the system in which she works. Regardless, setting expectations for what is and what is not appropriate in the way of appearance should be established from the outset of the rotation. Correcting fallouts will be much more comfortable if the expectation has been established a priori.

"But we will see the patients every day; seeing a patient is worth more than all of the other data combined. Before entering a patient room, and immediately after exiting a patient's room, we all need to either wash our hands or use the Purell dispenser. Even if you did not touch the patient, it is impossible for other people to know that you didn't. It's a good habit that I want you to have. If at any time someone doesn't wash their hands on entry or exit, I want you to remind them to do so—regardless of level on the team. And that includes me. It's that important."

The attending extends the "no-blame culture" by noting that no one, including himself, is above doing what is best for the patients—in this case, hand-washing.

"Before entering each room, I will ask you if there are sensitive data that cannot be discussed in front of the patient. If there are, we should discuss the patient outside of the room before entering.

If there are not, we should do all of our discussions in front of the patient. This will communicate that we are on the same team, eliminating any mixed messages or miscommunications that might have resulted from our different rounds. And it will teach the patient about his or her disease and condition, as well as show him or her how much intellectual effort is being expended on his or her care. It will also save us time. When we are in the room, let's all show the patient respect by standing attentively. I promise not to make the bedside sessions longer than they have to be. We will round as a team, just as you did on resident work rounds, so that each team member can learn about each other's patients, and be able to advance patient care if one team member is absent."

As will be discussed in chapter 3, rounding at the bedside is a useful technique to assess the learner's relationship with the patient (professionalism, patient care) and to help the team establish rapport with the patient (that is, the patient comes to recognize how much intellectual energy has been invested by the team on his or her behalf). Despite its benefits, however, bedside rounding is rarely done, and the attending should be prepared to provide the expectation and rationale so that the team is not shocked on the first day of rounds.

"When we are in the middle of a discussion, and definitely when we are at a patient's bedside, try not to leave the discussion to answer a page or your cell phone. The person in front of you deserves the same amount of respect that the person paging you from a distance does. If it is that urgent, we'll know by the way of the code pager or overhead announcement. Finally, let's all do out best to end at 11:45 a.m. each day. At that point, the interns and students should get to their conference; Moni and I will discuss the remainder of the patients, and if need be, Moni, I will see the remainder on my own. Attending conferences is an important part of your education, so I expect that you will not miss any of the conferences. This is very important to me."

The attending establishes a release valve for when time gets tight (the resident and the attending will round alone after 11:45 a.m.). The attending also recognizes that a mere admonishment to attend conference will fall into the avalanche of other similar admonishments from the chief residents, program director, et cetera. By making it personal and committing to a hard-stop end time for rounds, the attending provides much more gravity for the expectation that the interns will attend noon conference.

Afternoon Work and Teaching

> *"Paul and Stef, do your best to complete your progress notes in the afternoon. Stef, if you are in clinic in the afternoon, try to get here earlier in the day to make sure that the progress notes are mostly done, so that Moni is not left doing a lot of this work. Otherwise, just be sure that progress notes are done by the end of the day. I do not want you to spend your mornings writing about patient care; I want you to be actively involved in it as a part of resident work rounds. I also doubt the data you need for the progress note will be available by early morning, and I would rather that the note reflect a coherent plan after our discussions on resident work rounds and attending rounds."*

This expectation (when progress notes are to be completed) may vary by institution. It is, however, important to recognize that a system that prioritizes progress note completion in lieu of active decision-making (spending the morning writing notes instead of designing a plan) is at great risk for locking learners into the "reporter" stage on the reporter-interpreter-manager educator (RIME) developmental spectrum (see chapter 3 in *Teaching in Your Office*, another book in the *Teaching Medicine* series [4], as well as the original reference [5]).

> *"Stef, it is important that Paul have the first chance to write his own progress notes, but remember that each patient has to have a doctor's note each day, and Paul is not yet a doctor. I'll expect that you will write a full progress note as well as editing Paul's and giving him feedback. Moni, I do not expect you to write progress notes, but I do expect you, on occasion, to help Stef where he needs it in completing the notes. I also trust that you will read and edit Stef's progress notes and give him feedback. Where an additional addendum is required to clarify or correct a plan, I expect that you will do that. You are the team leader, and it is important that you assure that each patient care plan is accurate."*

The attending provides expectations not only for each individual team member but also for how each individual team member should interact with other team members. In doing so, he sends a message that both individual accountability *and* team-based patient care are priorities.

> *"For all of you, I expect that your notes will be legible and show pride in your work. Your notes are the touchstone upon which all other team members—nurses, social workers, consultants, and others—will use to contribute to the patient's care. I expect full*

sentences, not abbreviations; not everyone understands our jar-
gon and acronyms, and besides, sloppiness metastasizes. Sloppy
notes suggest sloppy care. People will not trust your data collec-
tion or assessment if it looks sloppy, and that means each consult-
ant has to re-do the whole history and physical, which is a waste
of their time."

The attending uses the act of writing notes as a step-off point to remind
the team that they are not alone in managing the patient: The needs of each
member of the multidisciplinary patient care team must be considered in
the learner's actions.

"Finally, Moni, particulary when I am not available in the after-
noons to do additional teaching, please try to find time to sit the
team down and teach them. I will help with you with that. Not
only is this the right thing to do, it is also a useful tool to help you
assess what you know and what you don't know. Teaching makes
smart physicians smarter, and that's what I wish for you, Moni."

End of the Day: Sign Out

"Stef, you should personally sign out each patient to the night
float intern. Moni, I expect that when Paul is in clinic, he will not
be returning after clinic, and that you will take care of this and
other duties that he normally would do. Stef, when you are in
clinic, I want you focused on your clinic patients and not worry-
ing about how soon you can get back to the wards. For both of
you, it is important to me that the patients are signed out in per-
son—not by phone, and not by leaving a sign-out sheet some-
where. The transition of care is where most mistakes happen, and
I want to do all that we can to provide good communication
between our team and the cross-covering team."

Call Days

"On call days, I will round with you briefly in the morning, start-
ing at 10 a.m. just like we usually do. I want to make sure that
rounds do not impair your ability to provide prompt patient care,
however, so our on-call rounds may be abbreviated. I will round
with you a second time on all on-call days, in the late afternoon
or evening. This will allow us to discuss any of the patients you
have already admitted, accelerating the discharge of a few, and
advancing the earlier care for all; it will also decompress our post-

call rounds a bit, so we'll have more time for teaching during both sessions."

The structure of the call day may vary according to the institution in which the attending works. Regardless, the attending should set explicit expectations for how the "call" or "admitting" days will vary from standard days.

"Moni, my job is to be your counselor and your coach. Call me on my cell phone at any time, day or night. If there is any question that you have, I want you to feel free calling me. I want you to have the latitude to make your own decisions, but if there is any doubt, call me. I definitely want to know about any patient that you plan on discharging, and a patient who dies or has a sudden and dramatic turn for the worse, and any patient who might be in the watershed between two services. For example, any patient that the emergency department wants to admit but you do not, or any patient that surgery wants to transfer to medicine but you do not. These are all high-risk times in a patient's care, and I would like to offer my additional experience in assuring that we get these decisions right. For conflicts between services, please call me. I know the attending physicians much better than you do, and I have a relationship with all of them. It will be much easier for me to navigate these political waters."

The attending establishes and encourages an open line of communication with the resident, a key step in ensuring patient safety. The explicit expectations outlined here establish a balance between autonomy and supervision. He anticipates that if he insists on a call for every decision, the resident will not develop into a true manager, which is where she needs to be on the RIME development spectrum (see above). He anticipates that if the resident feels intimidated in calling him, patient safety will suffer.

Post-Call Days

"Let's start post-call rounds at 7 a.m., and end by 11 a.m. This will give you time to act on our plans for each patient, and to leave the hospital by 1 p.m. Moni, I want you to guide me in determining the order in which we discuss patients, based on the three Ds: dire, diagnostics, and discharge. We'll start by discussing any patient who is in dire need of care—that is, the critically ill or those in need of ICU evaluation; then those who will need diagnostic tests that may take time to complete, radiology procedures, consultations, et cetera; and then patients who are ready for discharge.

*After that we'll discuss all other patients. Moni, if we run short of
time, we will release the team at 11 a.m., and you and I will finish
discussing the remainder of the patients."*

The single biggest difference between an intern and a second-year resident is the ability to recognize "sick" from "not sick," regardless of laboratory values. By establishing the criteria by which the team will sequence
the rounds, the attending not only ensures patient safety (dire patients
first) and efficiency (diagnostic and discharge patients next), but also gives
himself a measure to assess the resident or intern's ability to recognize
"sick" versus "not sick" (discovering a "dire" patient at the end of rounds
illustrates that the team might be coming up short on this important
assessment skill).

❖ The Supervision-to-Autonomy Spectrum: How Decisions Will Be Made

The inpatient ward team is a balance between a hierarchy and a group of
equals. Teaching on the inpatient wards is a balance between autonomy
and supervision. As illustrated in the preceding dialogue, the attending
physician can advance the effectiveness of the team by establishing the
expectations of how decisions will be made, and by creating an honest
vision for how the balance of autonomy versus supervision and hierarchy
versus a group of equals will change during the rotation.

Autonomy and independent decision-making are the keys to transi-
tioning from one level to the next, and only by active engagement in
patient management can this occur. Learning to make the best patient care
choices while in a supportive environment builds the confidence and ability
trainees need to make these decisions on their own.

As shown, the team should be instructed that they are expected to
make decisions, and that deferring decision-making to others, including
the attending, will stunt their growth in becoming independent physicians.
Day-to-day assessment of accountability, responsibility, and competence
will lead to either expanding or contracting their autonomy.

The resident for the team should be established as the team leader
because it is this individual who will spend most of the time as team leader
(assuming an 80-hour work week and 15 hours of attending rounds time
per week). The team should be encouraged to entertain open discussions
and debate about clinical decisions, but it should be made clear that in the
absence of the attending, where disagreement remains, the resident has
the final say with respect to patient care decisions. Likewise, the team
should be encouraged to have open debates on attending rounds, but if dis-

agreement remains after this debate, the attending physician will make the decision. In all situations, the residents and students should give their assessment of a situation before the attending expresses an opinion.

❖ Establishing Communication Expectations

Communication Between Team Members
Cell phone and pager numbers should be exchanged during the first session, and all members should have each other's contact information. To facilitate sharing of articles and reference materials, it is also useful to exchange e-mail addresses. This enables sharing articles in PDF format as opposed to having to make paper copies that inevitably find their way to call rooms or to an infinitely growing and daunting stack next to the resident's bed at home.

Establishing Expectations for Communication Within the Team
The attending should take the time to establish her expectation about how the team members should communicate with each other. While the attending should encourage open discussions between team members regardless of team rank, it is important that each member knows the importance of not "skipping ranks" in their communication—this can lead to fatal missteps when one team member is left out of the loop:

> *"I want all of you to know that Moni is leading this team. Paul, Stef, you are always free to ask me questions, but do not be surprised if I ask you to first talk with Moni regarding all management decisions. It is important that we not overstep any member of the team, and she needs to know what we are doing; not having that information might lead her to make a decision that would have adverse effects on the patient's care. For example, if we start a beta-blocker, she needs to know that before starting another antihypertensive agent. Moni, I'll trust that you will let Stef write most of the orders, and if there are orders written by you after rounds, that you will keep Stef in the loop such that he knows what has transpired. For all of you, if I write any orders, which will be rare, I will make sure that you know that I have done so. This will ensure that we are all on the same page."*

Oral Communication

The attending should establish her expectations as to the oral case presentation. Sample expectations for the oral case presentation are contained in chapter 4. The presentation is a good surrogate measure of a student's clinical reasoning and understanding of the medical decision-making affecting the patient's care. Outlining the specific expectations for the oral case presentation can be handled during the orientation session or be reserved for the first time that the attending and the team approach the task together, which is usually during the first oral case presentation given to the attending physician (the first rounds).

Communication Outside of the Team: Written Communication

As illustrated in the dialogue, the attending should clarify the expectations she has for discharge summaries, admission notes, and progress notes. As with the oral case presentation, sample expectations are outlined in chapter 4. Providing expectations for specific content and structure for admission and progress notes is best reserved for the first time the attending and the team encounter the medical record together, usually during the first walk rounds where the chart is reviewed. As the attending did in the preceding example, he or she should outline who is responsible for each note, when notes should be placed in the chart, and additional responsibilities as they pertain to reviewing, editing, and modifying notes. These expectations will vary by health care system, although a universal expectation should be established that team members should not remove content from the medical record.

Expectations for Tracking Patient Data

The attending should anticipate that medical students, and some residents, will not have a method for tracking patient data, and will resort to using progress notes, extracted from the chart, to present their patients on rounds. Team members should be instructed that removing progress notes or other documentation from the chart hinders other members of the health care team (nurses, social workers, consultants) from advancing the patient's care.

Team members should be expected to develop a method for tracking their patients' data because this enables them to detect trends in the data. A resident presenting from one progress note at a time will miss the drop in the hemoglobin that occurs at a rate of 1 g/L per day for 5 days. The method of tracking data—cards, books, personal digital assistant—is largely at the discretion of the team member; the attending's expectation should be to establish that each team member *has* a method that detects trends in patient data. (See chapter 5 on data organization for more information.)

❖ Establishing a "No-Blame Culture"

The single biggest advance in patient safety is the "no-blame culture," in which all health care team members, regardless of rank or degree, feel comfortable raising an issue of patient safety or quality if they believe it is in the patient's best interest. As the attending did in the dialogue, he or she should establish from the outset that no team member will be chastised for honestly admitting an error or admission. "No blame" does not mean "no accountability," however, and it is important that the attending clearly establish this distinction, as exemplified in the following dialogue:

> *"For all of you—Paul, Stef, Moni—let me say this. I expect that you will make mistakes. I do routinely, and so will you … for the rest of your lives. Medicine is just too tough and too complex to be performed perfectly. I promise that only if you disregard three rules will I become angry with you. If you follow these three rules, then I will always support you.*

> *"First, that you show up on time, both mentally and physically ready to care for your patients and to learn. I think I've already made those expectations clear. Second, that you be honest. For example, there are times when you will not have checked a lab value, and it will be tempting to say that you did because you are pretty sure that it was normal yesterday. Don't do that. Simply be honest and say that you didn't check it. At least that enables someone else on the team to know that it needs to be checked, and the patient doesn't get hurt. If you say that you did, we are going to trust that you did. And if you didn't do something and you lie about it, no one else will do it—and the patient gets hurt." Phaedrus pauses for effect. "Now, I may remind you that it is your responsibility to check the labs each day. We are all still account-able to fulfill our roles on this team. But I promise that I will not be angry with you if you are honest. The honesty is much more important to me than any one task that wasn't completed.*

> *"My third requirement is that you play as a team. Despite your 'ranks' on this team—resident, intern, student—and the impor-tance of fulfilling our roles to the team, we are a team. This is not about us—it's about the patients. There will be no reward for*

undercutting a teammate or selfishly doing only what is your typ-
ical role. Rewards will go to those who make the team better, who
take care of their teammates, and who chip in where needed to do
whatever has to be done. And that goes for me, too. If need be, I
still remember how to write a progress note or make phone calls
for appointments or whatever. I'm a little foggy on disimpactions,
though, so Stef, that's all you." The team laughs.

"Just kidding, I'll do that as well if it comes to it. Okay? Are we all
cool with that? Show up, be honest, play as a team."

At the beginning of the rotation, the ward team should be encouraged to question each other and the attending when a clinical issue is not clear. The attending physicians should explain the rationale: Only when learners stop deferring to others' opinions do they learn how to assess problems and make informed decisions on how to solve them. Defending their decisions forces trainees to analyze situations thoroughly. When performed in a safe learning environment, debate can advance the learning process not just for the individual resident or student but the entire team as well. The expectation that open and honest debate will not only be tolerated but also encouraged establishes from the outset a culture of "It's not about me (or my ego, or my rank), it's about the patient." From comfort in open discussions about medical decisions comes a culture in which any person, regardless of rank, would feel comfortable reminding the chair of medicine or hospital CEO to wash her hands if she did not do so.

❖ Establishing Expectations for Evaluation

Team members should be instructed that that they will be evaluated daily, with direct feedback (coaching) provided appropriate to the activity. Formal evaluation will occur at the midpoint of the rotations, and again at the conclusion of the evaluation. The complexity of the ward environment, and the seemingly unconquerable volume of information to learn, may weaken team member's self-esteem, causing even self-confident team members to misinterpret midrotation evaluation sessions, or even daily feedback, as indications of failure or disapproval. The emotionally charged nature of evaluation sessions can be mitigated by establishing from the outset of the rotation that daily, midrotation, and end-of-rotation evaluation and feedback is a regular and expected exercise that is important for every team member's development. Feedback and evaluating learner performance is addressed in greater detail in chapter 3 of *Theory and Practice of Teaching Medicine,* also part of the *Teaching Medicine* series (6), and in chapter 6 of this book.

❖ Conclusion

Setting expectations and goals for the rotation is a critical component of the ward rotation. Despite the time pressures of the inpatient ward, time must be reserved at the outset of the rotation to clearly establish the expectations for each team member, and for the team as a whole. At first, it may feel uncomfortable and demanding (for example, telling people what to do), but the attending should be assured that if the expectations are anywhere close to reasonable, the team will accept and appreciate the explicit nature of what has been conveyed. There is a psychological security for teacher and learner alike that comes with knowing precisely what is expected. The true discomfort comes with trying to correct behavior later in the rotation because an expectation had not been clearly established.

Expectations properly delivered establish the "no-blame" culture under which the team will operate, creating a learning environment that encourages open discussion and freely admitting mistakes; both components are central to patient safety and quality. By clearly outlining the goals and expectations for each team member, how each team member will interact and communicate with other team members, and by defining how decisions will be made (autonomy vs. supervision), the attending's expectations define the team-based mentality that will guide the rotation. Finally, the attending's expectations set up the midrotation and end-of-rotation feedback and evaluation (chapter 6), making this experience much more comfortable and constructive: Nothing will be a mystery to the learner during these sessions, as the expectations have been clearly defined.

REFERENCES

1. **Accreditation Council for Graduate Medical Education.** Outcome Project. Accessed at www.acgme.org/outcome.
2. **Litzelman DK, Cottingham AH.** The new formal competency-based curriculum and informal curriculum at Indiana University School of Medicine: overview and five-year analysis. Acad Med. 2007;82:410-21.
3. **Smith SR, Dollase RH, Boss JA.** Assessing students' performances in a competency-based curriculum. Acad Med. 2003;78:97-107.
4. **Alguire PC, DeWitt DE, Pinsky LE, Ferenchick GS.** Teaching in Your Office: A Guide to Instructing Medical Students and Residents. 2nd ed. Philadelphia: ACP Pr; 2008.
5. **Pangaro L.** A new vocabulary and other innovations for improving descriptive in-training evaluations. Acad Med. 1999;74:41-5.
6. **Ende J, ed.** Theory and Practice of Teaching Medicine. Philadelphia: ACP Pr; 2010.

3

Strategies for Succeeding as an Inpatient Attending Physician

Jeff Wiese, MD, FACP
Lorenzo DiFrancesco, MD
Neil Winawer, MD, FHM

As outlined in the introduction to this book, the life of the inpatient attending is laden with challenges. Yet from these challenges come unique opportunities in medical education. This chapter addresses several issues unique to the inpatient teaching environment. Inpatient attendings must have defined strategies to ensure that their diverse range of goals is accomplished and their equally diverse responsibilities are met.

When time gets tight, education is the first to be sacrificed, and with it goes the fulfillment intrinsic to teaching on the wards. This chapter identifies structural issues that should be of concern to inpatient attendings, regardless of their role in administrating the service. It also provides time management strategies that attendings can use to accomplish both their clinical and educational roles. The challenging issue of dealing with the heterogeneity intrinsic in each ward team is discussed next, followed by methods for assessing where learners are on the autonomy-to-supervision spectrum. Methods of successfully conducting ward rounds and dealing with successful transitions of care are also addressed. Finally, this chapter gives strategies for fulfilling the attending's financial obligations (coding and billing) while maintaining the educational environment.

KEY POINTS

- Inpatient attendings need to take whatever steps are necessary to ensure they have enough time to focus on patient care as well as teaching.
- Several specific strategies that will allow the attending physician to leverage his or her available time, including having an organized approach that assigns certain activities to different times of the day.
- Inpatient teaching attendings can more effectively relate to learners at different levels by addressing certain topics to individual members of the team, organizing teaching to fit learners' personal schedules, and being deliberate about granting autonomy.
- Several lenses are available through which the inpatient teaching attending can determine whether residents are ready to assume autonomy and greater responsibility for decision-making.
- Conducting rounds involves a series of decisions about the location of rounds (e.g., conference room vs. bedside), the order in which patients will be seen, and the content of rounds.
- Attending rounds should be a venue for teaching about transitions of care.
- Inpatient teachers need to be well versed in the requirements for documentation, coding, and billing on the inpatient service.

❖ Addressing Structural Issues

The attending has a large stake in ensuring that the structure of the rotation is conducive to education and clinical service. If it is not, accomplishing all of the goals and objectives of both clinical service and education will be impossible, and education will be lost. The critical components of a teaching service that are a concern for the attending include the following:

The attending should advocate that his time be protected to ensure that he can fulfill his primary responsibilities during the rotation: patient care and education. This will be particularly challenging for the traditional internist who still manages a clinic during ward teaching assignments, and for the subspecialist who attends on the wards but still has procedures to perform in the afternoon. Even for hospitalists who have additional job requirements (such as committees and preoperative care) this may be a challenge. Where possible, committee meetings should be rescheduled during the month and other professional responsibilities (writing papers, participating in conference calls, compiling business reports) deferred. The attending should advocate strongly for having protected time from these responsibilities when attending on a busy teaching service. While time is money, nothing is more costly than adverse patient events or loss of a training program's accreditation.

The attending physician should advocate that the residency and student programs construct a system that is time efficient. The ideal training environment should minimize fragmentation of the learner's time (for example, having residents attend morning report, then 1 hour of attending rounds, then noon conference, then wards, then clinic). The ideal schedule of the day should maximize the high-yield times of clinical decision-making (for example, mornings are not occupied by clinics or conferences). The resident and student schedules should be constructed such that the effect of learner absences is mitigated (so that all learners are not in clinic at the same time or have the same days off). On an attending's first teaching assignment, these issues will be out of his sphere of influence and the best of the situation has to be made. Over time, however, the attending physician should advocate for change to ensure that the hospital teaching environment allows for resident and student focus, which are requisite for successful patient care and teaching.

The attending physician should advocate for a rotation length that is conducive to accomplishing his goals. Too many consecutive weeks on an inpatient service may preclude office-based practitioners from inpatient attending, and will lead to a piling up of office work and outside duties. Conversely, the attending may lose the economy of scale that goes with assignments of 2 weeks or less. Time is wasted with frequent attending turnover as the attending tries to both learn the new patients and assess the needs of the team. Educational value is also diminished with short assignments because the attending loses track of what the team must be taught, where skills deficits might exist, and where remediation strategies might be required.

Regardless of the system, attendings should adapt by synchronizing their daily schedule with the residents' and students' schedules. Office hours should be truncated or blocked out. Committee meetings should be moved to the windows of time when the resident-student team is by definition without the attending (morning report, noon conference, or resident-only work rounds). Conversely, attendings may want to ensure that they are on the wards when the supervising resident is not (the resident's days off or clinic times). This will ensure efficiency and safety in patient care, as younger learners often defer management decisions when supervisors are not present. It is very important that attendings cancel all other obligations on the post-call days—the intensity will be high on these days, and the resident team will not be around to facilitate patient care in the afternoon.

❖ Time Management Strategies

Today's attending is faced with an unprecedented challenge in balancing the service requirements and ensuring educational excellence for her team. To accomplish this goal, time management strategies are a must.

For systems that allow remote access to the electronic medical record, the attending should invest in the software and home computer to enable "spying" on the patients' laboratory values from home. While "spying" sounds devious, it is important that the attending exercise stealth in observing laboratory data, lest the team come to expect that their failure to follow the laboratory values will be offset by the attending's doing the job. Upon waking up, the attending can gain insight into the service size and intensity, and can find answers to several questions that otherwise would consume the first part of the day at work: Were new patients added to the service? If so, how many? Did the patient's condition change? Are any patients ready for discharge? With these insights, the attending can mentally prepare himself on his ride into the hospital for how the rounds will be conducted that day, how much teaching time will be available, and what topics might be addressed in teaching sessions.

Attendings should round alone on early discharge patients. Upon arrival at the hospital, the attending's first task should be to visit patients who have a high probability of being discharged that day. This will allow the attending to start attending rounds with these patients and, if necessary (see below), splitting off one team member to quickly write the discharge order to get the process in motion. As with the laboratory values, the attending should exercise due stealth, lest the team lose the impetus for diligent rounding on their own.

Attendings should avoid splitting the team unless absolutely necessary. Team rounds (all learners present for all patients) instill the hidden curricular message of the importance of team-based care, enable all learners to expand their patient-care database, and enable the continuity of care when one team member is absent. Routinely rounding with only a portion of the team (such as just the resident and then just the intern) will appear to save time in the short run, but the time saving is largely offset by the confusion over team management that results. In the long run, especially when one team member has off, the time loss due to inefficiency will exceed whatever time was saved by splitting the team. However, when a quick task can be performed, as in a quick discharge order, allowing a team member to be temporarily absent to accomplish this task is time efficient. The exception to this rule may be on post-call days in systems that still use the 24-hour call system, especially on teams with more than one intern. Here all team members must leave within 6 hours of the call completion, and it may be most efficient to round with the resident, students, and one intern, allowing the other intern to complete patient care duties (and then vice versa with the second intern). This still maintains a core of the team while enabling the team to leave the hospital under the work hours regulations.

The attending can ensure her own time efficiency by teaching the team to be more efficient and independent. An efficient team will maintain patient throughput and provide the attending with the data necessary for her own clinical decisions (see the discussion of "Important vs. Urgent" in chapter 5).

For systems that provide time for the residency team to round as a unit before meeting with the attending, the attending should stress the importance of the team's arriving at attending rounds with a plan for each patient. Where there is diagnostic uncertainty, the team should arrive committed to a hypothesis about the diagnosis (see chapter 4). Nothing wastes time as much as a disorganized, undirected discussion about patients on rounds. Even if the team's decision or hypothesis was wrong, the conversation will quickly hone to the issues that need correcting.

The attending must know how to remediate deficits in oral communication. As stated above, disorganized and verbose student and resident presentations can destroy the efficiency of rounds. Chapter 5 includes specific suggestions for addressing this issue. As with time management training, the attending can be exponentially helpful in his efforts by teaching the residents these skills, with the directive that they are responsible for teaching the other team members.

Attendings should reserve billing, coding, and documentation for the afternoons and devote rounds to the education of the team. Using attending rounds as a venue where learners watch the attending document patients is painful, eroding the teaching time of the residents and destroying the team's morale. It also lengthens attending rounds, which pushes the residents' "action time" (where they actually do the tasks assigned on attending rounds) into the afternoon, outside of the window of efficiency for making things happen. The better approach is to reserve attending rounds for education and management decisions.

The billing, coding, and documentation requirements will vary according to the system in which the attending works. If the system allows, the attending should use linking notes that enable billing and coding from the resident's or intern's documentation. This will not only save time but also ensure that the attending is critically reviewing the resident's notes (see later discussion of documentation).

Attendings can offer to see patients twice. One of the perils of rounds is the time lost because of the verbose patient. Outside of patients with axis II mental disorders, verbosity usually has one of two causes: 1) The patient is having a hard time expressing what she wants to say and, feeling misunderstood, repeats the same information in different ways, or 2) the patient is nervous that he will have only one opportunity to talk to his doctor and, with pressured speech, tries to fit all questions and comments into one session. The result of this pressure, of course, can be a jumble of words that make the patient feel misunderstood; this, in turn, feeds back into the first cause of verbosity. The attending can offset both causes by three approaches. First, sitting or kneeling down while at the bedside gives the impression of greater time at the bedside and alleviates some of the pressure to "get it all in quickly"—a seated physician does not appear to be about to leave the room as a standing physician does. Second, the attending can assure the patient that whatever is not addressed in this session can be discussed in the afternoon session when he returns. This alleviates the pressure, allowing more linear speech with less anxiety. Finally, repeating the patient's message back to him assures the patient that he has been heard and understood, alleviating the verbosity due to the first cause.

The other advantage to seeing patients twice, even if the second encounter is just a brief visit in the afternoon, is that it enables a quick response to any changes in the patients' condition. It is more time efficient to catch and solve small problems early, before they become big problems. Patients who improve can be identified, and patients with diagnostic information that becomes available in the midafternoon (for example, a negative stress test result) may be eligible for discharge earlier, thereby decompressing the following day's rounds.

Late afternoons on post-call days are an optimal time to call the patients' primary care providers. The attending will be alone during such times because the team will have retired early (as a result of work hour requirements), and primary care providers are probably winding down their clinic schedule. Making calls at the end of the day can save time—there is a greater chance of talking directly to a primary care provider rather than playing phone tag. Not only is calling the primary providers important to begin the transition of care for patients recently admitted, but it can also prevent duplication of diagnostic tests and improve understanding of patient personalities and wishes in subsequent management.

Rounding a second time during on-call days can save time. This allows the attending to hear about patients admitted during the first 10 hours of the call day. Early discharge may be possible for some, thereby decompressing the post-call day. The resident team's presentations are likely to be more cogent than they will be after a night on call; the residents can establish a plan for these patients that only needs to be reviewed the following day. This, too, decompresses the time pressures of the post-call day. By instituting evening on-call rounds, the morning on-call rounds can be truncated, if necessary, permitting the team to deal with admissions earlier (instead of being tied up in morning rounds). This approach in turn accelerates patient care. Evening on-call rounds also enable a more relaxed teaching environment to address some of the more complex clinical issues (see the teaching dialogue on acid-base in section II of this book and on electrocardiograms in the online portion of this book, available at www.acponline.org/acp_press/teaching/).

After completion of afternoon rounds alone, it saves time to touch base, even if by phone, with the resident leading the team. Some patients might be eligible for discharge, and the ones who are close to discharge can be reviewed with the resident. This discussion enables the resident to make early-morning discharge decisions based on contingency plans: *"Mr. Panda looks much better. If his hemoglobin remains stable tomorrow morning, let's plan on discharging him during your morning work rounds."* Any late diagnostic information can be acted upon with the resident team, thereby advancing care a day earlier as opposed to waiting for the following day's rounds: *"Mrs. Phillips' CT scan came back nondiagnostic. I think we need to put her on the schedule for bronchoscopy tomorrow. Will you call the pulmonary fellow and do that?"*

❖ Dealing With Heterogeneity of the Team

As opposed to a teacher in the ambulatory environment, the inpatient teaching attending must regularly deal with the heterogeneity of her learner team. A range of leaner levels (ranging from students to residents) and interests (nonmedicine, general medicine, medicine subspecialties) will probably be present. There are three methods for addressing this heterogeneity.

Shifting Higher-Level Learners Into a Different Gear

The attending should not overestimate how much upper-level learners know. The nature of graduate medical education is that learning opportunities (patients) present randomly. Depending on the patients admitted during the call days, it is possible that a resident, despite 2 or 3 years of training, may not have seen even the most important inpatient problems (such as diabetic ketoacidosis). Further, even residents with solid foundations of understanding disease may have been corrupted over time by bad or sloppy methods. For this reason, the attending should not feel guilty about teaching even the most basic of internal medicine topics.

However, the attending should be sensitive to the resident's ego and her responsibility for maintaining a position of authority over the team. This conundrum can be easily escaped by leading into the topic by addressing the resident with, "Since you are a resident, I know you know this, but as I talk, I want you to think of how you would teach it." This shifts the resident into an ego-neutral gear, allowing her to indeed focus on the teaching method if she knows the topic, or to learn the topic (or relearn a proper method) if she does not.

Providing Progressive Learning That Is Proportional to Difficulty

For the middle-of-the-road topics, the attending can deal with the heterogeneity of the team by a progressive increase in the questioning that parallels the difficulty of the topic. During this process, it is important to recognize the team dynamics. Asking questions that are too difficult will naturally lead to wrong answers, embarrassing the learner. This is especially true for the team leader (the resident). If the leader is made to appear incompetent, it will destroy the team leader's morale and erode the team's effectiveness when the attending is not present. As the line of questioning escalates, it is important that lower-level learners (students) are not confused. The attending can offset this risk by asking the lower-level learners if they understand the content or by explicitly "mentally dismissing" the lower-level students by saying, "This is more at an intern/resident level, so don't worry if you don't get this." The teaching dialogues in section II of this book and on the companion Web site to this book, available at www.acponline.org/acp_press/teaching/, have examples on progressive escalation of questioning that is proportional to content.

Taking Advantage of Days Off, Clinic Absences, and Class Absences

In terms of team composition, the team will vary from day to day because of days off and clinic or class obligations. The attending can turn this curse into a blessing by selectively planning teaching topics on the basis of levels of difficulty. The day that the resident has off, for example, is the ideal time to talk about fundamental topics; on the intern's day off, the attending may choose topics that are directed toward the students; more complicated discussions can be reserved for days when only the resident is present. The point is, be adaptable, be able to improvise (see chapter 3 in *Theory and Practice of Teaching Medicine* [1], another book in the *Teaching Medicine* series), and, by all means, "teach to your learners."

❖ Assessing Where Learners Are on the Autonomy-to-Supervision Spectrum

Skillful physicians, regardless of specialty, have the ability to make decisions, especially the tough ones. But decision-making requires courage, confidence, and foresight, virtues that can be acquired only by the deliberate practice of actively making decisions. For this reason, it is vital that the attending foster an environment that encourages learners to actively manage their patients, as opposed to the passive environment, where the attending merely tells learners what to do. Further, active management inspires learners to take ownership of their patients, another central virtue for the professionalism development of the learner.

Balancing the need to encourage active decision-making and ownership of patients is the concern for patient safety; learners are not expert physicians, and the attending is ultimately responsible for each patient's management. This balance, the autonomy-to-supervision spectrum, varies according to the level of learner, with higher-level learners moving closer to the autonomy side of the spectrum. However, the appropriate level of autonomy afforded to a resident may vary widely even within the same level of training: Some residents are more adept at patient management than their peers.

To maximize learners' development on the autonomy-to-supervision spectrum, the maximum amount of autonomy appropriate to the trainee's ability should be assigned. To do this safely, however, the attending must be able to assess the trainee's patient management ability and his level of ownership of the patient. The following techniques are useful in assessing which learners are ready for increasing autonomy in their patient management.

Observe the Learner on Rounds

Assessing autonomy ability begins by observing the learner as she presents her patients on rounds. Learners who appear consistently nervous and disorganized during their presentations or continuously flip through papers to find clinical data may not be ready for more autonomy. The attending should pay particular attention to the presentation of the assessment and plan—learners may quickly master the reporter function on the reporter-interpreter-manager-expert progression but not yet have acquired management skills. As learners demonstrate progressive competence in designing and presenting assessments and plans, more autonomy can be provided.

However, caution should be used in relying on this standard alone in assessing a learner's autonomy ability because impaired performance could be due to a fear of public speaking, generalized anxiety, or a failure of supervising residents or interns to provide appropriate preparation. Conversely, well-appearing presentations may be solely due to exceptional preparation by supervising residents or interns, and the student's autonomy ability may be overestimated.

Observe the Observers
Observing senior-level team members during a student's or intern's presentations can also offer insight into the level of autonomy appropriate for a given resident. Say, for example, a resident is writing data down during a student's presentation, suggesting that he (the resident) is learning about these data for the first time. That suggests the resident has not taken sufficient ownership of the patient to ensure that the patient's management is appropriate. Conversely, residents who observe with confidence students' presentations, smoothly correcting inaccuracies and answering questions from the attending, are showing that they have ownership of the patient's condition and are ready to assume increased autonomy.

Observe the Patient: Bedside Rounds
Bedside rounds are a useful arena in which to determine the appropriate autonomy that should be afforded to learners. During bedside presentation, a patient who interacts primarily with the learner assigned to him is indicating that this learner has demonstrated responsibility and ownership for the patient and is probably ready for increased autonomy. Conversely, learners who appear nervous in front of the patient, or those whose presentations contain numerous inaccuracies as pointed out by the patient, probably have not taken appropriate ownership of their patient's condition and deserve no increased autonomy.

Assess the Quality of Notes
Like the spoken case presentation indicator, the admission note can provide insight into the learner's ownership of the patient's condition and ability in clinical decision-making. Well-organized, complete, and accurate notes indicate greater responsibility and warrant consideration of increas-

ing a learner's autonomy. Like the oral presentation, the assessment and plan, especially regarding the clinical reasoning shown therein, is the best indicator that the student has progressed to the "manager" level as opposed to just being a good "reporter." Unlike the oral case presentation, the admission note is not subject to the confounder of nervousness in public speaking. However, it is subject to the "protective bias," where excellent supervising residents can make less competent students look better than they are and vice versa. Further, some learners may appear better and more competent than they are by copying other physicians' notes; this is especially true in systems using an electronic medical record.

Separate Team Members
Protective bias is a considerable problem for the oral case presentation and admission note indicators. The attending can use the variability of the team's composition (for example, during a team member's days off) to isolate learners from their supervisors. Performance that remains consistent with previous observations indicates that the attending can be more confident in her assessment of the learner's autonomy ability; a learner whose performance dramatically worsens indicates that a protective bias was present.

Conduct Second Rounds
During an attending's solo afternoon rounds, patients should be asked, "Who is the doctor who is primarily taking care of you?" Learners whom patients indicate by name have probably demonstrated the responsibility and accountability to warrant increasing their autonomy.

Check Nurse Evaluations
With the exception of the patient herself, no one knows about the actual care of patients like the nurses. By being visible on the wards during the afternoon and by establishing relationships with nurses, the attending physician may gain valuable insight into each team member's responsibility and accountability simply by asking the nurses their opinions. This is especially true for the interns and residents; those who receive the nurses' endorsement are probably worthy of increased autonomy.

Use Afternoon On-Call Time With Learners (Individual Assessments)
The gold standard of assessing the appropriate autonomy that should be afforded each learner is direct observation. Although the time pressures of the inpatient ward do not allow direct observation of each learner each day, the attending should try to devote sessions to observing each learner performing independently. Afternoon on-call rounds are an optimal time to

conduct these evaluations; these rounds may not require more than merely asking a student, intern, or resident to talk through the details of a patient whom they have just admitted. Observing a learner conduct a history and physical examination is of even greater value should time allow. The attending can then use this gold standard to assess her accuracy with other indicators. Over time, this adjustment with the gold standard will improve the attending's assessment accuracy.

❖ Conducting Rounds

The timing of inpatient teaching rounds depends on the system in which the attending works. The attending should advocate for enough time to adequately advance patient care and to provide education in the process. That said, the attending should stay within the confines of the rounding time provided by the training program for which he works. Rounds should not infringe on organized education sessions.

The nature, character, and content of rounds will vary on the basis of the team's needs, the patients on the service, the team constituents (that is, which team members remain after days off), and the time requirements of the service. The attending should see the nature of teaching rounds as a daily choice, and he should read the circumstances of the teaching service in deciding which is the best course for that day. In making that determination, the attending must make several choices, including those related to location, sequencing, and emphasis of rounds.

Choosing the Location of Teaching Rounds

Conference room teaching has some unique advantages. It allows the teaching physician to use a whiteboard to diagram key pathophysiologic or complicated concepts for the trainees. It also enables frank discussions of patients' diagnostic and therapeutic plans, while occasionally allowing for light-hearted teaching opportunities (something that would otherwise appear inappropriate at the bedside of a sick patient). Even if conference room rounds are chosen, it is still important to spend a portion of the rounding time seeing a few select patients to ensure that the team is continually reminded that internal medicine is best practiced at the bedside and that all discussions and management should be patient-centered.

Bedside rounds offer specific advantages over conference rounds. They allow the patient to be viewed as an individual, someone who can actively participate in her own care. By taking this patient-centered approach, teaching physicians are more likely to observe, demonstrate, confirm, or refute aspects of the history and physical. In addition, pivotal secrets often emerge on bedside rounds (for example, the rash that was mysteriously not present on admission or the pericardial rub that was identified for the first time by the attending). At the bedside, teaching physicians can also reincorporate the human dimension of doctoring by allocating time to sensitive social or psychological aspects of a patient's illness. It also demonstrates to patients the valuable teaching function of physicians because patients get to experience first hand how physicians advise and instruct each other on rounds.

The choice between conference room and bedside rounds depends on the day-to-day circumstances of the team, and the attending should see this choice as part of his daily roster of decisions. For large services, bedside rounds are more time efficient for the attending. When services are small, conference room rounds can be used to address "whiteboard" teaching, while still enabling the team to see the patients afterward. Post-call conference room rounds should be evoked when the work from the previous night was particularly intense. This will allow the team to consume coffee or food while still addressing many of the management decisions from the night before. The teaching topics that the attending expects to address during the rounds may also determine the location. Obviously, physical examination teaching is best conducted at the bedside, while talks about abstract or complicated talks requiring diagrams are best conducted in the conference room.

Sequencing of Rounds

When efficiency is the priority (for example, on a large teaching service), the attending should choose bedside rounds because this limits the rounding episodes per patient to one (as opposed to conference room rounds, in which each patient is discussed initially and then discussed again at bedside). Further efficiency is the technique of *geographic rounding*; the sequence of rounds is based on each patient's proximity to the last patient. Efficiency can be enhanced by dispensing with the hallway discussions outside of each room and immediately proceeding to the patient's bedside to entertain the discussion. In doing so, it is important to ask the learner responsible for the patient if any sensitive issues cannot be discussed in front of the patient before proceeding.

Efficiency for the attending should not be confused with efficiency for the team. Note-writing on the part of the attending during rounds should be discouraged; even though this is efficient for the attending's day, it lengthens the overall time of rounds and thus delays the team's time to actually carrying out tasks assigned on attending rounds. Ultimately, this slows patient throughput. Efficiency should also not obviate autonomy; although it is more efficient for the attending to merely tell the team what to do, this defeats the purpose of teaching rounds because the learners fail to develop their clinical decision-making abilities.

When time allows, clinical reasoning should be the criteria by which rounds are conducted. The singular difference between an intern and a resident is the ability to determine severity of illness, that is, which patient is sick (regardless of the numbers or data) and which patient is not. By asking the intern or resident to choose the sequence of rounds, the attending can use the sequence as its own assessment of this ability. The team should use the 3Ds: dire, diagnostics, and discharge. Patients whose clinical condition is dire or who may need intensive care unit evaluation should be visited first, followed by those who need immediate diagnostic tests (radiographic or consultation) and then by those who are ready for discharge. Once informed of this expectation, the attending can provide feedback to the team on any patient who was out of sequence with this standard. This method is also useful in ensuring appropriate throughput and efficiency because it moves the team to act on diagnostic tests and activates the discharge process early. This teaches the team valuable lessons in time management (see chapter 5). It is also useful to sequence all patients with communicable diseases (such as infection with methicillin-resistant *Staphylococcus aureus*, vancomycin-resistant enterococci, or *Clostridium difficile*) to the end of rounds, decreasing the risk for patient-to-patient spread, and illustrating the importance of this principle to the team as manifest in the rounding sequence.

Rounding Techniques to Teach and Assess Clinical Reasoning

Encourage Students and Residents to See as Many Patients as Possible

Direct patient experiences enable learners to develop essential clinical knowledge about both typical and atypical presentations of disease. Attendings should role-model that the best way to become a good diagnostician is to carefully evaluate as many patients as possible, and then augment that knowledge through reading. The more patients with a given disease that a learner sees, the more likely she will be able to apply her knowledge to atypical presentations in a variety of contexts. Attendings should encourage team members to return to the bedside of patients after rounds, even if they are not "following" them to learn more about diseases with which they have limited experience. This practice will build an extensive set of mental models for many of the diseases commonly seen in internal medicine.

Teach Regularly About Epidemiology and Risk Factors

A learner's development from phase 3 clinical reasoning to phase 4 is contingent on integrating prevalence and probability into the learner's differential diagnosis. One of the attending's roles should be to highlight the relevant epidemiology of a given patient and compare and contrast it with the "textbook" presentation. This approach has particular strength in helping learners diagnose atypical presentations of common illnesses because knowledge of the epidemiology will enable them to recognize the salient disease, even though the signs or symptoms may be unusual.

Highlight Pathophysiologic and Basic Science Principles to Improve Connections Between Learners' Biomedical and Clinical Knowledge

Attendings should ask the student to explain the relationships of the clinical presentation to the underlying basic science and pathophysiology of the disorder when applicable. Inexperienced learners have a greater ability to recall and apply knowledge of diseases when they understand how the disease causes the clinical findings. This approach can help learners to strengthen their recall and attack more challenging diagnostic situations.

Use Evidence-Based Medicine When Possible

Role-modeling an evidence-based approach is an important part of teaching clinical reasoning. Role-modeling literature searches during rounds or in the afternoon is an effective way to help build the team's desire to strive for evidence-based practice. When evidence does not exist or a patient's chooses a non–evidence-based option, attendings should feel comfortable stating that reason, rather than substance, dictated the choice. Learners should be reminded that patient preference supersedes even the best evidence.

Special Considerations for Conducting Post-Call Rounds

On the post-call day, the attending will be saddled with the responsibility of learning about new patients. The attending should budget appropriate time based on the patient's complexity, and should begin rounds by asking the resident to give him an idea of how many patients fall into the following categories: category 1, simple (such as chest pain; ruled out for myocardial infarction); category 2, moderately complex (one primary problem; diagnostic reasoning required, but diagnosis has been determined); category 3, complex (multisystem disease, or the diagnosis has still not been determined). For most attending physicians, the time requirements to hear and discuss each will be as follows: category 1, 10 to 15 minutes; category 2, 20 to 25 minutes; category 3, 25 to 35 minutes.

As noted earlier, bedside rounds may be the best strategy for call nights that did not have a high work intensity or had a high volume of admissions (to augment efficiency). Call nights with high intensity warrant at least some time in the conference room for the team to rest and consume coffee or breakfast.

For teams with two interns, especially with a large volume of admissions, the attending may elect to split the team for post-call rounds by releasing one of the two interns to complete patient care tasks while the other intern presents her patients. The first intern then replaces the second in swapping duties. This may be necessary to ensure compliance with Accreditation Council for Graduate Medical Education work hours (24 hours of patient care plus 6 hours to finish duties).

❖ Teaching Transitions of Care

Attending rounds is the best venue for teaching transitions of care because it allows the attending to model the behavior of patient education, and it is the venue in which the decisions of accepting patients from other services and decisions of discharge are made.

During each patient encounter, the attending can emphasize the importance of communication with the patient's primary care provider by asking the patient who her primary care provider is. If the patient has none, the attending can ensure that the team begin arrangements to find her one. While the attending should make direct contact with the primary care provider (see earlier discussion), the team should be encouraged to actively participate in this process by regularly communicating with the primary care physician.

During each patient discussion, the team should be asked to identify the solvency issues for the patient. Solvency issues are problems that require resolution or, at the very least, a definitive plan for long-term management before discharge. The attending should anticipate that learners may have acquired bad habits as a product of their clinical experience and that these habits will have to be readjusted, particularly as they regard transition to the outpatient venue. The worst of these habits is the notion that problems the inpatient team does not "want" to be addressed can be "worked up as outpatient." Learners must be taught that although the team members are not responsible for resolving all issues during the inpatient stay, they are responsible for establishing a plan for resolving each unresolved issue in the outpatient setting. This entails arranging for clinic appointments and performing all diagnostic tests that will enable the most successful first outpatient visit. Finally, the attending should emphasize the importance of medicine reconciliation; the discharge visit to the bedside is the best time to emphasize the importance of this quality indicator: The patient must understand what medicines she is to continue taking at home and what should be discontinued.

❖ Documentation, Coding, and Billing: Linking Notes

It is useful to consider that in a nonteaching setting, the attending physician would perform all of the care, including the history, examination, and medical decision-making (the assessment and plan). In this case, he must document this care in the medical record. The billing code (the 992xx Current Procedural Terminology [CPT] code) should be based on the attending's documentation alone. Table 3-1 outlines the billing codes commonly encountered on an inpatient service and the criteria by which level of billing is met.

Table 3-1. Billing Codes Commonly Encountered on an Inpatient Service

CPT Code	History	Examination	Decision-Making
Admission			
99221	Detailed	Detailed	Straightforward
99222	Comprehensive	Comprehensive	Moderate complexity
99223	Comprehensive	Comprehensive	High complexity
Daily notes			
99231	Problem-focused	Problem-focused	Straightforward
99232	Expanded problem-focused	Expanded problem-focused	Moderate complexity
99233	Detailed	Detailed	High complexity
Discharge			
99238	30 min or less		
99239	30 min or more		
Consultations			
99251	Problem focused	Problem-focused	Straightforward
99252	Expanded problem-focused	Expanded problem-focused	Straightforward
99253	Detailed	Detailed	Low complexity
99254	Comprehensive	Comprehensive	Moderate complexity
99255	Comprehensive	Comprehensive	High complexity
Critical care			
99291	30–74 min		
99292	Each additional 30 min		

CPT = Current Procedural Terminology.

On a teaching service, however, where educational responsibilities exist, the preceding scenario is unlikely to be a tenable option. There is just not sufficient time to perform clinical responsibilities, document this care, and teach the residents and students. A better option is the *linking note*, which enables the attending to bill according to the resident's documentation.

Critical Elements of Linking Notes
There are three critical elements to linking documentation. At a minimum, the linking note must document 1) that the attending was present; 2) the attending participated during the critical elements of the history and examination; and 3) the service provided (that is, the assessment and plan). Once a linking note has been established, the attending can bill for the appropriate level of service as determined by the CPT system (Table 3-1). Medicaid rules will vary by state.

Disallowable Linking Practices
It is not sufficient to have the resident attest to the attending's presence and participation. The attending must document her presence and participation and the service rendered (that is, the plan of care). If the attending is going to use *any* part of the resident's documentation (for example, the history that the resident obtained; the patient's medical or family history or review of systems; examination; or assessment and plan), the attending must use the appropriate linking documentation. Statements such as, "Agree with above," "Rounded, reviewed, agreed," or "Discussed with resident, agree" are not acceptable because the linking note is missing the three critical components.

Linking to Student Notes
Attendings cannot link to student notes, with the following exception. Attendings can link to the student's documentation of the review of systems and past medical history, family history, and social history if the attending physician, or the resident, was physically present when this information was collected. Naturally, this must be documented (2).

Best Practices in Linking to Resident Notes
There are two possible scenarios by which an attending physician can link to a residents' note.

1. *The attending and the resident see the patient together.* In this case, the attending can link to the resident's documentation and does not have to do the documentation himself. The linking note should state that the attending was present during the performance of the critical or key portions of the service and that the attending was directly involved in the care of the patient: *"I was present with the resident during the history and exam. I discussed the case with the resident and agree with the findings and plan as documented in the resident's note."* The level of service that is billable is then contingent on the resident's documentation (see Table 3-1).

2. *The resident sees, examines, and documents the patient's care without the attending present.* For example, the resident admits the patient overnight, and the attending then sees the patient on the following day, post-call. The key difference from the first scenario is that the attending was *not* present when the resident performed the history and examination and designed the plan (that is, the medical decision-making). In this case, the attending's linking note should document that he personally saw the patient and that he performed the key or critical portions of the service (during attending rounds, he performed the key elements of the history and examination and participated in patient care by designing the plan with the resident). For example: *"I saw and evaluated the patient. The patient's history, exam, and assessment and plan were discussed with the resident, and I agree with the resident's findings and plan as documented in the resident's note, with the following exceptions…"*

The Educational Value of Linking Notes

The attending should anticipate that most residents see their documentation as perfunctory. In most systems, the residents know that their notes amount to little in the way of billing and coding. As a result, there is very little interest to improve proper documentation practices. The attending can improve this problem by creating an environment that motivates the resident to learn proper documentation practices (Tables 3-2 and 3-3). Once the resident's note is established as *the* documentation to record the patient's care, the motivation to learn proper documentation practices will improve.

Linking documentation not only saves the attending time but also provides a teaching opportunity for the learner. Regardless of her ultimate spe-

Table 3-2. Elements of History of Present Illness

Dimension	Definition	Examples
Frequency/timing	How often do the symptoms occur? When does the patient experience the symptoms?	Chest pain worse at night; always occurs after exercise
Associated signs and symptoms	What other symptoms accompany the main symptoms?	Nausea, diaphoresis, dizziness
Character/quality	Description or characteristics of the symptoms	Pressure pain, radiating pain, dull pain
Onset/timing	When did the symptoms start? What regularity/frequency of occurrences? What time of day?	Stomach pain worse after eating, worse at night, always occurring after exercise
Location	Where is the problem located?	Left chest, lower abdomen, right leg
Duration	How long has the patient experienced the signs or symptoms?	Pain began 3 days ago
Severity	What is the severity, degree, or intensity of the symptoms? (Scale of 1–10)	5 on a scale of 1–10
Context	What precipitated the symptoms, or what was the patient doing when the symptoms started?	Chest pain while climbing stairs
Exacerbating/ relieving (modifying) factors	What has improved or worsened the symptoms?	Nitroglycerine relieved the pain, cocaine worsened the pain

cialty, billing and coding will be a prominent feature of the resident's career. Although most residency programs will devote some curricular time to proper billing and coding (systems of care teaching), the attending should anticipate that the resident is unlikely to retain much of this information. Billing and coding is an active skill, and by establishing linking documentation as the practice, the attending is in a position to coach the residents in their day-to-day documentation skill. Providing written supplementation to the note, where documentation deficiencies exist, is an effective method of teaching the principles of documentation and providing feedback to the residents as to their documentation skills.

Table 3-3. Critical Elements of the History and Examination

Variable	Chief Complaint	History of Present Illness	Review of Systems	Past/Family/ Social History*	Examination Criteria
			Historical Criteria		
Problem-focused	Yes	<4 elements	0 systems	0	1 body area or organ system
Expanded problem-focused	Yes	<4 elements	>1 system	0	Limited examination of the affected organ plus 2–7 body areas or organ systems
Detailed	Yes	>4 elements	2–9 systems	At least 1 in 1 category	Extended examination of the affected organ plus 2–7 body areas or organ systems
Comprehensive	Yes	>4 elements	All 10 systems	At least 1 in each category	A general multisystem examination (more organ systems)

*Past history includes previous illnesses, injuries, operations, and hospitalizations; current medications; allergies; and immunization status. Family history includes the health history of parents, siblings, and children. Social history includes marital status; living arrangements; occupational history; drug, tobacco, or alcohol use; education level; and sexual history.

REFERENCES

1. **Ende J, ed.** Theory and Practice of Teaching Medicine. Philadelphia: ACP Pr; 2010.
2. **Centers for Medicare & Medicaid Services Transmittal 1780.** Supervising Physicians in Teaching Settings. Accessed at www.med.ufl.edu/complian/Q&a/CMS_Transmittal_R1780B3.pdf

Teaching Clinical Reasoning on the Inpatient Service

Joseph Rencic, MD, FACP

Richard Kopelman, MD, FACP

Jeff Wiese, MD, FACP

Without discounting the value of teaching about a specific disease or clinical diagnosis, inpatient attendings need to appreciate that if they are doing their jobs well, they should be teaching clinical reasoning. The challenge here is that physicians are often not consciously aware of how they think—they just ... do. Expecting learners to pick up clinical reasoning through observation as an apprentice to the expert physician is unrealistic. Clinical reasoning takes place inside the expert's brain and by its nature is not apparent to the observer unless the attending physician effectively articulates her internal thought processes. Casual, unplanned language may not capture the reasoning process that occurs internally; even if it does, it may not capture all that went into the final decision or action.

❖ The Attending

The first step in addressing this challenge is for the attending physician to recognize that her clinical reasoning is "tacit"—she has done it for so long, she may have forgotten how she first learned how to do it. Much like learning to add or subtract, the act of clinical reasoning may come easily, but instructing people how to do it may be difficult. It's just so natural that it's hard to imagine why everyone doesn't just do it. It is tempting to presuppose that everyone is thinking at that same level.

KEY POINTS

- The inpatient setting provides an opportunity to teach not only clinical medicine but also clinical reasoning.
- The inpatient attending can assess learners' clinical reasoning skills in several ways, including direct observation, but also through the admission note and spoken case presentation.
- Learners' clinical reasoning skills develop through multiple phases, from the early stage in which students focus only on symptoms to more advanced phases in which they can synthesize clinical presentations and begin to use both nonanalytic and analytic approaches to diagnosis and treatment.
- Expert clinicians frequently use intuitive reasoning, pattern recognition, and other forms of nonanalytic reasoning. Although appropriate for them, this form of clinical reasoning introduces potential for errors, as described by common heuristics, and may not allow the clinical novice to appreciate the full process required to reach a correct diagnosis or treatment plan.
- Principles of clinical epidemiology are instrumental in the inpatient setting for developing a proper differential diagnosis but also for understanding thresholds for treatment.
- Bayesian theory provides inpatient attendings with an opportunity to teach analytic clinical reasoning in an orderly, concrete fashion, using the actual clinical cases encountered on the inpatient setting.

Moreover, attendings need to appreciate that their learners will be at different levels in terms of clinical reasoning skills, and that what may be effective for the advanced resident may not be effective for the less experienced student. The "learn by proxy" method implies that it is fine for novice physicians to jump to the expert level without first learning the fundamentals necessary to get to that point. The reality is that learning clinical reasoning, like any complex task, is contingent on learning successive blocks of "fundamentals," specifically, deep and comparative knowledge of diseases *and* a strong analytical approach. Failure to develop either of these skills will lead to significant deficits in the student's long-term clinical reasoning skills. On the other hand, the more clearly the abstract skill of reasoning can be made concrete, the easier it will be for the student to acquire the skill, and the easier it will be for the expert to assess the student's progress and provide corrective action.

Observation of a student admitting a new patient followed by discussion (question and answer) has the most value in assessment of clinical reasoning skills. Although the former (observation) may be difficult to accomplish because of time constraints, the latter can easily be done on attending rounds on the post-call day. More information about surrogate measures of clinical reasoning, including the admission note and the oral case presentation, is discussed later in this chapter.

❖ The Clinical Reasoning Process: How Experts Think Diagnostically

As described in chapter 1 of *Theory and Practice of Teaching Medicine*, another book in the *Teaching Medicine* series (1), experts use both analytic (hypothesis-based deductive reasoning) and nonanalytic (pattern recognition) reasoning flexibly to make diagnoses (2). Consider an elderly patient who presents with low-grade fever, nonproductive cough, and hypoxia. On the basis of the clinical symptom complex, or pattern, a physician would probably diagnose pneumonia. However, if after 2 days of antibiotics the patient develops worsening hypoxia and tachycardia, the physician will analyze the case and reconsider it, possibly realizing that she may have missed a pulmonary infarction that could have the same symptom complex as pneumonia. In most cases, the initial diagnosis would have been correct and the patient would be quickly discharged, but the astute clinician will recognize when to implement analytic reasoning. Physicians may implement analytic reasoning in at least two situations: 1) when no clear pattern emerges from the clinical data or 2) when it seems appropriate to double-check or verify that the reasoning in a specific case makes sense. Furthermore, physicians often will use both processes simultaneously in the diagnostic process.

Given this, teaching attendings need to address both nonanalytic and analytic approaches in clinical reasoning. From the nonanalytic standpoint, attendings should focus on highlighting key aspects of disease presentations, especially epidemiology, so that students develop accurate and detailed mental constructs of diseases. These mental constructs have been termed "illness scripts." Teaching in this manner is quite natural, once the attending begins to verbalize her thought processes.

Attendings must also be adept at teaching analytic reasoning, and this may not come as easily to them. It requires knowledge of the accuracy of tests and Bayesian reasoning.

From a pedagogical perspective, while it is advisable for teaching attendings to balance their focus on nonanalytic and analytic reasoning, stressing analytic, quantitative methods over nonanalytic/pattern-recognition approaches is advisable. The human brain is evolutionarily designed to recognize patterns. Students will develop pattern-recognition skills (nonanalytic reasoning) through experience, regardless of clinical instruction. Analytic reasoning, however, is not as intuitive or as readily acquired, and will usually develop only with active coaching. Practical approaches to teaching analytic clinical reasoning will be discussed in later sections of the chapter.

❖ The Evolution of a Learner's Clinical Reasoning

Many theoretical constructs have been created to explain how diagnostic reasoning develops (see chapter 1 in *Theory and Practice of Teaching Medicine* [1]). The following section highlights five phases of development.

Phase 1: Symptom-Only Diagnosis

Medical students start by learning biological and physiologic principles that allow them to understand the causes and consequences of specific diseases (3). Faced with a clinical problem in this period, students tend to focus on one symptom and consider its biological and physiologic causes. The student has difficulty seeing the unifying pattern of a specific disease amidst myriad symptoms and signs. Thus, the early student's clinical reasoning may be characterized by an approach that separately addresses one symptom at a time. For example, the student will address edema, then dyspnea, and then paroxysmal nocturnal dyspnea, but he will not identify the three symptoms linked together as a presentation of congestive heart failure. The processing of data will often be slow and filled with many irrelevant details (4–7).

Phase 2: Symptom-Cluster Pattern Recognition

As students gain clinical experience, their knowledge begins to become condensed, or "encapsulated." Students merge pathophysiologic and disease details and group related symptoms into syndromes. Students rely less on pathophysiologic knowledge and more on symptom patterns to aid in diagnosis (3). For example, the student now recognizes that a combination of shortness of breath with paroxysmal nocturnal dyspnea and lower-extremity edema is a pattern seen in congestive heart failure. This clinical reasoning is effective for common or uncomplicated presentations, but students will return to pathophysiologic reasoning or biomedical knowledge if they don't recognize an obvious syndrome or other clinical pattern. In this phase, students have not yet developed a thorough knowledge of the epidemiology and risk factors for diseases, which can lead to diagnostic uncertainty or error.

Phase 3: Combining Symptom Clusters With Narrative Stories

In the third stage, the student's knowledge is further encapsulated into narrative structures. These "illness scripts" are mental groupings of words or images that describe the story of a disease, linking symptoms, signs, and laboratory results, as well as risk factors and other epidemiologic considerations. These scripts can vary from the memory of a specific patient's presentation of a certain disease (such as Mrs. Mandrake's case of congestive heart failure) to an abstract synthesis of the presentations of multiple patients and textbook descriptions of a given disease. Included in the development of these illness scripts is knowledge of "enabling" or predisposing conditions (for example, demographic characteristics and risk factors), which allow students to rapidly exclude categories of diseases (7–10). For example, a phase 3 student will exclude influenza in diagnosing a patient with fever and myalgias in the summer by knowing that flu season occurs only in winter; a phase 2 student might continue to entertain the diagnosis because it meets with the classic symptom cluster. As students advance through these stages, pattern recognition becomes a more prominent aspect of their clinical reasoning.

Phase 4: Analytic Reasoning: Hypothetical Deductive Reasoning

In the fourth phase, students begin to use analytic or hypothetical deductive reasoning. This adds another dimension of flexibility to the students' clinical reasoning skill, a dimension that is important for attendings to encourage. Initially, the physician develops a hypothetical diagnosis based on preliminary information and then, through a careful history, examination, and data analysis, refutes or proves these hypothetical diagnoses. Through an iterative process, the correct diagnosis emerges.

The first step of this process is hypothesis generation. By using the patient's age and appearance, the character of the chief complaint, and the time course, hypotheses are generated, often through pattern recognition. The hypotheses prompt targeted questions, which attempt to evaluate each hypothesis being considered. Additional data may confirm or eliminate the hypothesis, and may even trigger new hypotheses. As the differential diagnosis narrows, more careful discrimination is required to reduce the number of possible diagnoses, and additional testing, such as laboratory or radiologic studies, is targeted on the basis of the hypotheses being considered. This final step of the process (analogous to the assessment and plan) is the diagnostic verification. In this step, physicians assess the adequacy and coherency of the diagnoses. An "adequate" diagnosis is one that explains all the patient's clinical findings, and a "coherent" diagnosis is one that fits the altered pathophysiologic state of the patient. After completing these steps, physicians choose a working diagnosis or diagnoses. Despite remaining uncertainty, they begin to manage the patient's illness (11). Table 4-1 summarizes this clinical reasoning process. Although these analytic skills probably arise in parallel with less analytic forms of diagnostic reasoning, they may remain rudimentary without clinical instruction and emphasis from a knowledgeable attending.

Phase 5: Transition From Novice to Expert: Appropriately Choosing When to Use Analytic and Nonanalytic Thinking

Although experienced physicians frequently use the nonanalytic method of diagnosis, and although it is often effective (especially for simple presentations or diseases), attending physicians tasked with coaching developing learners need to encourage learners to use analytic reasoning. Realizing that pattern recognition is the default pathway that students will use regardless of teaching, attendings must role-model the analytic approach so students become comfortable with the terminology and the process of deductive reasoning, as well as medical decision-making. This will help to ensure that students can use either process, depending on the clinical scenario. If an attending recognizes that she or the student has used pattern recognition in the diagnosis of a patient, she can make this explicit by discussing the key aspects of the clinical presentation that elucidated the diagnosis. A key element to this would be to carefully compare the top two or three conditions in the differential diagnosis and articulate why one diagnosis stands out as correct relative to the others. Through this process, the attending and learner would focus on epidemiology and risk factors as a key way to determine the likelihood of a disease. The attending can incorporate frequency tables of symptoms and signs of the diseases in the differential diagnosis, as well as actual prevalence numbers, to demonstrate how this type of in-depth analysis strengthens the clinician's ability to make diagnoses. Students who practice such an analytic approach over years will build a much more robust knowledge of diseases. Through experience, the diagnostic process will become more intuitive and nonanalytic, although a significant part of its foundation derives from the analytic approaches used early in the process.

Table 4-1. Sample Phase 4 (Hypothetical Deductive) Clinical Reasoning

Anatomic Area	Long List: Diagnoses That Fit the Patient's Chief Complaint	Smart List: Diagnoses That Fit the Pattern of the Patient's Presentation	Ranked Smart List: Probability of Each Diagnosis Based on the Pattern of the Patient's Presentation and the Prevalence of Disease	Smart List 2: After Further Questions, Physical Examination, and Laboratory Testing
Stomach	Gastroenteritis Peptic ulcer	Gastroenteritis	Gastroenteritis (40%)	Gastroenteritis (20%)
Duodenum	Duodenal ulcer			
Liver/bile duct	Cholangitis Cholecystitis Hepatitis	Cholangitis Hepatitis	Cholangitis (5%) Hepatitis (20%)	
Pancreas	Pancreatitis	Pancreatitis	Pancreatitis (5%)	
Intestine	Bowel obstruction Appendicitis Diverticulitis Bacterial colitis	Appendicitis Diverticulitis	Appendicitis (25%) Diverticulitis (5%)	Appendicitis (80%)

❖ Heuristics in Clinical Reasoning

As discussed, expert clinicians frequently use intuitive reasoning, pattern recognition, or their "instincts" when making simple diagnoses but also in more complicated cases in the hypothesis-generation phase of analytic reasoning. The rapid, nonanalytic mental shortcuts that humans use to recognize and categorize things are called *heuristics*. In many cases, intuitive, or nonanalytic, reasoning may be accurate. But there is the potential for errors in nonanalytic reasoning. Heuristics can lead to an inaccurate diagnosis, and because the error is at the unconscious level, the mistake may not be recognized. Learners need to be made aware of these types of diagnostic errors and encouraged to verify diagnoses with analytic reasoning approaches (for example, the verification step mentioned in the hypothesis-deductive reasoning section to minimize the potential for diagnostic errors associated with nonanalytic reasoning, some of which are discussed below).

1. *The representational heuristic* describes a mental shortcut by which the unconscious mind rapidly categorizes the patient's illness into a pattern (such as a disease or syndrome) that it recognizes from previous experience, excluding all other information. The representational heuristic ignores the principle that it is more likely to have an atypical presentation of a common disease than it is to have a typical presentation of an uncommon disease (that is, prevalence).

2. *The availability heuristic* refers to the idea that physicians tend to diagnose diseases that are either very familiar or striking because these are most easily recalled. An example is a student's predilection for diagnosing pheochromocytoma for any patient with hypertension, despite its tiny prevalence, merely because the disease is such an interesting diagnosis that learners easily recall it.

3. *The recency heuristic*, similar to the availability heuristic, is the mind's predilection to unconsciously assign a greater probability that a disease is present because it was recently seen (for example, the superstition that things "come in threes") or read about: *"I just read about myeloma in the journals, and today I diagnosed a case. That's weird."*

4. *The dramatic heuristic* refers to the nonanalytic assignment of probability to diseases that are scary or dramatic. Although scary diseases (that is, diseases that can kill you) warrant lower testing and treatment thresholds (see below), they are not more prevalent because of their scariness. The statement *"We have to exclude pulmonary embolism in all*

patients with shortness of breath because it kills people" is
an example. Although the potential mortality of pulmonary
embolism warrants a lower testing or treatment threshold,
this mortality does not make the disease more likely. The
absurdity is captured in considering smallpox, a disease
that has excessive mortality but is not routinely excluded
in patients with a skin rash.

5. *The anchoring heuristic* refers to the predilection of physicians to give more credence to data that confirm a diagnosis
   established early and less credence to data that do not, even
   when subsequent information argues to the contrary. The
   anchoring heuristic begins with either premature closure (a
   diagnosis that was established too soon without consideration
   of alternative diagnoses) or referral bias (a diagnosis made by
   another physician that, once established, takes on greater
   mental weight) (12).

6. *The positive test result heuristic,* in which physicians
   unconsciously give more weight to positive than negative
   test results (13).

❖ Using Bayesian Theory to Make Clinical Reasoning More Concrete

The limitation to hypothetical deductive reasoning is that the process of
confirming or excluding the hypotheses (the diagnoses) remains nebulous.
If a wrong decision is made, it is difficult to dissect the process to determine where the error occurred. One of two outcomes results for the learner: 1) The learner ignores the error and clinical reasoning does not improve
or 2) the learner internalizes the error and overcompensates for subsequent patients to prevent the error from happening again. This may cause
additional errors (the dramatic heuristic: the learner misses a pulmonary
embolism and subsequently overdiagnoses and administers anticoagulant
therapy to a subsequent patient with this condition, leading to a fatal hemorrhage).

The Bayes theorem states that the pretest probability of a diagnosis
directly affects the post-test probability of that disease (14). Using this theorem helps make concrete the abstract process of assigning probabilities to
the diagnoses being considered (the mental "ranking" of conditions being
considered in the differential diagnosis).

In the Bayesian theory method, numbers replace the physician's
gestalt (Table 4-2). Should an error result, the physician can inspect the

Table 4-2. A Sample Bayesian Theory Calculation

Step 1	Step 2	Step 3	Step 4	Step 5
Establish pretest probability for disease	Convert to pretest odds	Multiply by LR to get post-test odds; use positive LR if test result was positive, negative LR if result was negative	Convert post-test odds back to probabilities: top/(top + bottom)	This is your post-test probability
60% appendicitis	60% yes/ 40% no	CT of abdomen is positive; positive LR for appendicitis is 10.0 (multiply 60 by 10.0)		
60%	60/40	600/40	600/(600 + 40)	**94%**

CT = computed tomography; LR = likelihood ratio.

numbers assigned to each step of the process (the pretest probabilities and the data used to test the hypotheses) to determine where the error resulted (Figure 4-1). With this method, the physician uses initial patient data to establish a list of hypotheses, but instead of using gestalt about the likelihood of disease, she uses the prevalence of disease and the narrative pattern to assign *pretest probabilities* to each diagnosis being considered. Subsequent data are then obtained (such as physical examination and laboratory data), as directed by the hypotheses being considered. However, instead of relying on her gestalt as to the tests' accuracy, she uses the test characteristics, such as sensitivity, specificity, and likelihood ratios (15), to determine the post-test probability.

Step 1: Assigning Numbers for Pretest Probabilities

The initial step of hypothesis deductive reasoning is to acquire the preliminary information (the character of the chief complaint and the time course narrative) to establish the hypotheses (the differential diagnosis). On the basis of this information, each diagnosis has a probability of being correct. Because the method works on deductive reasoning, the sum of these probabilities must add up to 100%. As with a multiple-choice examination, eliminating one diagnosis increases the probability of other choices as its pretest probability is added to other diagnoses. The Bayesian theory assigns numbers to each of these diagnoses.

Because this is a developmental stage for the learner (recognition 2), it is important to tell learners that they will rarely see expert attendings assign numeric probabilities to their diagnostic hypotheses. Otherwise, they will dismiss the method as merely a style preference inconsistent with what they have seen before. They should be told that using the numbers and doing the math is something extra that will help them learn how to clinically reason accurately and help them to identify and shore up weaknesses in their reasoning. See the following dialogue:

"Paul, I'm going to ask you to use the following method when you evaluate your patients. I'll be honest with you in saying that assigning numeric probabilities to each diagnosis is not something that physicians routinely do ... but this exercise will help make your clinical reasoning more concrete. Are you up for it?"

"Sure," Paul replies.

"Okay, here is what I want you to do for the patient you admit on call tonight. I want you to go in and interview the patient, but I want your history to be disciplined. I want you to focus only on establishing the time course of the chief complaint and the character of the chief complaint. I want you to use the 'FAR COLDER' mnemonic in prompting you to ask the questions that adequately characterize a chief complaint." Phaedrus writes out the mnemonic as he speaks: **f**requency, **a**ssociated symptoms, **r**adiation, **c**haracter, **o**nset, **l**ocation, **d**uration, **e**xacerbating and **r**elieving factors.

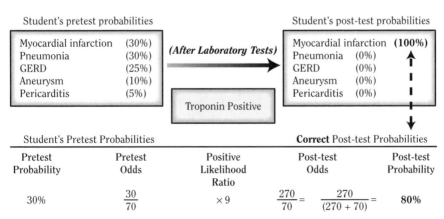

Figure 4-1 Using Bayesian theory to isolate a mistake. GERD = gastroesophageal reflux disease.

"I've got that. That's what they told us to do in Physical Diagnosis."

"Right. But here's the new wrinkle … and Stef, I want you as the intern make sure that Paul does this. Okay?" Stef nods, clearly keeping track of the method as well. "Then I am going to ask that you write all of this down. When you go to write up your admission note, this will be the first paragraph of your admission note. Just this, and nothing more. After you have that initial information, I want you to think about a differential diagnosis for the chief complaint—a list of all of the diagnoses that could explain the patient's symptoms. Over the course of the month, I am going to coach you on the methods that go with building a differential diagnosis for each chief complaint. But for tonight, since we don't know what you might admit, Stef will help you."

"Okay," says Paul. "I get the time course and the chief complaint, then I build a differential diagnosis."

"Correct. And on that sheet of paper where you wrote out your differential diagnosis, I want you to write a number next to each diagnosis. This number should be the probability that the diagnosis is correct. It should be somewhere between 1% and 100%. For now, we are going to presume that the patient has only one disease explaining all of his symptoms, so all of these numbers, Paul, have to add up to 100%. As you assign the numbers, I want you to think about the prevalence of the disease for the age and gender of your patient and how well that first paragraph of information (the time course and chief complaint) fits the pattern you would expect for each disease you are considering on your differential diagnosis."

"Okay. I get the paragraph 1 information. Then I build a differential diagnosis, then I write down a number next to each diagnosis. But what if I'm wrong?" Paul asks.

"Don't worry about that for now. Just right down the numbers. Tomorrow, when you present the patient, I want to see the list you initially came up with after doing the 'paragraph 1' data collection, and the numbers you assigned for each."

Step 2: Teach the Student to Use the Differential Diagnosis to Drive the History, Examination, and Laboratory Testing

It is important that the learner see the value of the second paragraph: the focused line of questioning inspired by the differential diagnosis. Students who close down the history early do so because they do not see the utility of asking more questions. They have seen "expert" physicians come into the room and ask only a few questions, and they are modeling this behavior. The difference is that the student is not an expert, nor does he know what knowledge allowed the expert to ask so few questions. The expert, using nonanalytic reasoning, knew why she was asking these questions (on the basis of her mental differential diagnosis) and that afforded her targeted, brief questions in obtaining the history. But not being privy to the attending's thought process, the student does *not* learn that a targeted line of questions based on the differential diagnosis allows both thoroughness and concision. The only thing the student learns is that it's okay to ask just a few questions and call it a day. Students who excessively expand the history are really no different: They are doing so because they do not know which questions to ask. They hunt and peck, hoping to stumble on something relevant. Either way, the history atrophies in the hand of the student who does not understand clinical reasoning. Asking the student to do the exercise of comparing the pretest probabilities after the "first paragraph of information" (that which generated the differential diagnosis) and again after the "second paragraph of information" (that which the differential diagnosis inspired) will consolidate the importance of using the differential diagnosis to drive the history in a rational manner.

> *Phaedrus continues. "Okay, Paul, then what I want you to do is this. I want you and Stef to ask questions that evaluate each of the diagnoses on your list. This will help you structure your interview such that you are asking questions that are relevant. And Paul, I want you to understand that from this point going forward, when I say the word 'relevant,' that is what I mean. 'Relevant' means that it helps us with our differential diagnosis. Okay?" Paul nods. "Paul, what's the definition of 'relevant'?"*

> *"Something that helps us evaluate our differential diagnosis."*

> *"Well done. So for example, Paul, if you have a patient with chest pain, myocardial infarction might be on your list, so you would ask questions such as, 'Do you smoke? Do you have a family history of heart disease? Have you been told you have high cholesterol?' Does that make sense?"*

> *"Sure," says Paul. "But what if I have a pretty good idea of what it is? Do I have to do this for every diagnosis on my differential?"*

> *"Someday you will have the luxury of not using this method, Paul—when you are an expert. But for now, I want you to do it*

just as I say. I promise you that this will help you develop the experience necessary to have that luxury. And Paul, if you happen to make a mistake, it will help me figure out where the error was so I can improve your method of thinking. So, yes … you have to ask questions about each diagnosis on your list. And after you have finished that, I want you to write another number out to the side of each diagnosis. This is the pretest probability of the diagnosis after this second line of questions. When you go to write up your admission note, I want the answers to these questions outlined in the second paragraph of your history. Just these answers, nothing more, nothing less. Sound good?"

"Sure," Paul replies.

"Great. I look forward to seeing this tomorrow."

Step 3: Converting Pretest Probabilities to Pretest Odds

The next step is to ask the student to practice converting pretest probabilities (use the probabilities obtained after paragraph 2) to pretest odds (Figure 4-1). This will enable the next link in the iterative thought process: how diagnostic testing affects clinical decision-making.

Step 4: Assigning Numbers for Test Characteristics

Each test (physical examination, laboratory, or imaging) has a sensitivity and specificity for detecting each disease. For any given test, the sensitivity and specificity vary from disease to disease. Electrocardiography, for example, may be very sensitive and specific for diagnosing myocardial infarction but not sensitive or specific in diagnosing pneumonia. The problem is that because we are interested in both excluding and confirming diagnoses in this deductive method, both the sensitivity (ruling diagnoses out) and specificity (ruling diagnoses in) are important. In the Bayesian mathematical method, we need a number that incorporates both.

Likelihood ratios are the numbers used to assess a test's characteristics in the Bayesian method (15). A positive likelihood ratio is used when a test result is positive. It is the sensitivity (true-positive/[true positive + false-negative]) of the test divided by 1 minus the specificity (false-positive/[false-positive + true-negative]) of the test. Looking at the actual equation, it becomes clear that the positive likelihood ratio is a ratio of true-positive results over false-positive results. Naturally, a test with a high positive likelihood ratio is valuable because there will be few false-positive results (that is, a positive test result is very likely to be a true-positive result). Positive likelihood ratios are always 1 or greater, and when multiplied by the pretest probabilities (actually, the pretest odds) they increase the probability of that disease being the correct diagnosis. Intuitively, this should make sense: a positive electrocardiogram increases the probability of myocardial infarction. The negative likelihood ratio is used when the test result is negative. It is 1 minus the sensitivity (false-negative/[false-negative + true-positive]) of the test divided by the specificity (true negative/[true-negative + false-positive]) of the test. Looking at the equation again, it becomes apparent that the negative likelihood ratio is a ratio of false-negative to true-negative results. Therefore, a very low number for the negative likelihood ratio indicates a valuable test because it means there are very few false-negative results relative to true-negative results (that is, a negative test result is very likely a true-negative result). Negative likelihood ratios are therefore always 1 or smaller, and when multiplied by the pretest probabilities (actually, the pretest odds) they decrease the probability of that disease being the correct diagnosis. Intuitively, this should make sense: A negative electrocardiogram decreases the probability of myocardial infarction.

The advantage of likelihood ratios is that it allows the physician to numerically assess the magnitude of a test's ability to increase or decrease a disease's probability rather than relying on the gestalt. The greater the positive likelihood ratio, the better the test is in diagnosing that disease. The smaller the negative likelihood ratio, the better the test is in excluding that disease. A weak likelihood ratio suggests that the test neither confirms nor excludes a disease. Hence, this type of knowledge has the potential to offset the tendency of learners to weigh "objective" but insensitive/nonspecific tests (for example, an intermediate-probability ventilation–perfusion scan that has a likelihood ratio of 1.0) more heavily than their history and physical examination. Learners may ask why the likelihood ratio should be used rather than the positive or negative predictive value. The attending should clarify that these values are derived from the prevalence of a disease in the given study population, whereas likelihood ratios are not affected by prevalence; they can be directly applied to the specific individual patient for whom a pretest probability has been calculated on the basis of patient characteristics and presentation.

"Okay, Paul. Yesterday you said the pretest probability of MI [myocardial infarction] was 30%. The troponin was positive, and I asked you to tell me what the post-test probability of MI was based upon this test result. You said it was 100%. Is that right?"

"Yeah, that's what I had. The test was positive, after all."

"Okay, and I asked you to look up the sensitivity and specificity of a positive troponin in diagnosing MI. What did you find?"

"Well, the troponin is 90% sensitive and 90% specific. But there were lots of different kinds of troponins."

"Indeed, Paul. Seems like it's not so simple to just rely upon a lab test, is it?"

"Yes. It's more vague than I thought."

"But for the sake of this coaching session, Paul, let's say those are the right numbers. Since the test is positive, which likelihood ratio will we use? Let's see, positive test … is it the negative likelihood ratio or the POSITIVE likelihood ratio?"

Paul smiles. "The positive likelihood ratio."

"Okay, Paul. The positive likelihood ratio is the sensitivity divided by 1 minus the specificity. If we were going to calculate the negative likelihood ratio, which we won't since the test was negative, we would just move the '1 minus' to the top of the equation. And remember, Paul, for both equations, 'sensitivity' goes on top; alphabetically, it comes before 'specificity' so it should be on top."

"So the positive likelihood ratio would be 90% divided by 1 minus 90% … or 90% divided by 10%. Is that right?" asks Paul. "We are using percentages as a 'point 9-0,' right?"

"Yes, 90% would be point 9-0. So 90% divided by 10% would be…"

Step 5: Putting Pretest Probabilities and Likelihood Ratios Together
In simple format, the Bayesian theory states that the pretest odds of a diagnosis, when multiplied by the likelihood ratio of the diagnostic test chosen, will determine the post-test odds of that disease. The actual math can be calculated (see Table 4-1).

"So the likelihood ratio is 9. So 9 times as likely to be an MI?" asks Paul.

"Not exactly, Paul. Let's go back to your pretest probability of 30% and work through the math. I know this is tedious, but it will help you learn the lesson, and later it might help you figure out where a mistake was made. So what are the pretest odds if the pretest probability is 30%?"

"Well, from what you taught be earlier ... 30% would be on top ... divided by 1 minus 30% on the bottom ... so, let's see... 3/7."

"Correct. Now I want you to multiply the 3/7 by the 9. What do you get?"

"Nine times 3 is 27... divided by 7.... So 27 over 7."

Likelihood ratios can be "stacked" if each test is a unique test (that is, the likelihood ratios of troponin and the electrocardiogram can both be used, but the likelihood ratios of two electrocardiograms cannot be used). As the pretest odds are multiplied by the likelihood of the first test, continue to multiply the second likelihood by that number, and so on. Then convert the post-test odds back to post-test probability.

Over time, physicians can accumulate likelihood ratios for common physical examination findings and diagnostic tests, memorizing them, storing them in a "peripheral brain," or just searching for them in the literature (15) or on the Internet as need be. By using the simple rules and these likelihood ratios, physicians can rapidly assess the utility of a test in affecting the post-test probability, and they can avoid falling into the trap of thinking that tests are more valuable than a good history and physical examination in determining the likelihood of diagnoses.

Step 6: Ask Students to Calculate Post-Test Probabilities

After the student has multiplied the pretest odds of a diagnosis by the likelihood ratio of the test, ask the student to convert this post-test odds value back to a probability. To convert the post-test odds to post-test probability, use the "top over top + bottom" (that is, odds/odds + 1) formula. A post-test odds of 1/2 is a probability of 1/(1 + 2), or 33% (top number divided by the "top plus bottom" number). A post-test odds of 3 is 3/(3 + 1), or 75%.

"Indeed. Now convert back to post-test probabilities. Do you remember how to do that?" Paul has a look of mental constipation on his face. Phaedrus continues, "Okay, remember it is 'top' over 'top plus bottom.' So 27 over 27 plus 7 ... or 27 divided by 34 (27/34). Do the math, Paul. What's the post-test probability?"

"About 80%. Wow, that's a lot less that I thought. How is that possible?"

Now, ask the student to compare the actual post-test probability to what the student "guessed" the post-test probability was on that post-call day. Although the math seems tedious, it will consolidate the lesson (see Figure 4-1).

Step 7: Ask Students to Identify Where They Made Errors

Here is where the tedious effort of walking through the math involved in Bayesian theory pays off. The discrepancy between what the student thought the post-test probability would be and what it actually was will reveal the importance of the two components central to diagnostic accuracy: accurate pretest probabilities and accurate assessment of the diagnostic power of the test. Box 4-1 lists the common diagnostic errors. Doing this

---

Box 4-1. Types of Errors in Clinical Reasoning

History

> **Error 1. You overestimated the pretest probability of a wrong diagnosis.** Example: You were overconfident in the diagnosis of tuberculosis because that patient had once spent time in a jail.

> **Error 2. You underestimated the pretest probability of the correct diagnosis.** Example: In a patient with dyspnea, you failed to note the patient's history of an around-the-world airplane flight as a risk factor for pulmonary embolism.

Examination and Laboratory Tests

> **Error 3. You overestimated the power of a diagnostic test whose results were positive.** By overestimating the test's positive likelihood ratio, you suggested the wrong diagnosis. Example: You thought it was definitely a urine infection because there were 0 to 5 white blood cells in the urine.

> **Error 4. You underestimated the power of a diagnostic test whose results were positive for the *correct* diagnosis.** Example: You discounted the T-wave inversion on the electrocardiogram as a sign of myocardial ischemia.

> **Error 5. You overestimated the power of a diagnostic test whose results were negative (i.e., a negative likelihood ratio) for the *correct* diagnosis.** Example: You excluded sepsis because the first blood culture was negative.

> **Error 6. You underestimated the power of a diagnostic test whose results were negative (i.e., a negative likelihood ratio) for the *wrong* diagnosis.** Example: You persisted in believing it was endocarditis despite the negative transesophageal echocardiogram.

> *continued*

> ## Box 4-1. Types of Errors in Clinical Reasoning (continued)
>
> ### Treatment
>
> **Error 7.** You correctly estimated the post-test probability of the disease, but you withheld treatment from a patient who needed it because you **set the treatment threshold too high**. This occurs because of **overestimating the potential risks of the therapy** or **underestimating the potential benefits.** Example: You established a reasonable probability of appendicitis, but you did not take the patient to the operating room because you overestimated the potential complications of the surgery or you underestimated the potential benefits of the surgery.
>
> **Error 8.** You correctly estimated the post-test probability of the disease, but **you gave treatment prematurely because you set the treatment threshold too low.** This occurs when a physician clearly sees the benefits of potential treatment but does not see the potential harms. Example: You established a reasonable probability of myocardial infarction, so you gave the patient thrombolytics (blood thinners), resulting in a fatal gastrointestinal hemorrhage. You failed to note the history of a bleeding stomach ulcer 1 month prior. Although the treatment threshold may have been appropriate for most patients, the potential risks were much higher in this patient. In turn, the treatment threshold was also much higher; to justify therapy, the probability of myocardial infarction would have to be almost certain.

six-step process early in the month will enable valuable discussions as the month continues. As mistakes are made, the team can discuss why they were made.

"Well, Paul, it illustrates the important lesson I want you to know. There are only two variables in this equation: the pretest probability and the likelihood ratio of the test. If you ever make a mistake, which we'll define as either overestimating or underestimating the post-test probability of a disease, it is due to one of two errors: either you over- or underestimated the pretest probability of the disease, or you over- or underestimated the diagnostic power of the test."

"But Dr. Phaedrus, these pretest probabilities, they are ones that I just made up. How do you find the actual pretest probabilities? Is there a book somewhere?"

"No, Paul, that's why some day you will have a job. Only the human mind can estimate pretest probabilities because only the human mind can process the infinite number of variables that come with an infinite number of different patient types, ages, genders, with an infinite number of comorbidity combinations, and with a multiple number of diseases to be considered. There is no book. This is your clinical reasoning, and it's why I'm spending so much time on it with you. It is THE attribute that distinguishes excellent diagnosticians from average diagnosticians. The better you become at accurately assessing pretest probabilities, the better a diagnostician you will become. It's that simple. All physicians use the same CT scanner. It's the clinical reasoning ability to accurately predict pretest probabilities that separates the two. It's also the reason I'm making you learn this math, Paul, so that you can see the lesson."

"Hmm.... But how do I know it was an error in my pretest probability?" asks Paul. "Maybe it was an error in how much weight I gave to the test."

"Indeed. But just as you did last night, Paul, you can always look up the sensitivity and specificity of the diagnostic test. Just remember that you have to look it up for the disease you considering." Phaedrus pauses. "Paul, here's the lesson. If you ever make a diagnostic mistake, I want this to be your method. Look at the tests that you ordered, get a mental idea of how much weight you gave to the test result in your clinical reasoning, and then go to the literature to see if that matches up with what you thought. If it does, then the only other diagnostic error was in your pretest probability. Then go back to the initial history and think about what might have gone wrong there. What data did you give too much credence to in assigning your pretest probability? What data should you have given more credence too?"

"Wow. This is really helpful. Can we do this again at some point?"

"Indeed, Paul."

❖ Incorporating Clinical Reasoning Into Teaching on Rounds

At the outset of this chapter, three steps were outlined to teach clinical reasoning: 1) recognize the "tacit" quality of an attending's clinical reasoning, 2) recognize that this is a developmental stage for the learner, and 3) recognize that for the abstract process to be instructed and assessed, it has to be made more concrete.

A useful method for teaching clinical reasoning is to sequentially "walk through" a clinical case with a learner, pausing at certain junctions in the presentation to ask questions that illustrate the clinical reasoning principles. This prospective approach more closely mirrors the actual process that clinicians go through as they see a patient. This method is similar to the *New England Journal of Medicine*'s clinical problem-solving cases, wherein the discussant is given "chunks" of information in a piecemeal fashion and the expert's diagnostic process is explicitly stated. Presenting a case in its entirety has the potential to introduce too much retrospective, or "hindsight," bias. The following narrative will illustrate this "walk-through" method of instruction. The narrative begins with the team at the bedside of a patient who was recently admitted. The student (Paul) admitted a patient with syncope, and is presenting the case to the attending (Phaedrus), the resident (Moni), and the intern (Stef).

> *"Paul, rather than giving a traditional presentation where you go all the way through, I'm going to ask you to present small chunks of the presentation and then we'll pause to discuss it. I want to focus on how to think through a case. So can you start by giving me his relevant history? Remember our discussion yesterday— the definition of 'relevance' is that information that helps us in assessing our differential as we move towards a diagnosis."*

By using this method, the attending will role-model the clinical reasoning that goes into each segment of the history and physical examination.

> *"Sure. Mr. Hutt is a 35-year-old man with a history of hypertension, hypercholesterolemia, and morbid obesity, who presents with a first-time syncopal episode while standing at church this morning, associated with some lightheadedness. By a witness's report, he had loss of consciousness for about 1 minute."*

> *"Okay. Let me stop you there, Paul. Based on the chief complaint, what were your initial thoughts about what could have caused his syncopal episode?"*

The attending is assessing early hypothesis generation.

"Well, my differential includes vasovagal syncope, orthostatic hypotension, cardiac causes, such as an arrhythmia or valve problem, medications, and psychiatric causes."

"Great. It's reasonable when first learning about the case to think broadly about the differential so you become familiar with the differential, but once you have done that, it is equally important to start narrowing down your differential early in the evaluation. This will allow you to actively confirm or refute diagnoses based on the patient's symptoms, signs, and studies. So I'll ask you to change your approach now and give me the diagnoses that you think are most likely with specific numbers assigned to them based on the history and physical exam that you obtained."

The attending emphasizes that as the case evolves, the student needs to realize that the initial long differential diagnosis must be prioritized in a probabilistic manner because a clinician cannot exclude every diagnostic possibility. In this manner, the attending is encouraging the student to commit to a diagnosis.

"I guess I would focus on vasovagal or cardiac causes given my evaluation. I would say, a 30% chance of vasovagal syncope and a 70% chance of a cardiac cause."

"Great work, Paul. I agree with your differential. So how do you distinguish between vasovagal syncope, or what is called neuro-cardiogenic syncope, and cardiac syncope?"

The attending is probing the learner for his understanding of the typical clinical presentations, that is, his illness scripts, for the diagnoses on the initial differential diagnosis. He is also making the diagnostic process more concrete by having the student use numbers.

Paul says, "I think of cardiac syncope as occurring suddenly without much warning, as opposed to neurocardiogenic syncope, which is less abrupt."

"That's an excellent place to start. So what questions might we ask to distinguish these two categories of disease, Paul? And as a reminder, Paul, this should be the data you incorporated into 'paragraph 2' of your admission note."

The attending is asking the student to compare and contrast in order to clarify the discriminating features of the presentations of the diseases. This approach may help him to identify the reason for a potential diagnostic error.

Stef jumps into the discussion. "People usually have warning symptoms like light-headedness before neurocardiogenic syncope, unlike cardiac syncope where they can have pretty severe injuries."

"That's right, Stef. Expand on that a bit. What are some specific symptoms a patient with neurocardiogenic syncope might have?"

"Well, they usually feel light-headed, warm, and diaphoretic, and I think sometimes have nausea."

"Great. Any predisposing factors that we should consider in our history? Moni, what do you think?"

The attending is guiding the team to consider predisposing conditions, which might affect the pretest probability of an illness.

Moni replies, "I know stress can be a precipitant for neurocardiogenic syncope. I think coughing and eating can be, too."

"Good. These are important things to ask about in the history. I would add prolonged standing as a precipitant as well. Epidemiology is not so helpful for neurocardiogenic since anyone can get this type of syncope. So is any of this history present, Paul?"

"Actually, yes. He had been standing for a while, and had light-headedness, diaphoresis, and nausea before the episode. He lost consciousness for about a minute based on his wife's report, and when he woke up, he was still nauseated but rapidly became oriented."

"So at this point what is your leading diagnosis?

The attending asks the student to commit to a diagnosis.

"Based on the history I am thinking neurocardiogenic syncope is now 80% and cardiac causes are 20%."

"I agree, Paul. What would you look for on physical exam to confirm or refute the diagnosis?"

The attending is stressing diagnostic verification and demonstrating that the physical examination can be valuable in this exercise.

"Signs of trauma, vital signs, especially orthostatics and tachy- or bradycardia, and a careful cardiac exam to listen for murmurs," Paul replies.

"Perfect. Paul, did you find anything significant on his exam?"

"Well, he was not orthostatic, his heart rate was 76, and his rhythm was regular, but he did have a 2/6 systolic murmur best heard at the base."

"Nice work with the physical examination. But tell me, did that finding change your differential?"

"Well, I know syncope can be associated with aortic stenosis and the murmur sounded like aortic stenosis to me. He had been standing for a while in a hot, crowded church before it happened. I know aortic stenosis patients are preload-dependent, so this might have led to less left ventricular filling and precipitated the syncope. So I thought that's the most likely diagnosis now."

"Good. Give me a number. How probable is the diagnosis based on that reasoning, Paul?"

"I would say aortic stenosis is 80% and vasovagal syncope is 20%."

"So why don't you tell me a little more about what you know about the epidemiology and clinical findings in aortic stenosis?"

"I know the murmur is a crescendo-decrescendo murmur best heard at the aortic position. I don't know much about the epidemiology," Paul says.

"Okay, Stef, can you help out Paul?"

"Sure," Stef replies. *"I think exertional angina occurs before syncope in terms of symptoms. The murmur usually radiates to the carotids and the carotid pulse may be diminished and slow. It is a disease of older people but young people can get it if they have a bicuspid valve."* Stef pauses. *"But he seems a little too young."*

"Those are some really great points," says Phaedrus. *"It's important to learn the details about diseases, especially the epidemiology of them. When you mentioned aortic stenosis, I thought, 'Pretty unlikely,' because aortic stenosis tends to occur in patients in their sixties and seventies, and even though it can occur in people younger with bicuspid valves, bicuspid valves are quite rare. So based on epidemiology alone, my suspicion for AS was very low. In addition, as Stef mentioned, there are features of the cardiac exam that can help to increase or decrease the likelihood of aortic stenosis. I Googled the likelihood ratios for aortic stenosis*

*findings last night and found out that if a murmur does not radi-
ate to the right clavicular head, the negative likelihood ratio for
aortic stenosis is 0.1. The prevalence of bicuspid aortic valve is
about 2% to 4% in men. Can you calculate the post-test probability using Bayes theorem, Paul?"*

The attending teaches epidemiology to help the team prioritize the differential on the basis of probability. He also introduces evidence-based literature regarding the physical diagnosis of aortic stenosis to help the team
incorporate physical signs into their clinical reasoning. Finally, he continues using numbers to make the clinical reasoning process more concrete,
asking the student to perform a Bayesian calculation.

*"I can try." Paul looks at his piece of paper and begins to do the
calculations. Phaedrus watches at each step to ensure he is on the
right track.*

*"If we use the prevalence number of 4%, the pretest odds would be
1/1-p, or 0.04/0.96 = 0.042. I can now multiply pretest odds and
the negative likelihood ratio, 0.042 × 0.1, which would lead to a
post-test odds of 0.0042. Converting it back to post-test probability using odds/odds + 1, I get a post-test probability of 0.4%, which
would seem to more or less exclude aortic stenosis."*

*"In this case, with such a low pretest probability, we probably did-
n't need to go through the calculation." Phaedrus pauses. "But it
does make the point, doesn't it? The negative likelihood ratio
made us even more comfortable in excluding aortic stenosis."
Phaedrus pauses again. "Paul, can you see the power of knowing
epidemiology? Even if you had no idea what the murmur of aortic
stenosis sounded like, you could have pretty much excluded that
on your differential diagnosis just based on epidemiology alone.
Let's go into the patient's room now and examine the patient
together."*

The attending has the student explicitly calculate a post-test probability to concretely demonstrate the power that epidemiology and the physical
examination can have in excluding disease in certain cases.

*After examining the patient, the team returns to the hallway.
Phaedrus continues:*

*"Okay, so Paul has pretty much ruled out aortic stenosis as a
cause of this patient's syncope. So how many of you would get an
echo on this patient?" They all raise their hands.*

"Okay, so all of you would get an echo. It's common practice to get an echo in patients who have syncope to make sure you are not 'missing' any structural heart disease. But we should ask the question, 'Is it necessary?' In the setting of a patient with no known heart disease, a normal physical exam, and normal electrocardiogram, the likelihood of an unsuspected finding on echocardiography is only 5% to 10%. This case is different since we have discovered a murmur. So given that you all wanted to get an echo, what do you think it will show? Write down your answers on a piece of paper and hand them to me."

The attending models the act of using evidence-based literature in clinical decision-making. He also uses the competitive nature of the team members to increase participation and create a fun learning environment

Phaedrus counts the votes. "Well, it looks like everyone voted for hypertrophic cardiomyopathy except for Moni and me. Moni, why did you think it would be normal?"

"Well, the story is very good for vasovagal syncope, and after going to the bedside with you, we learned that the murmur had benign characteristics and did not change in intensity when we had the patient stand and squat. Innocent systolic flow murmurs are very common and so is vasovagal syncope, but hypertrophic cardiomyopathy isn't, even in people who present with syncope."

"I agree with your reasoning. I think it's quite natural when you have less clinical experience to rely on additional diagnostic testing to try to confirm your diagnostic impressions, particularly if a test is safe and easy to obtain. However, if it seems like your leading diagnosis is quite likely, then it's worthwhile to stop and assess the testing characteristics, such as the likelihood ratios or sensitivity/specificity, of your next study. You should really try to figure out how much more information it would give you. Given the very typical history for a neurocardiogenic cause of syncope and the very low prevalence of hypertrophic cardiomyopathy, which makes our pretest probability less than 1%, I think an argument can be made to forego the echo in this patient. If you thought it would show nothing, why did you still vote to get the echo?"

The attending challenges the resident to defend her management decision given a contradictory diagnostic opinion. He is also asking the resident more advanced questions, which are more likely to engage her than the earlier questions, thereby teaching to the level of the learner.

"Well, it's a noninvasive test, and hypertrophic cardiomyopathy is a potentially life-threatening disease, so weighing the risk of the test versus the potential benefit of diagnosis, I thought the echo was reasonable. In addition, the murmur was in the aortic position as opposed to the left upper sternal border, where most benign murmurs are heard."

"Well done, Moni. I think most physicians would agree with your reasoning. I just wanted to hear you say it."

❖ Teaching Management Decisions: Treatment Thresholds

At the end of the hypothetical deductive reasoning process, the physician decides whether to perform further testing or begin treatment. Both problem-solving and decision-making exist in an environment of uncertainty, and the expert physician's decision to treat depends directly on her diagnostic confidence. When a diagnosis is highly likely, efficacy of the therapy is high, and risk is low, then no further testing is necessary and treatment should be undertaken. On the other hand, if the diagnosis is very unlikely and the treatment is not very effective or is risky, the patient should not be treated. The challenge in medical decision-making is the gray range where the diagnosis is not definitive, treatment is questionably efficacious, more than one treatment is appropriate (a "toss-up"), or treatment is somewhat risky.

Step 1

Remind the learners that the point of the *diagnostic* clinical reasoning method was to establish the probability of *each* diagnosis being considered. At the end of the diagnostic process, more than one diagnosis may and, in fact, probably will, still be in play. The learner needs to understand that all diagnoses that still remain may be important (this will explain step 4 below).

Step 2

The student should be instructed that management decisions are based on a combination of the potential costs and risks versus the expected benefits of the treatment. The combination of the two defines the treatment threshold. If the benefits are high and the risks (for example, the costs) are low (such as treating suspected pneumonia with antibiotics), the probability needed to start antibiotics for a patients suspected of having pneumonia is low (20%). If the potential costs are high and the benefits are low (for example, chemotherapy), we have to be absolutely certain the diagnosis is correct (100%). It is important to emphasize that although the risks and benefits are unique to each patient, the treatment threshold for that patient is independent of the probability of her having the disease. That is, the safety/efficacy profile of aspirin does not change according to the probability that Ms. Jones is having a coronary intervention.

Step 3

Instruct the student that when the probability of disease exceeds its treatment threshold, treatment should be given, even if you are not 100% sure that the patient has the disease. If the probability remains below the threshold, treatment should not be given (Figure 4-2). This will help alleviate the anxiety that goes with the uncertainty of clinical medicine (acting before you are 100% sure) and explain the variability from diagnosis to diagnosis (for example, why you must be 99% sure to give chemotherapy but only 20% sure to give antibiotics).

> *"Dr. Phaedrus, I'm a little confused as to why we decided to start Mr. Richardson on warfarin."*

> *"Okay, Paul, let's talk through it." Phaedrus draws a rectangle and labels the left part of the box as 0% and the right part of the box as 100%. He continues. "Let's say we were considering treating a patient with antibiotics for a urinary tract infection. What would the risks be?"*

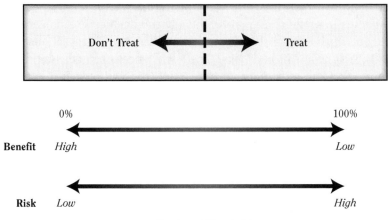

Figure 4-2 The dashed line dividing the "don't treat/treat" rectangle moves to the left when benefit of treatment is high and risk is low; it moves to the right when benefit of treatment is low and risk is high.

"Not that high."

"Indeed. And what would the benefits be?"

"Pretty good, I suppose."

"Okay, so how confident would you have to be to give a patient antibiotics to treat a suspected urinary tract infection?"

"Well, it would depend on the probability of him having a urinary tract infection."

"No, not really. Think about it." Phaedrus pauses. *"Would the risks of the antibiotics change based on his probability of having the disease? If so, we need to notify the manufacturer of the drug that they need to keep this guy healthy?"*

Paul laughs. *"No, I guess not."*

"Would the benefits of the antibiotics change based on the probability of him having coronary disease? Same gig … if it does, we need to notify the manufacturer of the drug."

"No."

"So we can say that the risks and benefits of a therapy are independent of the probability of him having the disease." Paul nods in agreement. *"Okay, so back to your question. If the risks were low and the benefits high, how confident would you have to be?"*

"Not very confident."

"Draw a vertical line on this box, somewhere between 0 and 100 percent, to indicate how confident you would have to be to treat the suspected infection with antibiotics." Paul does as instructed, drawing the line at 20 percent.

Phaedrus continues. *"Okay, now let me ask you this. How confident would you have to be to give a patient chemotherapy for a suspected mass in the lung?"*

"Well, more confident. The benefits aren't that great, and the risk is much higher."

"Indeed, Paul, you're catching on. So draw another vertical line for me on the box indicating how confident we would have to be." Paul draws a line at the 90% point.

"Great. So here's the lesson: The treatment threshold is defined by the risks and benefits of the therapy. Riskier interventions, such as chemotherapy, and/or interventions that do not have that much benefit, will have thresholds that are very high. Low-risk interventions or treatments that have high benefits will have thresholds that are very low. If your pretest probability for a disease crosses that threshold, we will treat. If it sits to the left of that threshold, we don't treat."

Step 4

Anticipate the problems that learners will have with this method. Even if these questions are not asked, learners will ask themselves these questions eventually. Novice physicians will not understand why some patients, even with the same probability of the disease, will receive treatment and others will not. The answer is that the risk versus benefit assessment changes according to the patient. The best method is to give the student a few theoretical examples of a clinical decision applied to different patients; each could have the same probability of having the disease, but with different risk profiles. It is important that the student understand that 1) the patient's individual probability of having the disease *is independent* of the treatment threshold but 2) the patient's individual risk/benefit profile *is unique* to that patient. Failure to explicitly teach the student that the risks and benefits vary from patient to patient, and that is the reason for the patient-to-patient variability in the management, may result in students "copying" what was done on the last patient with the disease to the next patient with the same disease. It is also very important to point out that ultimately the patient makes this decision, and patient preferences may lead to additional variability in the treatment plan.

"Dr. Phaedrus, I get the treatment threshold concept, but I don't understand why we treated Mr. Dhaliwal with warfarin for his atrial fibrillation and why we didn't treat Mr. Shlipak for his last week. They both seemed to have the same probability of having atrial fibrillation."

"That's a very astute question, Paul. The answer is that the treatment threshold changes from patient to patient." Paul looks confused. "Let me put it to you this way. I'll give you two patients and you tell me if you would start warfarin or not. Let's assume that both have the same probability of atrial fibrillation. I'll begin with a 60-year-old man with hypertension, diabetes, a previous stroke,

and atrial fibrillation. He has no bleeding risks. Would you give him warfarin?"

"Yeah, sure. He has three of the CHADS criteria; the benefit will be high and the risk is low."

"Great, so the treatment threshold will be low, maybe 20%. Is that correct?" Paul nods in agreement.

Phaedrus continues. "Okay, how about a 50-year-old woman with diabetes and alcoholic liver disease. She has had frequent falls, one of which has caused a subdural hematoma in the past, and she has had one episode of variceal bleeding. Would you give her warfarin?"

"Well, no. The risk would be way too high."

"But the efficacy would be good, right? We would prevent a stroke," says Phaedrus.

"Yeah, but the risk is still too high. I'd put the threshold at 80% or so."

"Good thinking, Paul. Do you see how even with the same probability of having atrial fibrillation, the treatment threshold changed with the patient?"

"I understand that now."

Variability Due to Patient Preferences
Treatment thresholds can vary significantly from patient to patient on the basis of physiologic variables (for example, a patient's risk for hemorrhage in deciding when to use anticoagulation), but can also vary according to the patient's personal values and beliefs. Management decisions vary by patient preferences, and while this is intuitive to the expert clinician, it is not necessarily intuitive to the novice. It is important for the attending physician to alert learners when standard management has been altered to incorporate patient values and preferences; otherwise, they believe that there is no standard management plan for a disease or condition and that all management decisions are merely "style."

Multiple Diseases
The deductive clinical reasoning process works on the presumption of Occam's razor: Statistically, the patient will have *one* disease that will explain all of the symptoms that prompted presentation to the hospital.

However, the attending should be on guard for areas in which students may be confused. The following are commonly seen:

1. Finding a Unifying Diagnosis

The attending should be aware that despite Occam's razor, early learners may struggle to find a single diagnosis that explains the multiple symptoms. Students should be taught the principle of Occam's razor (parsimony) and to look for a disease syndrome (such as heart failure) that might explain the presenting problems (for example, edema, dyspnea, and weakness). The use of Venn diagrams in addition to teaching the pathophysiology of the disease (see the dialogue on congestive heart failure in section II of this book) can help students cross symptoms into a single syndrome.

2. Hickam's Dictum

It is important to be honest with students, however, and there are patients, especially the elderly and the immunocompromised, who will present with two distinctly different diseases at the same time (Hickam's dictum: a patient is entitled to have as many diseases as he pleases). In these cases, it is important to explain to the student that this is the exception and not the rule, lest the student lock into phase 1 clinical reasoning (that is, assuming that their n-of-1 experience with one of these rare patients is the rule).

3. Comorbid Conditions

Novice physicians sometimes see comorbid conditions (such as hypertension, diabetes, and chronic obstructive pulmonary disease) as having equal weight to the presenting problem, exerting the same amount of time and energy (including diagnostic time) as they do for the presenting problem. If not explicitly addressed, this may result in one of two bad outcomes: 1) The student will treat all problems (that is, the admitting diagnosis) and each comorbid condition (even if not active) with equal allocation of time and energy, thereby diluting the attention available for the primary problem; or 2) the student will ignore all the comorbid conditions entirely. To address this problem, attending physicians should instruct students to exert most of their time and attention (80%) to the primary problem. The attending should also explain that not every issue must be solved on the first day of admission; long-standing comorbid conditions can be addressed during the rest of the hospital stay. Finally, attendings may find it useful to instruct students on the concept of "solvency issues." As described in chapter 3, issues should be addressed, or "solved," as part of a definitive plan of action by the time of discharge, not necessarily on day 1.

"Paul, how is the admission note coming?"

"Well, okay, I guess. I understand the two-paragraph approach to the history, and how to write up the past medical history, examination, and laboratory values, but I'm not sure how to do the assessment and plan. I know you said that you want me to organize the assessment and plan by problems and that I should commit to a hypothesis as to the diagnosis and support that. I know I should talk about what my differential was and how we excluded those, but should I use the same approach for every problem?"

Phaedrus looks at Paul's admission note in progress. It's clear Paul is trying to use the same method of diagnostic explanation for every problem. The note is five pages long, and he is stuck on the differential diagnosis for the problem of "diabetes." Largely because there is no differential diagnosis for the patient's long-standing diagnosis of diabetes (it just exists), Paul is stuck.

"Paul, let me clarify this for you. First, I want you to devote most of your time and energy to the primary presenting problem, let's say 80%. This is not a get-it-all-done-now-or-not-at-all event. We'll have some time during the patient's hospital stay to address in detail his other comorbid conditions, such as hypertension and diabetes. For this first day, let's just make sure that we have a plan for each of these to at least keep him safe, and then we'll address the details on subsequent days." Phaedrus pauses.

"Second, let me explain the theory behind the method used to present the assessment and plan for the primary problem. There is a diagnostic uncertainty there, and that is why I am asking you to outline the hypothesis, the differential, and the supporting or refuting data. This is to show me, and anyone else looking at the chart, where your line of reasoning has been. It is also to help you clarify your thoughts about the case, especially at this stage of your development." Phaedrus pauses again. "Now look at your problem number three, there ... 'Diabetes.' Is there any diagnostic uncertainty there?"

"No, I guess not," says Paul. "So I don't have to do the full assessment and plan method for these issues?"

"No, Paul, you do not. I want everything you to do to have a reason—if there is no diagnostic uncertainty, and it's just management, then I want you to switch your focus to defining the management and anticipating any consequences of that management.

On the first day, set a course for the management and keep him safe. We can spend time later fine-tuning the issue before his discharge."

4. Treating Two Diseases Simultaneously While Diagnosis Continues
Finally, there are times when more than one diagnosis is being treated. Learners coming from an environment of certainty may have a hard time understanding why, when the goal is to establish the *one* diagnosis, the attending may elect to treat two diseases at once. The attending should anticipate the question, making it clear to the student that if the probabilities of both diseases have crossed their respective treatment thresholds, both diseases should receive treatment.

> *"But I have one other question," says Paul. "Why is it that we sometimes treat more than one diagnosis? Why not just treat all of the diagnoses, or just treat one?"*
>
> *"The answer, Paul, lies in the treatment threshold for each diagnosis being considered. Certainly, if a diagnosis has no probability remaining after our history, then it should be treated. But let me ask you: Let's say we had a patient who had a 50% probability of having pneumonia. Based on the risks and benefits of antibiotics, would you treat that patient?"*
>
> *"Well, it would depend upon his personal risk and benefit profile." Paul pauses for the approbation for having incorporated the last lesson in his response, which Phaedrus obliges with a nod of the head. "But assuming that it was a standard risk-benefit profile, I would definitely treat. The risks are low and the benefits are high."*
>
> *"Great thinking, Paul. I like it. Now let's say the other competing diagnosis for this patient was an exacerbation of COPD [chronic obstructive pulmonary disease], and let's say that it too was of 50% probability. Based on the risks and benefits of inhaled steroids and bronchodilators, would you treat that patient?"*
>
> *"Well, I suppose I would. The probability of COPD would be above the treatment threshold as well since the risks of steroids and bronchodilators are not that big, and the benefits could be huge if that was the diagnosis."*
>
> *"There you go, Paul. It's all about each diagnosis being considered, and whether its probability is above its respective treatment threshold."*

❖ Using the Admission Note to Assess Clinical Reasoning

The admission note documents the results of the history, physical examination, and laboratory data collected. As noted earlier, learners should be instructed that it is vital for team care of the patient: Other team members (nurses, techs, social workers, other physicians) can quickly gain access to the obtained information without redoing a full history and physical examination. For this reason, learners must be made aware that the note must be accurate and neatly documented. Further, they should know that neatly written notes that use proper grammar and punctuation convey the measure of thoroughness that was expended in collecting the information: Professionally appearing notes convey a professional and accurate history and physical examination. Anything less is likely to prompt other team members to recollect the data on their own, wasting the team's time.

The admission note, however, has an additional purpose in assessing a learner's clinical reasoning if the following method is used. Because no hospital attending will have the time to observe, from start to finish, each student's history, physical examination, and clinical reasoning synthesis of the data, this method allows the attending to use a surrogate to assess the student's clinical reasoning. (This works in the same way a creatinine level is used as a surrogate measure of renal function.) It also allows the attending to make this assessment on her own time, for example, on afternoon solo rounds as she reviews the chart. Intermittently through the month, the surrogate measure (this method) should be correlated with the gold standard (actually observing the student in this process).

Step 1: Ask The Student to Construct the Admission Note in the Same Way as the History

1. The first paragraph of the note should outline the time course and characterization of the chief complaint.
2. Ask the student to routinely make a second paragraph; the data in this paragraph should correspond to the questions he asked in evaluating his diagnosis, without explicitly listing this differential diagnosis in the text. It may be useful to ask early learners to also list their differential diagnosis in the margin of the note to make the evaluation more explicit.
3. The past medical history, the review of systems, and the physical examination should be written as is standard practice.
4. Instruct the student to write the assessment and plan in the following format to allow for assessment of the clinical reasoning. The assessment and plan should be grouped by problems. The discussion of the assessment and plan should focus on the

general problem (for example, shortness of breath), with careful consideration of qualifiers unless the diagnosis is obvious; in that case, the assessment and plan can be organized around the diagnosis.

For each problem, the student should explicitly state the hypothesis by using active words (such as "We believe this is..."), not passive words (such as "Would consider..."). A sentence or two to support the hypothesis should follow. The student should then list the other diagnoses considered and any data that supported or refuted these diagnoses. The student should then state the plan, again using active verbs (such as "We will treat with antibiotics"), not general ones ("We will consider using antibiotics").

Step 2: Look for Errors in Clinical Reasoning

A slim paragraph 1 might be a clue that the student is succumbing to premature closure, is locked in an anchoring heuristic, doesn't know what to ask of the patient or feels uncomfortable with the patient, or is lazy.

A slim or absent paragraph 2 might be a clue that the student has not advanced to using the differential diagnosis to drive the subsequent history. It may also indicate that although the student understands the utility of the differential diagnosis to drive the questions, he does not know what to ask for each.

A physical examination that looks like a liturgy (for example, the same physical examination for every patient) *or a code* (for example, VSS, EOMI, PERRLA, RRR, CTA, grossly normal) might be a clue that the student is not using the differential diagnosis to distinguish physical examination maneuvers that are relevant to the case but rather is merely following a template. He has memorized the method for obtaining and writing the history but doesn't understand it. Caution should be used in saying the word "relevant" to students because this presupposes they understand what relevance is. For the clinical reasoning process, "relevance" refers to data that are useful in evaluating the differential diagnosis. The physical examination should include both positive and negative findings, provided that they assist in evaluating the differential diagnosis.

An assessment and plan-by-problems that has a new differential for each problem (symptom), but does not link comments to other problems (for example, the discussion of "edema" should link in some way to the discussion of "dyspnea" in a patient with heart failure) might be a clue that the student is interpreting each symptom as its own problem; he is not making the move to seeing syndromes.

An assessment and plan that does not contain a committed hypothesis or features passive, noncommitted words suggests that the student has merely collected the data. On the reporter-interpreter-manager-educator (RIME) scheme (16), he is locked in the reporter mode.

An assessment and plan that provide a hypothesis with no supporting data suggest that the student is just guessing or has succumbed to taking another's opinion as fact without evoking supporting or refuting diagnosis (anchoring or blind obedience heuristics).

An assessment and plan that address only one diagnosis, with no commentary on what else was considered in the differential diagnosis, might indicate that the student has succumbed to an anchoring heuristic or premature closure.

An assessment and plan that provide a hypothesis with supporting data, but no commentary on the differential diagnosis, might be a clue that the student has succumbed to premature closure—only one diagnosis was considered.

An assessment and plan that frequently reference other members of the team suggests that the student has succumbed to a blind obedience heuristic.

Even if all of the above are accurate, it is possible that the student has just been well coached. This is why it is important to directly observe the student do the whole process at least once or twice per rotation (see chapter 3).

❖ Using the Spoken Case Presentation to Assess Clinical Reasoning

This same approach can be used to assess clinical reasoning by way of the spoken case presentation, although additional deficits (discussed in chapter 3) may confound the assessment (17). The value of using the same organizational structure for both the spoken case presentation and the admission note is that doing so sends the message that all three components (*obtaining* the history, physical examination, and laboratory data; *writing down* the data in the admission note; and *speaking* during the spoken case presentation) should follow the same format. This format should be the clinical reasoning process outlined in Box 4-2. Students who make, or who are coached to make, the link between each of the three components will find an upward spiral of competency in their clinical reasoning. As the student writes the admission note in this format, it will prompt him to think of the questions that he should have asked. As he presents the patient orally, it will prompt him to think of what he should have written down in the admission note. As he takes the history on a subsequent patient, he will be thinking about what data he needs to complete the admission note. This makes the difficult link between the theoretical concept of clinical reason-

---

Box 4-2. Clinical Reasoning by Using the Seven-Step Approach

History

1. Take a history.
2. Create a list of possible diagnoses (four or five).
3. Ask questions about each of these diagnoses.
4. Mentally assign a pretest probability to each diagnosis.

Physical Examination

5. Perform a physical examination. Focus the examination on the diagnoses you are considering. Change the probabilities of each diagnosis on the basis of the examination results. Reorder the diagnoses.

Laboratory Tests and Other Studies

6. Order laboratory and other studies. Focus these tests on the diagnoses you are considering. Change the probability of each diagnosis on the basis of the laboratory test and study results. Reorder the diagnoses.

Assessment and Plan

7. Make an assessment and plan on the basis of the remaining diagnoses.

---

ing to the more tangible skills of writing the admission note and doing the oral case presentation. It also enables the attending to see the clinical reasoning in a more tangible way and to provide targeted feedback to improve the student's clinical reasoning.

Many students will have mimicked the physicians they have previously seen, and this method will seem onerous and foreign to them. It is best to acknowledge that this method is useful in developing and assessing their clinical reasoning at this stage of their development. The attending should acknowledge that they may not be required to use this method later in their career as they develop experience and become more adept at pattern recognition, or as analytic methods become integrated as habit in their thinking. Failure to do so may lead the student to summarily dismiss the analytic methods and, dangerously, the clinical reasoning process they support. *"This is only what Dr. Phaedrus does ... other physicians I've seen don't do this!"* As described earlier in chapter 1, that kind of presumption may impede students' development of advanced clinical reasoning skills.

❖ The Anatomy of a Mistake: Using Mistakes to Advance Learners' Clinical Reasoning

Mistakes are inevitable on the clinical wards, especially as students learn and practice their clinical reasoning skills. These frequent occurrences, where the student thought one thing (the wrong diagnosis or the wrong management plan) and the attending thought another, are excellent teaching opportunities to diagnose and fix the deficits in the learner's reasoning process, thereby moving him to the next level in his reasoning abilities. For this to work, however, learners must be encouraged to "put their nickel down" in actively using the clinical reasoning process and committing to the diagnosis and management plan. Valued physicians of any specialty share one common denominator: the ability to make decisions. But only by actively making decisions can a learner develop this level of competence. When a mistake is made, the learner should be rewarded for her courage in putting ego aside and making a decision. The error in the learner's clinical reasoning should then be identified and categorized (Box 4-2) and the student "talked through" each step of the clinical reasoning process in a manner that clarifies where and how the error was made, and how a similar case might be better handled in the future.

❖ Final Thoughts

The inpatient service provides an enormous opportunity for teaching attendings to appreciate and advance students' clinical reasoning skills. The more the attending knows about clinical reasoning, and the more attention she gives to this critical aspect of clinical expertise, the more likely it is that her students will develop as skilled physicians. And is that not what inpatient teaching is all about?

REFERENCES

1. **Ende J, ed.** Theory and Practice of Teaching Medicine. Philadelphia: ACP Pr; 2010.
2. **Eva KW.** What every teacher needs to know about clinical reasoning. Med Educ. 2005;39:98-106.
3. **Schmidt HG, Rikers RM.** How expertise develops in medicine: knowledge encapsulation and illness script formation. Med Educ. 2007;41:1133-9.
4. **Rikers RM, Schmidt HG, Boshuizen HP.** Knowledge Encapsulation and the Intermediate Effect. Contemp Educ Psychol. 2000;25:150-166.
5. **Schmidt HG, Boshuizen HP.** On the origin of intermediate effects in clinical case recall. Mem Cognit. 1993;21:338-51.
6. **Boshuizen HPA, Schmidt HG.** On the role of biomedical knowledge in clinical reasoning by experts, intermediates and novices. Cognitive Science. 1992;16:153-184.

7. **McLaughlin KJ.** The Contribution of Analytic Information Processing to Diagnostic Performance in Medicine. Rotterdam: Erasmus Univ Pr; 2007.

8. **Custers E, Boshuizen HP, Schmidt HG.** The role of illness scripts in the development of medical diagnostic expertise: results from an interview study. Cognitive Instruction. 1998;16:367-398.

9. **Custers EJ, Boshuizen HP, Schmidt HG.** The influence of medical expertise, case typicality, and illness script component on case processing and disease probability estimates. Mem Cognit. 1996;24:384-99.

10. **van Schaik P, Flynn D, van Wersch A, Douglass A, Cann P.** Influence of illness script components and medical practice on medical decision making. J Exp Psychol Appl. 2005; 11:187-99.

11. **Kassirer J, Wong J, Kopelman R.** Learning Clinical Reasoning. 2nd ed. Philadelphia; Wolters Kluwer; 2009.

12. **Saint S, Drazen J, Solomon C.** NEJM Clinical Problem Solving. New York: McGraw-Hill; 2006.

13. **Eddy DM.** Probabilistic reasoning in clinical medicine: problems and opportunities. In: Kahneman D, Slovic P, Tversky A, eds. Judgment Under Uncertainty: Heuristics and Biases. Cambridge, United Kingdom: Cambridge Univ Pr; 1982.

14. **Tversky A, Kahneman D.** Judgment under Uncertainty: Heuristics and Biases. Science. 1974;185:1124-1131.

15. **McGee S.** Simplifying likelihood ratios. J Gen Intern Med. 2002;17:646-9.

16. **Pangaro L.** A new vocabulary and other innovations for improving in-training evaluations. Acad Med. 1999;74:1203-7.

17. **Wiese J, Varosy P, Tierney L.** Improving oral presentation skills with a clinical reasoning curriculum: a prospective controlled study. Am J Med. 2002;112:212-8.

5

Teaching the Important Nonclinical Skills on the Inpatient Service

Jeff Wiese, MD, FACP

T he time pressures, the interpersonal complexities, and the mass of clinical data on the inpatient ward can make teaching challenging. Yet these also represent opportunities for attending physicians to empower their learners with life-long skills that will improve clinical performance. This chapter addresses the strategies to teach the skills that lie outside of clinical knowledge, yet still are important for a physician's performance. The chapter begins with strategies to improve learners' time management and data organization skills. Next, strategies to improve learners' interpersonal skills are considered, followed by suggestions for teaching learners how to read the medical literature and for inspiring them to do so. Finally, the chapter discusses strategies for how to improve learners' communication skills, both written and oral.

❖ Teaching Time Management

The time pressures of the clinical wards provide an ideal laboratory for learners to assess and improve their time management skills: As a skill is taught, there is near-immediate feedback about whether the skill has been mastered. Mastering time management is not only a valuable skill for the long-term performance of the learner but also of great value to the attending physician: The more adept the team is at time

---

KEY POINTS

- The inpatient setting provides an opportunity to teach life-long skills, including time management, data organization, interpersonal skills, and strategies for continuous practice-based learning.
- There are several strategies that students and house officers can use to help with time management, including understanding the difference between important and urgent and general rules for prioritization.
- Learners become more efficient when they are encouraged to organize their schedule of activities, keep lists, use down-time effectively, and be sure that clinical data are organized.
- Given the complexity and intensity of the inpatient service, it is not surprising that this venue provides an opportunity for attendings to focus on their learners' interpersonal skills, which can be seen as directly related to their effectiveness and their ability to resolve conflicts.
- Habits for reading and self-directed learning can be shaped on the inpatient service, particularly if the attending emphasizes the practice of reading each day, organizing reading around clinical cases, and taking steps to mitigate the natural decline in skills that comes with time.
- Case presentations provide inpatient attendings with an opportunity to focus on learners' communication skills and address deficits in length of presentations, students' level of discomfort, and, finally, students' sense of discomfort about their own roles.

---

management, the more efficiently the ward service will run. This investment in teaching time management skills—early in the month—will enable better patient care and more opportunities for teaching in general.

The attending should assume, until proven otherwise, that most learners do not have essential time management skills and that they will succumb to three deficits that waste time: the failure to prioritize, the failure to see "windows" of time, and the inability to consolidate tasks and limit fragmentation. These and related time management skill deficiencies are the most important learning needs for students and house officers on the wards.

Teaching Prioritization: Urgent Versus Important

The key to time management is prioritizing tasks according to their *relative* importance and their urgency. *Importance* is defined internally, by the learners themselves, indicating tasks that are considered mission-critical in advancing patient care and learning. *Urgency* here is defined externally, by other peoples' agendas. Learners should be taught to categorize tasks on the basis of whether the task is important, urgent, both, or neither.

Priority 1: Important and Urgent Tasks
The learner should be coached to prioritize and focus first on tasks that are important (advancing patient care) *and* urgent (the needs of other team members caring for the patient). Examples of important and urgent tasks include 1) ensuring that a patient gets to a procedure that he needs (important) and that the procedure team is prepared to do the procedure right now (urgent) and 2) completing a discharge form for a patient who is leaving right now (important) and that the social worker needs to have completed immediately (urgent). It is worth asking team members, as the month ensues, to identify whether the task they are doing is important or urgent, both, or neither.

Priority 2: Important but Not Urgent Tasks
Tasks that are important but not urgent should be done next. Competing with this level of prioritization are urgent tasks that are not that important. The learner should be coached that she is not alone; everyone is dealing with this same dilemma: *"Do I do what I know needs to be done first?"* (importance) or *"Do I do what other people think should be done first?"* (urgent). It is worth being honest with learners by simply stating the facts: Everyone believes that his or her task is the most important, and these people will create a sense of urgency to get you to do their tasks first. Learners should be told that these people are usually well-intentioned, but they may not see the relative importance of their task in comparison with other people's requested tasks. It is the physician's job to assess all requested tasks and then to prioritize them *not* on the basis of who wants it done first (urgency) but according to what is most *important* for the patient.

Say, for example, that an intern who is seeing a patient gets a page. It is a nurse saying that a verbal order already carried out needs to be signed right away. Although neither task is important and urgent, the intern should stay focused on the patient in front of her. That task is clearly important, and while the nurse is instilling a sense of urgency about the verbal order, it is not as important as the patient right before her. Caution should be exercised in this instruction because learners may get the wrong impression that they need not do tasks if they do not find them that important. The verbal order still needs to be signed; it is just that this task is assigned a lower priority in the sequence of the day.

Rounding with a team affords great opportunity in teaching this lesson, especially when pagers or cell phones go off while the team is standing around a patient's bedside. The attending should take the time to tell the team that unless the code pager is going off, they need to stay focused on their important task (the patient they are with right now), and deal with the urgent task (the person on the other end of the pager) after they are through.

Another example might include what to do during prerounds. There is no external pressure (urgency) on the intern to see patients and write orders during prerounds, but this task does have considerable importance: It advances patient care early in the day and prepares the resident for meaningful resident/attending rounds. Conversely, the consulting team might want the intern to spend prerounds completing all of her progress notes so that they can bill more effectively and easily. A nurse or social worker may want the intern to spend her time on prerounds filling out forms for patients who will be discharged tomorrow. Both are urgent tasks (someone else's agenda), but because there will be time to complete the task just as well later in the day, it is not as important as seeing the patients and advancing patient care.

Priority 3: Urgent but Not Important Tasks
After all the important tasks are done, the resident should then focus on completing urgent tasks. This sequence follows naturally: After the team member has completed the important tasks, the urgent tasks (those driven by the external environment) receive his attention. However, the attending should look for learners who focus next on tasks that are neither important nor urgent: for example, the resident who is surfing the Internet for a car he can't afford instead of using the time to complete discharge summaries. It is worth recognizing that professionalism at its core is not a measure of appearance or speech but instead the willingness to consistently place the needs of the patient and the team over self-interests.

Anticipating Problems in Time Management
Students and interns may have a difficult time with time management, especially in a setting that is constantly in flux, with no day the same as the day before. Learning to separate urgent from important tasks will be difficult at first, and all team members should be encouraged to ask for a second opinion if they do not know how to prioritize tasks. Instead of asking, *"What should I do next?"* which is passive deference of time management decisions, they should be advised to ask after they have made their best effort. *"I have prioritized my list of things to do today. Can you tell me how you would have prioritized them?"* or *"I have two things to do, and I have*

an idea of which of these tasks I would do first. Can you tell me if I've made the right prioritization?"

Be patient. Continuous feedback and coaching will be required to develop the habit of prioritization. The attending can yoke the strength of his senior team members by instructing them directly in how to teach and assess time management skills. This is a great topic for the first day that the intern has off. Thereafter, the resident should be instructed to regularly ask her more novice team members (the interns and students) how they are prioritizing their tasks.

Students and interns should also be instructed that the team's priorities may not always be the same as theirs, but when it comes to sequencing tasks, their team leader (the resident) is the general on the top of a hill: She has a better perspective on the whole battle plan, and they should trust the team leader in defining importance.

Using Time Management Instruction to Consolidate Professionalism

Correctly presented, teaching time management can provide lessons in professionalism. Time management, after all, is an exercise in continually prioritizing important tasks (that is, patients' needs) over other people's agendas, including those of the learner himself. The wards provide an opportunity for continual practice in this principle. If the coach can consistently direct and redirect the teammates to this principle, eventually the hidden curriculum of "patient first" becomes ingrained.

Maintaining Interpersonal Relationships While Managing Time

Prioritization may be misinterpreted by others as selfishness or laziness, especially by those whose urgent tasks are not completed first. The attending needs to sensitize his learners to this misunderstanding, so common on a busy inpatient service, and provide his learners with an approach that will maintain interpersonal relationships even as tasks requested by others are deferred. The lessons here should be quite explicit, as in the following example:

> *"So, Stef, that should give you an idea of how I want you to prioritize tasks in your day. Start with the important and urgent tasks, then do the important tasks, then do the urgent tasks, and then everything else that remains. Let me ask you, what are you going to do when you are completing an important task and someone comes to you with an urgent but not important task? Say you're seeing a patient and talking about his prognosis, and someone comes to you to fill out a request for medical records. What are you going to do?"*

Stef looks confident in his naiveté. "I'll tell them I'm doing something important and I'll do that later."

"Good, you have the priority correct. But how would it make you feel if someone said that to you? I'll rephrase if for you. 'What I'm doing is more important that what you want done.'"

"Well, not that good, I suppose."

"So let me give you a strategy such that you can have your cake and eat it too, a strategy for how to maintain your priorities in the day, while still 'winning friends and influencing people.'"

"Sounds great."

"Okay, step 1. Recognize that everyone finds their agenda most important, and they link that with their persona. When you tell them that their agenda is not number one, they feel you are saying that they are not number one. That hurts." Phaedrus pauses. "So your first step is to validate their need, which will validate them as a person. Be genuine now, no sappy, insincere talk—people feel manipulated by that. Just say, 'You know, I can see that task is very important. It needs to get done.' Let me hear you say it, Stef."

Stef replies, "You know, I can see that completing the form for medical records is very important. It needs to get done."

"Fantastic. Now you've done two great things. One, you have validated their work and needs as important, and you have assuaged their greatest fear—the fear that the task is not going to get done. Remember that since all anger is fear turned inward, you have now offset the anger of not doing their task first.

"Okay, second step. Tell them what you are currently doing. As physicians, we just assume that everyone knows that we are doing important things, and that should be enough. But not everyone knows that. So, for example, tell them, 'I'm with a patient right now who really needs me. As soon as I'm finished with this patient, I'll be right there.' Now take the first line and put it with this one. Say it for me."

Stef obliges. "You know, I can see that completing the form for medical records is very important. It needs to get done. I'm with a patient right now who really needs me. As soon as I'm finished with this patient, I'll be right there."

"Now that's the easy part. It's harder if they are right in front of you, and it will be very tempting for you to just respond to the immediacy of their demand, forgoing your responsibility of completing your important task. When that happens, I want you to pull out your card with your checklist, and I want you to say the first two lines. Even if you are not seeing a patient right then and there, tell them what you are currently doing and why it is important. Then let them see you write down the task on your checklist. Put a star out to the side of it. This will give them some perspective on how many things you have to do, it will assure them that their task is in the queue for getting completed. And, since it has a star to the side of it, it will have some priority."

Stef asks, "Do I have to do that starred item next?"

"No. That's to make them feel better. You should still complete all of your important tasks, and when you get to the tasks that are urgent by not important, then feel free to do that one as well."

Anticipating and Preventing the Jet Wash

The coach should also anticipate the "analysis paralysis" that can result from the busy hospital wards. Like flooding a car by pushing on the accelerator too much, the condition known as "status pagerous" on the wards can paralyze the learner if too many requests come at once. That overload results in anxiety that reduces performance, which, in turn, increases the list of things to get done and leads to more anxiety, and so on. Once in the tailspin, the learner may not get out. The attending can offset this by training the learner to sometimes expect it and to provide a strategy for getting out of it—much like a flight instructor teaches a pilot to expect jet wash (a form of turbulence) and prepares her with the strategy to get out of it.

"One last thing, Stef ... and this will be important for your sanity. There will be times during the day when the requests just don't seem to stop. It will feel endless, and you will start to freak out. It will begin with anxiety, and then guilt, and then frustration, and then hopelessness. When you start to experience those feelings, just go to the bathroom and enter a stall. Sit there for 10 seconds and tell yourself, 'Whatever happens, they can't stop the clock. Eventually, I will go home, and until that point, I will do my best.' Then wash your hands."

Stef smiles. Phaedrus continues: "And then come back out. Pull out your to-do list card, and fill in the list of tasks as they come. Inefficiency results from being overwhelmed, and at moments like these, you can't afford that. Then, reprioritize the day, and get task number one done. Then task number two, and then task number three. Just keep working. Almost all tasks will eventually get done. Some might have to be put off until tomorrow, and some you might have to ask your resident or students to help with. But it will all eventually get done. If you have taken care of your patients—the important stuff—no one will die. All of the rest is just details, and believe it or not, Stef, it's not the end of the world if some things, especially the unimportant things, get rolled over until tomorrow. And believe it or not, the storm will end. Other people go home, too, and as they do, their requests go with them."

Stef smiles. It's weird how Phaedrus knows what he is thinking.

Teaching Time Windows

One hour is not the same as every other hour on the wards. There are windows of opportunity, and starting a task within one of these windows will lead to a quick time to completion; once the window closes, the task takes exponentially more time to complete. For example, a magnetic resonance imaging (MRI) examination ordered at 8 a.m. may be completed by 10 a.m. because no one else was on the schedule when the test was ordered. That same MRI ordered at 10 a.m. may not be read until the following day. Learners will fail to recognize this principle, and this will limit their ability to prioritize correctly. The easiest way to instruct learners in this principle is to use the analogy of rush hour traffic: If you hit the interstate at 6:55 a.m., the commute is 10 minutes; at 7:01 a.m., the commute takes an hour.

Some tasks have a longer "wait time" than others. For example, the reading of an MRI may take a couple of hours, while the reading of a chest radiograph may take only 30 minutes. The easiest way to instruct learners in this principle is to use the analogy of cooking a Thanksgiving dinner: You always start with putting the turkey in the oven first; it will take 5 hours to cook, while the mashed potatoes may take only 30 minutes. Time-expensive tasks should be "placed in the oven" at the beginning of the day.

General Rules for Assigning Time Windows

Although assignments should be based on the day-to-day needs of the service, it will help learners if they have a general overarching strategy. Learners should be coached to categorize patient care issues by using the three Ds: dire, diagnostics, and discharge. Then, other patient care issues will fall into place.

Dire. The first priority always goes to patients who are acutely ill, for example, need to go to the intensive care unit.

Diagnostics. Next, focus on radiographic tests, consults, and procedures. The MRI example noted earlier is a case in point. Getting an order placed early in the morning may yield a result by noon; if not, the "read" may roll to the next day. Learners should be encouraged to call the requested procedure or consultation team instead of just writing an order. Merely writing the order will mix that order in with all of the others written during the morning.

Subspecialty consultation services usually round in the mid-afternoon. The team should be coached to call for consults early in the morning to allow the consulting resident or fellow to see the patient so that he can be addressed during their rounds. As with radiology diagnostic tests, if the consult is prepared in time for the afternoon rounds, an answer will be available for which a second action for that day can be made. Waiting until the afternoon will force the consultation to be rolled over to the next day's rounds for discussion.

Discharge. Social workers, nurses, and the patient's family need time to plan. Emphasize to the team that the fewer the patients in the hospital, the fewer the small, distracting calls the team will receive during the day. An understandable concern is whether a discharge plan should be initiated before the attending sees the patient. Discharges, regardless of when the plan is initiated, are unlikely before attending rounds. It is easier to call off a discharge during attending rounds than it is to start a discharge process after attending rounds.

Beyond the Three D's
Orders. The sooner orders are written, the sooner they are executed. Because most services will be rounding in the morning, expect that the nurses will be flooded with orders at noon. If the team's orders are placed by 9 a.m., they are likely to be executed that morning.

Procedures. Procedures, such as paracentesis or central line insertion, should be performed later in the day, largely because the team will not want to have important tasks immediately after a procedure. If the procedure goes awry, they will not want to be under pressure to finish prematurely (a safety issue), or to have to put off the next task because the procedure went long. Learners should be coached on not wasting time for procedure trays. If they anticipate a procedure, they should write the order "please bring the lumbar puncture tray to the patient's bedside" early in the day.

Family Conferences. These should be scheduled later in the day. They can become very time intensive, and the learner does not want to be in a position of having to cut a family conference short because another task needs to get done. However, she also does not want to have to cancel the next commitment because the family conference went long. The best solution, therefore, is to plan for family conferences in the afternoon, and allow for an appropriate amount of time.

Progress Notes. Writing notes can be delayed until later in the day. It is important to emphasize to learners that "playing the game is more important that talking about it." Progress notes can take a good amount of time. The highly active morning hours are better spent on other tasks. Moreover, the data to complete a well-done progress note are unlikely to be available in the morning anyway. Notwithstanding the pressure to "get the note in the chart before the attending comes around," in fact the progress note is most important to the night-float physician trying to maintain continuity of care. That physician will need that note from the end of the day, providing all of that day's data and decisions.

Sketch Out the Day

Once team members understand that different tasks are better suited for different times in the day, team members should be instructed to think through their day while heading to work. This will offset the mental preparation that usually eats up the first 30 minutes at work. It is also the time to mentally assemble the list for the day. Once at work, the team should be instructed to take 5 minutes to sketch the day.

> *"Paul, here is what I want you to do. I want you to start the day by anticipating what needs to be done, and how the day might play out. Start with a 3 × 5 card and divide it down the middle with a vertical line. The left column is the morning, and the right is the afternoon. Then draw three horizontal lines. This will give you four rows, one for each hour in the morning and the afternoon. Remember that tasks are like a gas, not a solid: they will expand to fit the time/space allotted to them. Assign each task an expected amount of time. You will be inaccurate with this at first, but this is how you will learn how much each task requires. Take note of tasks that you underestimated... Plan accordingly next time."*

> *Paul nods.*

> *Phaedrus continues: "And Paul, beware of the easy tasks. It is not time-efficient to do all of the easy tasks first. There are a hundred easy tasks, and doing one leads to another. The task is easy for a reason: Anyone can do it. Given enough time, a percentage of these will be done by someone else."*

Team-Based Consolidation of Tasks

Efficiency is lost when people get overwhelmed. The team should be encouraged to work as a team in assigning tasks because this will prevent duplication of efforts, encourage teamwork, and ensure that no one person becomes paralyzed by being overwhelmed. The team leader (the resident) should be instructed to ensure that each set of rounds (resident rounds and attending rounds) ends with the team coming together to create a to-do list. Each item on the list should be specifically assigned to one person at a time on the team such that there is no ambiguity about responsibility. Assignments should be made according to ability. This will ensure that there is no duplication of effort, and it will allow the team leader to identify learners who are having a difficult time completing tasks. Further, this method will decrease fragmentation and enable consolidation of tasks (for example, one person to check on the radiograph reports), instead of multiple team members wasting time as they individually trek down to the radiology reading room. For this method to work, the team leader must establish a rally point and time such that each team member can report on what was and was not completed, and the results of the tasks that might be needed by other team members (for example, the intern might need the radiology report collected by the student).

Fragmentation

Fragmentation is the act of doing one part of one task and then another part of another task, and so forth. This is a huge risk to efficiency on the wards, and a huge temptation: The incessant demands of multiple people on the wards will pull team members in multiple directions. Attendings can mitigate this risk by anticipating that fragmentation will be the default unless they prepare their learners to overcome it. Teaching prioritization is the first step, but it is equally important that the attending emphasize to the team the importance of completing one task, at least to its natural stopping point, before proceeding to the next task. For example, a resident should be trained to complete the current task before answering the pager (unless it is the code pager), lest the page request distract him to another task. The risk of fragmentation of space should also be taught: for example, the team should complete the tasks on the fifth floor ward before moving to the seventh floor ward.

❖ Teaching Data Organization

Medicine is not a game of checkers, where the player merely reacts to the opponent's play. It is a game of chess, where the player must see six or seven moves down the game before making a move. The internist has to anticipate not only the expected reaction from an intervention (for example, that the angiotensin-converting enzyme inhibitor will improve cardiac function) but also all of the potential consequences (the blood pressure may drop, there might be a drug–drug interaction, the creatinine might increase) and the order in which they will appear. To do this effectively requires seeing trends because trends in data enable predicting the future much better than a single data point does.

The attending should anticipate, however, that most novice physicians will not understand this principle of internal medicine, and the way in which they organize their patients' data will reflect that. Thus, the attending will probably have to teach learners how to organize their patient data so they can see trends in their patient's progress (for example, the slow but steady drop in hemoglobin). In doing so, the coach has the opportunity to ensure that they learn this important lesson of internal medicine. The coach can also ensure that the manner in which the team organizes patient data enables them to make good decisions by predicting where the patient's condition will be in time.

Finally, the method by which learners organize and store their data must ensure that the integrity of the chart is not violated. This is less of an issue in systems with electronic medical records, but it still remains. Novice learners will enter the clinical wards with tunnel vision: *"It is me and my patient, and at the periphery, perhaps, the other members of the medicine team."* The learner may not see the other people who are equally a part of the patient's care team (nurses, social workers, technicians, other physicians). Even if he does, he many not realize how important the medical chart is as a touchstone for other team members plans.

The following dialogue captures the essential principles of instructing learners in data organization.

"Paul, that was a great presentation, but I noticed that you are presenting off of your progress note from yesterday."

"Yes, I'm sorry, Dr. Phaedrus, I haven't had a chance to complete my progress note for today."

"I'm not so worried about that, Paul. There will be time to do that, and you know my feeling—I would rather have you actively caring for patients early in the day as opposed to just writing about it." Phaedrus pauses. *"Paul, how are you keeping track of your patient's data?"*

"Well, I guess I just use the progress note."

"Hmm ... let me talk you through this, Paul, and I'll make it quick. First the expectation, and then I'll give you the rationale for it. Hopefully I'll be able to persuade you that the method I'm going to suggest might be a better plan for your patients.

"First, I want you to come up with a method that doesn't rely on taking things out of the chart. Once we get our electronic medical record, this will be less of an issue, but for now, remember that there are multiple nonphysicians—and other physicians—who are a part of the team caring for this patient. They need to know what our plans are to coordinate with their own."

"Okay," Paul responds.

"But there's another reason that we need to get you a method other than using the progress note. The progress notes allows you to see only what has happened in the past 24 hours. One point in time. We need a method, Paul, that allows you to see the trends in a patient's data. For example, if the patient's hematocrit is 28% today, well, that might not be that big of a deal if it was 28% for the past 2 days. But if it was 38% yesterday, then that's a very big deal. The same would go for a patient's blood pressure, creatinine ... in fact, pretty much any laboratory value. And there are two important points about internal medicine that you need to know, Paul. First, we care less about where a value is than we care about where it is going. If we have a data organization method that allows us to see the trend over the past few days, then we are in a much better position to predict where it will go next—you know, will it continue to improve, or is it continuing to worsen? The second lesson in internal medicine, Paul is this. Calculus."

"Calculus?"

"Yes, calculus—DP/DT. It is the rate of change over time, and not the change itself, that is risky to internal medicine patients. Some patients will come in with a blood pressure of 180 over 100, and they'll look fine because they have been at that blood pressure for some time now. We still need to treat it, but we have some time to do so. Other patients will come in with a blood pressure of 170 over 90, a blood pressure less than the first patients', but these patients will be having headaches and chest pain because their blood pressure yesterday was 120 over 70. As I said, it is the rate by which a variable changes that is important, not necessarily the change itself. And it is the sudden change of any variable that kills

patients, because the body cannot accommodate and compensate for the change. But to see that, Paul, you have to be able to see trends."

"I can see that. I guess I hadn't thought of it that way."

"That's okay, as long as you see it now. What I'm going to suggest is that you get a patient-tracking card. Or you can make your own—something that allows you to 'flow out' the laboratory findings and vital signs from day to day. The other advantage to this method, Paul, is that it will keep you disciplined. Just like in sports, big let-downs come when people get tired and cut corners. This method will force you to fill in the squares each day, reminding you to check the vital signs or a laboratory value that you forgot to check.

"And on the other side of that card, you can write a few details of the patient's history, though I want you to move toward the goal of being able to memorize your patient's stories. At any point as you walk through the halls, I want you to be able to catch one of the consultants that we need and present the patient's story. Perhaps without all of the details, but I want you to be able to present the story."

"For all of my patients?" asks Paul. "That seems impossible."

"It seems impossible, but eventually you will be able to do it. In a reverse fashion, if you have set an expectation to memorize your patients' stories, it will force you to listen intently as you take the history, and that will make you a much better physician. Moni, am I correct?"

Moni reaffirms the expectation: "You are correct. I thought it would be impossible, too, but as a resident, it's pretty much what I do now."

"She's a good role model, Paul, and we are both going to help you with that goal. The card will allow you to record the details that are unreasonable to expect that you could remember, including the patient's medications and doses, social history, other diagnoses, et cetera. There might also be room on the card to construct a to-do list of things that need to get done, and a list of his 'solvency issues' to keep us focused day-to-day in making sure we are addressing the issues that stand between him and discharge.

"Since the card will always be with you, it will allow you to be portable with the patient's details, able to talk about the patient to whomever needs to know for his care—radiology, a social worker, a consultant, or whomever—without having to go back and get the chart."

"Okay, I'll work on that."

Phaedrus hands him one of the cards he uses to track the data, modeling the behavior (Figure 5-1). *"Here, Paul, take this home and look at it. It's what I use. You don't have to use this method— you can use your own provided that it accomplishes the principles."*

❖ Teaching Interpersonal Skills

One of the unique challenges of teaching on the inpatient wards is the complexity and intensity of interpersonal interactions. However, this is also an opportunity for clinical coaches to empower their teams to develop life-long skills that are effective in interaction with the multiple personalities on the wards. The hospital wards provide an "interpersonal skills laboratory" where interventions can be taught and quickly evaluated.

Unfortunately, there is no shortage of interpersonal skills "opportunities" on the wards, and part of the attending's role will be to simultaneously smooth over these confrontations and teach learners better approaches to interpersonal skills to prevent these situations in the future.

Effectiveness

Instruction of interpersonal skills begins with an unvarnished acknowledgment of reality. Interpersonal relationships on the wards are complex: Everyone has an ego, everyone is insecure.

Dealing with people on the wards can be difficult, especially if the student forgets the first rule of interpersonal skills: *"This isn't about you. It's about your patients."* The best care for present and future patients comes when the student focuses not on determining who was right and who was wrong but instead on strategies of being effective.

"Phaedrus, I need to tell you about a nurse on 5 West." Stef looks indignant.

Phaedrus laughs. "Okay, what happened?"

"It was completely inappropriate ... I wrote the order for an EKG and he told me had 'too much to do,' and that I should just do it myself." Stef pauses and shakes his head. "Can you believe that?"

Name				#		Name				#
History				Meds: 1. 2. 3. 4. 5. 6. 7. 8.		History				Meds: 1. 2. 3. 4. 5. 6. 7. 8.
PMH:				9. 10. 11. 12. 13.		PMH:				9. 10. 11. 12. 13.

All:_____ ETOH:_____/d Tob_____pk/yrs Drugs_____ All:_____ ETOH:_____/d Tob_____pk/yrs Drugs_____

Physical Exam

Problems/Assessment
1)_____ 2)_____ 3)_____ 4)_____ 5)_____
*
*
*
*
*

Day 1	Day 2	Day 3
Day 4	Day 5	Day 6

Physical Exam

Problems/Assessment
1)_____ 2)_____ 3)_____ 4)_____ 5)_____
*
*
*
*
*

Day 1	Day 2	Day 3
Day 4	Day 5	Day 6

Date						
BP						Echo:_____ EF%
Pulse						
T max						
RR						
Sat %						
Weight						Cath:_____ LAD
						_____ RCA
HCT						_____ Circ.
WBC						
PLT						CT:
PT						
PTT						
Na^+						
K^+						
Cl^-						
$HCO3^-$						
BUN						
Creat						
Gluc						
Trop						
AST						
ALT						
Alk. P						
T. bili						
UA						
Cultures						

Date						
BP						Echo:_____ EF%
Pulse						
T max						
RR						
Sat %						
Weight						Cath:_____ LAD
						_____ RCA
HCT						_____ Circ.
WBC						
PLT						CT:
PT						
PTT						
Na^+						
K^+						
Cl^-						
$HCO3^-$						
BUN						
Creat						
Gluc						
Trop						
AST						
ALT						
Alk. P						
T. bili						
UA						
Cultures						

Figure 5-1 Sample data cards.

"Did the patient get the EKG?"

"Well, eventually the nurse did it—like 30 minutes later. There was no way I was going to do that, and I told him as much. Then he threatened to call you and my program director, and then I threatened to write him up. People like that shouldn't work here."

"Well, Stef, you might be right. But let me tell you what I know about people. Before I do, let me ask you … It sounds like you won the fight with that nurse, but was this effective in advancing your patient's care? I mean, it sounds like it took 30 minutes to get the EKG."

"No, it wasn't effective, he should have..."

Phaedrus interrupts. "No, I'm not asking about who was wrong. Your first assessment was probably right—I just want to know if it was effective or not."

"No, it wasn't effective." A sense of humility begins to come over Stef.

"So let me ask you, what matters more to you—being right and winning fights that end up with your program director being called, or being effective?"

"Being effective. I remember what you said, this isn't about me … it's about the patients."

"Well, said, Stef. So let me see if I can give you a better strategy for when this happens next time. First, remind yourself: Effectiveness begins by doing whatever it takes to reach your patient's goals. Start each day by identifying what you want to happen for your patient, and then appreciate that you do not care how your patient reaches these goals, as long as he reaches them. As long as your patient reaches his goals, you have succeeded." Phaedrus pauses for effect. "Next, Stef, recognize that the people who will help your patient reach his goals care mostly about how decisions/actions reflect upon them. That's just human nature. They care nothing about your opinions. If you want their help, you have to invest them in accomplishing your patient's goals."

"But how do I do that if they don't care about my opinions?"

"Good question, and that's the holy grail of winning friends and influencing people. We'll get to that in a moment. But now I'm going to draw you a picture. There are three players here: the per-

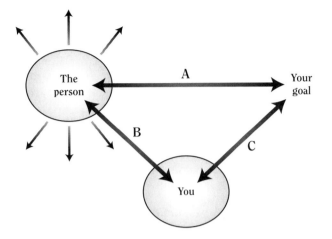

Figure 5-2 Motivating other people to join in your goal. A = Integrating the other person's motivations to your goal (most effective); B = focusing on the other person only, ignoring your goal (less effective); C = focusing on your goal only, ignoring the other person's motivations (least effective).

son whose help you need, you, and your patient's goals."
Phaedrus sketches out a diagram (Figure 5-2) *as he speaks. "If*
you focus only on your patient's goals, point C here, you exclude
the person whose help you need. Because that person will see
nothing in it for him, he is unlikely to move along line A. That's
what happened to you, Stef. You focused only on the EKG. Your
focus didn't include the nurse at all. By the way, what was his
name?"

"I forget."

"Hmmm, that might be the problem." Phaedrus pauses. "So
option two, if you focus only on the person whose help you need—
point B—your focus will be diverted away from your patient's
goals. You may have a great talk about football, but your patient
will suffer.

"And then there is the third option." Phaedrus points to point A.
"The only way to be effective is to get the person whose help you
need to focus on your patient's goals. He will move along line A
only if he has reason to do so."

"But again, how do I get him to want to do the EKG?"

"Well, now you are asking the right questions. But first, Stef, I
promised to be honest with you. So here's the honest truth. For

the most part, people are about themselves. This is not to say that they do not want to help other people. They do. But their interest is in how they are involved in helping people and how it reflects on them. Helping your cause without being recognized is not interesting to them."

"Okay, but again, how do I get the task to reflect on them?"

"Second lesson, people have values in life; not everyone has the same values. You will respect the values that correspond to your own; you will disrespect those that do not. And in the grand scheme, there is no proof that your values are any more impor-tant than anyone else's. What you respect and disrespect does not matter when it comes to being effective, Stef. Your interest in the other person's values is only that you can understand what will appeal to him as you try to get him moving in the direction of your patient's goals."

"So how do I figure out his values?"

"The second correct question in a row, Stef! Well done. Life's about asking the right questions." Phaedrus extends his hand for a handshake. "Figuring out his values is not easy because values that are not socially noble will not be made overt. For example, if the nurse values getting out of the hospital as soon as possible to spend time with his family, I doubt he will tell you that outright— because as a value it is not as flattering as self-sacrifice for the welfare of the patient." Phaedrus pauses. Stef is in suspense.

"So here's the trick, Stef. Listen carefully to casual conversations and you will determine values. Get to know people, become gen-uinely interested in them as people. Find out what they respect in others. This is what they respect the most in themselves. Ask them whom they most respect in the hospital. Ask them why—this is whom they want to be. Ask him what he likes about his job—this is what he values. Ask him why he chose to be a nurse—these are the values that are shaping the decisions in his life."

"So I'm supposed to ask him all of that while I'm asking for the EKG?"

"No, Stef. By then, it's too late. All you can do at that point is plead for his help. All of this starts long ago, and that has to be your strategy going forward. Become genuinely interested in peo-ple around you. Think about what motivates them, think about

what they value." Phaedrus pauses. "This part is important, Stef. Do not judge their values. Judge people based on their own standards. There is nothing to say that your values are any better than theirs. Just accept it for what it is, and know that when it comes time for the task that you need done, your goal will be to coach the request in the other person's values."

"I think I get that." Stef replies. "But what do you mean by couching the request in the person's values?"

"Well, Stef, let me give you an example. Let's say the nurse values efficiency. He just hates how people sit around on the ward waiting for discharge. You might phrase the request as "Rob, I know you are very busy, but I need your help. If I can just get this EKG for Mr. Phillips, I can get him ready for discharge."

"Ah, I see. So you are working his values into the request."

"Indeed, Stef. Appeal to the person as a person, and nothing says that like appealing to his values.

"That's fantastic. Any other tips?"

"Sure ... here're a few. Always interpret people in the context of their environment. Merely recognizing the pressures put on the person as part of your request will increase the probability that he will buy in to getting your patient's goals accomplished.

"Next, Stef, recognize that your request adds to the person's taxing environment. When you make a request, you are adding something to the person's plate, which is already full. Where possible, try to take something off the plate. If you can't do that, at least offer to make the addition small. Do as much of the task as you can, then ask for help with only the part that you cannot do alone."

"So how could I have done it better?"

"Well, you could have tried this: 'Rob, I know you are very busy— the wards are crazy right now, and I can see you're taxed. But I need your help. If I can just get this EKG for Mr. Phillips, I can get him ready for discharge. I can get the machine in there if you can help me with the leads and the print out.'"

Diffusing Conflicts

The clinical wards are full of tired, stressed, and often frustrated people. Many times, it is not the resident who initiates an interpersonal crisis, it's someone else. The resident makes it worse, however, by inappropriately responding to it. Conflicts on the wards are opportunities to teach residents how to diffuse conflict.

The first step begins with teaching residents that the first rule of arguments is that *both people are partially correct, and partially incorrect*. If the other person thought that the resident was overwhelmingly right, he wouldn't have engaged in the argument. There is probably a hole in the resident's case somewhere, and she is about to find out where. The focus must not be on pointing out how *"I am right and you are wrong"* but instead on *"Where is he right, and where am I wrong?"* Every argument is a warning that the resident needs to step back and carefully examine her position.

The second step is teaching residents the second rule of arguments: *Even if you win, you lose*. The other person thinks she is right, and she will have invested herself in her position. Her position and ego have become one. The only way to win the argument is to destroy her position, which also destroys her ego. This, in turn, will destroy her motivation to help you. A nurse that huffs away from the nursing station because of an argument (even if the resident is right) is still walking away from the nursing station. She cannot help you; you remain alone with your patient.

> *"Dr. Phaedrus, I just had it out with the surgery attending!" Moni exclaims. "They are just refusing to take care of Mrs. Halstead. I'm sure you'll hear about it because there was a lot of yelling."*

> *"Hmm ... lots of yelling, huh? That doesn't sound good." Phaedrus smiles.*

> *"It's not funny. These surgeons only care about themselves, and I told him as much. He's not professional."*

> *"Do you feel alone, Moni?"*

> *"Dr. Phaedrus, I mean it. This was completely inappropriate."*

> *"Okay." Phaedrus returns to a serious demeanor. "I do agree with you. Whenever two physicians are yelling at teach other, it is completely inappropriate. Can you imaging what Mrs. Halstead thinks?"*

> *"Well, I hadn't thought of that."*

"Listen, I don't mean to break you down over this. It's unfortunate that it happened, and I'm sorry that it happened to you. Perhaps I can give you a method for resolving conflicts in the future."

"That would be great," replies Moni.

"Okay, Moni. First rule. Whenever you get into an argument, it's because the other person thinks that he is right. If you were overwhelming right, there would be no argument. Put it this way, if Mrs. Halstead had amputated her arm and blood was squirting everywhere, would there be an argument about going to the OR?"

"No, definitely not."

"Indeed. So the first rule in an argument: You are both partially correct. You task is not to be right—your task is to either figure out where you are wrong or to figure out where the miscommunication occurred such that the other person believes he is right."

"How do I do that?" asks Moni.

"In a minute … but first, the second rule of arguments. Even if you win, you lose. Take the argument today. I'm guessing, for as smart as you are, you were able to clearly establish why Mrs. Halstead needs to go to surgery. And for the record, I agree with you, and I'll talk with the surgeons." Phaedrus pauses. "But I'm also guessing that as we sit here right now, as persuasive as you were in the argument, that Mrs. Halstead is not going to surgery right now."

"Well, you are right. The surgeon just huffed away after the argument."

"Indeed. Here's what happened, Moni. The surgeon had a position, and he believed he was correct. He integrated that position into his persona. So when you started attacking the position, you were actually attacking him. When it was all said and done, there was no way that he was going to help someone who had just attacked him."

"Yeah, I guess I didn't see that. I did refer to him as 'you' and 'your' position' a lot."

"Exactly, and that's one of the cardinal 'no-no's' in conflict. Never use the word 'you' or 'your.' You will only make the bond between the person and the position tighter.

"So here's your strategy. Try it out and see if it works. If it doesn't, then feel free to do something else. First, Moni, this isn't about you. It's about the patient, and that's just business. You want to do whatever needs to be done, regardless of who is right, to do the right thing by your patient. So the first step is to eliminate all emotion. Remember, anger is just fear turned inward, and you have nothing to fear. You may care deeply about this, but emotion will not make you effective. If an argument can be won, it is rational thought that will convince the other person of your position. Emotion is the antithesis of rational thought. A conflict is like a small fire: Any emotion is gasoline for the fire. Even an eyebrow or a stare can ignite a fire that will consume you both. Your first step is to control yourself."

"Okay. No emotion."

"Second, stand up straight with your arms to the side. Crossing your arms says you are recalcitrant to their ideas. Gesturing wildly is threatening. Arms at your side ... and then talk quietly in one tone of voice." Phaedrus pauses. *"But most important, Moni, your strategy is just to listen to their position. Do not interrupt. Do not rebut. Do not think about what you are going to say next. There will come a time for you to talk. No one is going to invest energy in a rant and then be denied a rebuttal. So let the other person burn himself out in his position. Remember that I told you that you were both partially correct and partially incorrect?"* Moni nods. *"So, there is a hole in his position somewhere; let him wander around in his talking until he is aware of it. And remember, too, that there is probably a hole in your position. If there is, it is because you have bad or incomplete information, and your best chance of figuring out where you are wrong is to listen to his position. This is your chance to learn this information before putting your foot in your mouth."*

"Yeah, I guess I didn't do that. I was just thinking about what I wanted to say next."

"Okay, as you listen to his position, I want you to be thinking in two tracks, thinking about two things at once. First, what is he saying? Second, what is prompting him to say this? Consider that there may be something else in his environment that is motivating him to engage in this, like a recent patient death or a fight with his significant other. If this is the case, you cannot win whatever you say: There is nothing you can say about Mrs. Halstead

going to surgery that will bring back that last patient who died, or resolve the fight with the significant other. This second track I want you to keep to yourself—never insinuate that this argument is a product of something else. Saying, 'I know you are having a hard time with your girlfriend' will explode the situation."

Moni laughs. "Okay, I get the point. I need to think about the person as much as the argument."

"Exactly, now let's say he has had his say, and it's your turn to talk. This is what you do: Look for areas of agreement. Point these out first. End by saying, 'So it appears that the only thing on which we differ is x. But we do agree on a, b, and c.' Keep emphasizing areas of agreement."

"Well, we do agree that she has a small bowel obstruction and that this isn't getting better. We just disagreed on whether she should go to surgery or not."

"Now you are getting it. Once you shift the argument away from 'me versus you' and toward 'us'—and what are you are both going to do to fix this small bowel obstruction—you are 90% there.

"And you can get to the last 10% by doing two things. First, disarm your opponent by admitting your mistakes and that you are frequently wrong because you do not have all of the data. Make it clear that truth matters to you more than being right. And then, two … Give him a way out. I'm guessing that he had not seen the CT we ordered early this morning. Am I right?"

"Exactly right, and I brought that up toward the end."

"And right now, Moni, he's probably in radiology looking at that CT. And right now, he's probably realizing that you were right. But he's not calling you right now because you pinned him into a corner, and he's fighting to get out." Phaedrus pauses. "Know this about people, Moni. People do not want to change their minds. They believe they are right, and they have married their position with their ego. If you can figure out a way to allow them the opportunity to divorce this association by adopting a new position—that is, if you could have given him a way out of the argument—Mrs. Halstead would be on her way to surgery right now. In fact, let's try this. Do you have the surgeon's number?"

"Sure, here it is," Moni replies.

Phaedrus dials the phone and waits. "Stone, this is Phaedrus, the attending on medicine. Listen, I want to apologize to you for my lack of communication. Regarding Mrs. Halstead, we obtained a CT scan this morning, and we didn't let you know about it." There is a pause as Stone speaks, loudly at first, and then tapers to a normal voice. Phaedrus continues: "You are absolutely right, and I have already spoken with her about it." Phaedrus winks at Moni. "In any event, I just want to call and apologize because we didn't let you know about the new CT scan, and I know that you would have liked to have had that before rounding on her today."

Phaedrus pauses as Stone speaks. "No, I haven't seen it yet … is that right?! Potentially a perforation?" Phaedrus pauses again. "Well, we're fine with her going to surgery, especially if you think it's the right thing to do." Another pause. "Okay, thanks, Stone. Always a pleasure. I'll see ya."

"I can't believe it. She's going to surgery?!"

"Moni, we all knew she had to go to surgery. She has a perforated bowel." Phaedrus pauses. "Your error was not in the assessment— your error was in not being effective. You got caught up in right and wrong versus being effective. The effective move, especially when you are right, is to give the other person an emotionally neutral way out of being wrong."

"So that's why you apologized about not telling about the CT?"

"Yes, and I know what you are thinking. You're thinking, 'Well, it's his responsibility to read the CT,' aren't you?" Moni smiles sheepishly. "But the issue is not 'his responsibility.' The issue is being effective for your patients. So Moni, lessons learned. Next time, stand still with your hands and your side, truly listen to the other person, think about him as much as you are about his argument, look for areas of agreement and emphasize those, if you are wrong, then admit it and go on. And if you are right, look for an emotionally neutral way of allowing the other person out of the corner."

"This is very helpful, Phaedrus. You're not going to put that on my evaluation, are you?"

"I'm your coach, Moni, not your scorekeeper. And besides, you just received my evaluation. I think we'll let this one go."

Moni smiles. "Okay, well, there is an issue with Mr. Johnson in the ER."

❖ Teaching Learners to Read

There is much to learn in medicine, and the busy wards hardly provide sufficient time. The student has to read. And while the teacher, in the traditional sense, has little accountability for the student's reading, the coach does. If the clinical coach does not motivate the student to read and to take stewardship over how she reads, performance will suffer in the long run. Several coaching strategies will encourage a student to not only read regularly but also smartly.

The simple admonishment "You should read more" is not effective. It is not as if there is a student out there who is confused about "reading more" versus "reading less."

Recognize that *students have developed bad reading strategies. Correct those strategies.*

In the preclinical years, the student was assigned a fixed amount of knowledge to learn (for example, the lecture material for the biochemistry course). Memorization and short-term memory techniques were successful because the knowledge set was finite, and the goal was to regurgitate the knowledge for the final exam. There was no need to apply the knowledge, nor was there a need to integrate the knowledge into other courses. To succeed in *clinical* rotations, however, the student has to switch paradigms. The coach should emphasize that studying for clinical medicine is about mastering the broad strokes of diseases, comparing and contrasting them to other diseases, and visualizing application of the knowledge on the wards.

Inspire Students to Develop the Habit of Reading

Children are encouraged to save not because a few pennies in the bank will amount to much money but because it develops the habit of saving. Later in life, the habit of saving equates to vast sums of money for retirement. So it is with reading. The knowledge the student acquires now will be trivial compared to what she will learn over a lifetime. The coach can do this simply by asking each day, *"Paul, what did you read last night?"* and by role-modeling the behavior by saying each day, *"You know what I read last night?"*

Get Students to Stop Binge-Reading

Reading is like training for a sport. The student cannot put off lifting weights and running until the night before a big game. The student has to know that the brain can assimilate only so much long-term knowledge per study session. Once it has reached this limit, the rest pours into short-term memory and will quickly fade. Long-term memory is the student's goal. To achieve this goal, he has to *read something every day*. The coach should make it clear: *"Paul, listen, I don't care how much you read each day. I just care that you read something each day. The volume does not matter. Even if it is one sentence from one paragraph, do not let the day go by without reading something.*" There is power in time: one sentence will come easy, which facilitates one paragraph, and then one article per day.

Teach Students to Read About Diseases in the Same Way They Watch Movies
The student should be trained to see each disease as its own movie. It has a cast of characters (that is, symptoms or signs), a plot (disease progression, management), and a conclusion (outcomes or prognosis). We cannot understand the movie unless we know each of these. The student should be instructed that once he starts reading about a disease, he should not move to the next disease until he understands these three components.

Ensure the Student Does Not Become Obsessed
The student's predilection will be to stay with one topic that he knows well, reading about anemia over and over. There is comfort there, and there is discomfort in discovering what he doesn't know in other topics. The student must be instructed to learn the basics of the disease (see above), and then move on to the next disease. Encourage the student to be guided by a textbook, and to use the table of contents to keep him moving from topic to topic. Because the table of contents will be organized by similar diseases, this will juxtapose diseases that have similar presentations (such as lupus vs. rheumatoid arthritis), allowing the student to compare and contrast diseases as he reads. This is the goal to enable the phase 4 clinical reasoning of assigning probabilities for the differential diagnosis (see chapter 4 of this book). It is as important for the student to know why a patient's symptoms are *not* lupus as it is to know why they are rheumatoid arthritis.

Teach Students to First Build a Foundation and Then Add to It
The attending should anticipate that the student's predilection in reading will be to master absolutely every detail about a topic before moving on to another topic. This is how he was trained to read in the preclinical years: The difference between an "A" and an "B" was in the details. The problem is that he will lose perspective and will not be able to compare and contrast diseases. The following dialogue describes the "skeleton, flesh, and skin book" approach to reading.

> *"Paul, what textbooks are in your personal library? That is, what are you reading?"*
>
> *"Well, I just read* Harrison's.*"*

"Okay, that's a pretty good book. But let me give you this approach. It might make it easier to cover a broader landscape in medicine. There are three types of books: skeleton books, flesh books, and skin books.

"A skeleton book has short chapters that quickly outline a disease. These books are like Cliff's Notes*: They cannot substitute for the real book, but they will keep the topic in perspective so that you do not lose sight of the forest for the trees as you start the flesh book chapter.*

"Flesh books have greater detail than a skeleton book, though not as much as a skin book, like Harrison's*. The chapters of flesh books are longer, but if you have read the corresponding skeleton book chapter, you will be able to navigate quickly through the details without getting bogged down.*

"Skin books have the details you need for presenting a topic—like Harrison's*—but the level of detail is too much. You'll get bogged down in reading about only one or two diseases without seeing how they compare to other diseases." Phaedrus pauses. "So, Paul, here is my reading strategy for you … try it out, and if it doesn't work, then you can try something else. Use your patients to guide your reading. As you see a patient with diabetes, for example, go home that night and read about diabetes. But always start with the skeleton book. These chapters are short, so it should take only 5 minutes to do so. Then, if you have time to continue reading, read the corresponding chapter in the flesh book."*

"Why not just read the flesh book?"

"Because you'll lose perspective. The skeleton book will give you the broad strokes so that you at least cover all the critical components of the disease—you know, the movie. This will then allow you to have the framework on which to hang the details that come from the flesh book. In the margins of both, Paul, I want you to write something about the patient you saw: her name, what she looked like, et cetera. Later, when you come back to the topic, having forgotten a lot of it (which is natural, by the way), the patient's face will bring all of the details back. You'll remember the patient."

Phaedrus pauses to think. "And the other reason this is a useful strategy, Paul, is that it will keep you focused on real prevalence.

The prevalence on the wards will match the prevalence of your reading."

"What if I want to read on my own? You know, like on a Saturday or something like that?"

"That's an excellent habit, Paul. On those days, when you have time to read even more, follow this strategy. Start by reading in the same way you would see a patient. Start with a symptom, not a disease. For example, start with chest pain, and then visualize yourself seeing a patient with chest pain. This part is very important, Paul. Always visualize yourself using the data as you acquire it. Make the dream as glorious as you like: from a humble contribution to a discussion on rounds, to the key contribution in saving a patient's life. If you can't visualize yourself using the information, then you are probably reading the wrong stuff. Move on to something else.

"Okay, so start with the symptom, visualize yourself taking care of the patient with that symptom, and then list the diagnoses that could cause this symptom. Just like we do in real life, Paul. Make a differential diagnosis. Then turn to your skeleton book and read about each of those diagnoses. Compare and contrast them, see what historical, examination, and laboratory data distinguish one from the other. And then think about your method of approaching the problem."

"Where do I get the method?"

"Right here, Paul. And that's how the wards interface with your reading. First, use what you see here to determine what you will read each night. And second, use the methods of approaching problem that you learn here from our team to organize your vision as you read about a symptom."

"That's a pretty good approach."

Teach Students How to Mitigate Skills Decline
As noted in chapter 2, all knowledge fades; skills decline, which is a natural feature of learning. The student's reading strategy should have a method whereby he can regenerate knowledge later. There are many strategies for coaching this; the following dialogue offers one such strategy.

"One last thing, Paul. I want you to buy a blank book. Number the pages ... numbering every other page is sufficient. And then I want you to assign a general topic to every 10 pages. So for example,

cardiology for the first 10 pages, endocrinology for the next 10 pages, et cetera. Then, I want you to buy several 3 × 5 cards and put them in your pocket with you on the wards. Or you can buy a moleskin or something like that."

"Okay, some cards and a blank book," Paul repeats.

"Here's the gig, Paul. You are going to hear many lectures on the same topic. Some of these talks will speak to you, some will not. When you find a talk, or a chapter or an article, that really speaks to you, really makes sense to you, record these notes in your blank book so that when you have forgotten the chapter or the talk, you can quickly come back to and regenerate in 2 minutes what it took you 2 hours to initially learn."

"So should I bring the book to rounds?"

"No, no, no. When you go to write in the book, I want you to synthesize the data into a format where you can understand it. Rounds are too fast for writing and synthesizing. As you hear something in our discussions on rounds that makes particular sense to you, write it down on one of the cards. When you get home, reflect on what you have learned, and then neatly transcribe it. Don't be compulsive about including every detail on the topic. Focus on the broad outline and only those things that really made sense to you. As you read on the side, do the same for articles or chapters.

"Do not transcribe every detail, but instead focus on the broad outline of the topic and the details that make sense of the topic. As you transcribe, focus on your method for approaching the problem. As you transcribe the data, visualize yourself using the method to take care of a patient. It is not necessary to have a perfect table of contents. As long as you can flip through your book and find the page on 'thyroid disease,' you are okay. The art of this method, Paul, is in not being compulsive. Record only the big points, and only those that make sense to you."

"Thanks, Dr. Phaedrus. Believe it or not, no one has ever told me how to read before."

"I believe it, Paul," responds Phaedrus.

❖ Remediating Oral Case Presentations

Learning on the clinical wards hinges on the premise that learners will collect information, process that information, make decisions, and then receive guidance from their supervising physician on how to do this better (1, 2). But all of this hinges on the ability of the two parties, the learner and the attending, to communicate, and the ability of the attending to precisely identify what elements of the student's clinical performance needs to be improved. For this reason, and because the fast pace of the clinical wards prevents directly observing each learner performing each component of clinical medicine, the spoken case presentation is a vital component of assessing and teaching clinical reasoning. As noted in chapter 3 of this book, listening to learners present on rounds, taken in aggregate, is a major component of the attending's day. Time-efficient presentations allow more time for teaching. On the other hand, disorganized presentations sap valuable teaching time, and everyone's energy. The attending should expect that some oral presentations are going to be just terrible. You know it when you see it, but how do you fix it?

First, the structure of the oral presentation should be based on the Bayesian method of clinical reasoning (see chapter 4 of this book), with a paragraph one (time course and chief complaint); paragraph two (answers to the questions the student asked to evaluate her differential diagnosis); the past medical, social, and family history; and, finally, the physical examination and laboratory and study data. The assessment and plan should finish the presentation. This serves three purposes: 1) It consolidates the learner's mastery of the clinical reasoning method (each iteration of the history, admission note, and oral case presentation follows the same clinical reasoning method); 2) it allows the attending physician to assess the student's clinical reasoning by identifying where deficits exist; and 3) it trains the student to present information in a fashion that allows the attending (and other members of the team) to formulate an accurate assessment of the patient's problem. By presenting the history first, the listener develops a differential diagnosis of his own, and then follows along as the order of the data presented parallels his clinical reasoning.

With this method, the spoken case presentation can therefore be a good surrogate measure for a student's clinical reasoning. As noted in chapter 3, however, the confounder is that the student may be suffering from weak presentation skills, masking his true clinical reasoning ability. These skills deficits are damaging in their own right because unless corrected, the student will not be able to communicate effectively with colleagues, diminishing collaborative team-based care.

Correcting a generic presentation (communication) deficit begins with identifying the major problem. A terrible presentation will probably have more than one deficit. The attending should select the major problem and focus on improving this problem first. Other problems should be disregarded; they can be corrected later.

The Deficit: Presentations That Are Too Long

A student should be able to present even the most complicated case within 5 minutes. Aside from wasting the team's time (thereby eroding into time that could have been spent teaching), the long presentation exceeds the audience's attention span. Even data that were presented are missed (during the audience's day dreams), resulting in a series of questions after the presentation that wastes even more time.

The Cause
The deficit results from one or more of the following causes: 1) The student fears not presenting all the patient data, 2) the student cannot prioritize information, or 3) there is too much unnecessary commentary throughout the presentation.

The Treatment
Begin by giving the student the "60% rule": *60% of the patient's data presented fluently is better than 100% presented nonfluently.* Remind students that it is not the act of speaking but the act of hearing that defines communication. Release him from the compulsion of having to include every detail.

Emphasize relevance. Remind the student that not all data contribute equally to understanding the patient's current admission and that he should become comfortable leaving out data that are not relevant. It is not sufficient, however, to tell a student, "Just present the relevant data." This command presumes that students understand what defines relevance; the fact that they do not is often the problem. Remind students that the definition of relevance is data that help the physician evaluate the differential diagnosis being considered. Data that are occasionally expendable include the review of systems; some past medical, social, or family history; and physical examination and laboratory data that do not help with assessing the differential diagnosis. To ensure that there is no confusion, emphasize that it is good to have these data in the admission note but that the oral presentation should focus on prioritized data, as in the following example:

"Paul, that's a fine presentation, but we need to hone it down. I want you to think of going on a vacation. You don't pack all of

your possessions to go on vacation, do you? You pack just what you need for the vacation—the essentials. Am I right?" Paul nods. "And when you to Hawaii, and you decide to take a day trip to go backpacking, you don't bring all of your luggage, do you? You pack just the very essentials—a change of clothes. Am I right?" Paul nods again.

"Well, see the patient's information, all details of his life, as the possessions in your house. See the information relevant to his illness as the luggage you packed on your vacation. That's the information that I want in your admission note. And see your oral case presentation as that day-pack—just the very essentials."

"I think I understand," Paul says.

"Okay, great. Here is what I want you to do. Look at your admission note. Now, in the margin, I want you to write down the differential diagnosis you considered. Now, go through the admission note and highlight the data that would help us evaluate the diagnoses on your list. I am going to allow you to choose up to 20 pieces of data from the history, physical examination, and the laboratory tests. Underline your top 20. Now, begin the presentation again, starting with the first line. But thereafter, Paul, you are allowed only to present the top 20 pieces of data."

Paul does as instructed. When he is finished, Moni notes, "Wow, that was pretty good."

"There you go, Paul," Phaedrus says. "That was a great presentation. I think you're getting it. And not a moment too soon. The airlines are charging a lot these days for the luggage you bring on board."

The Deficit: Use of Distracting Expressions
Presentation marred with frequent "uhs," "ums," and "likes" are so distracting that the audience loses concentration and communication is lost. These distractions also lengthen the presentation time.

The Cause
The student is using the fillers for one of two reasons: She is 1) having a difficult time thinking and talking simultaneously and uses the "uhs" and "ums" to think about what she wants to say next, or 2) she is concerned she will be interrupted during periods of silence.

The Treatment

Regardless of the pain associated with the student's presentation, the attending should not interrupt, or let others interrupt, a student's presentation, lest the student (or other learners) resort to using fillers to hold their place in the conversation. It is better to let the painful presentation continue until its end than to interrupt and allow the problem to perpetuate in future presentations.

Begin each presentation by telling the student that neither the attending nor anyone on the team will be allowed to interrupt the student until she is finished. The student should be told that presenting on rounds is not like her normal conversations. In normal conversation, when you stop talking, someone else starts. The presentation is much more like being on stage in a play. No one is going to interrupt you until you have finished your lines.

Remind the student about the "60% rule" (see above). The student is using the "uhs" and "ums" because she is afraid she has left something out.

Teach the student how to tell a story. Memorizing a set of facts is difficult, and the student is pausing to trying to recall the facts, filing these uncomfortable pauses with the distracting fillers. The attending should focus the intervention on teaching the student how to tell a story, which is a much easier way to link together a set of data, as one piece of data prompts the next.

"Paul, good presentation, but I want to coach you for a second. Is that all right?"

"Sure, Dr. Phaedrus. What can I do better?"

"I want to get rid of the 'uhs' and 'ums' that are littering your presentation—they are distracting your audience, and that's causing people to tune you out. You are using those to think about what you are going to say next, aren't you?"

Paul thinks for a moment and then nods.

"Okay, first, remember that 60% of the data presented fluently are better than 100% presented nonfluently. Next, I want you to think of this patient's presentation as a story, just like you were telling your best friend about it. Link everything together in time. For example, 'The chest pain first began 1 year ago. At that time, the patient was experiencing the pain only with vigorous activity. This changed about 3 months ago, when he noted that the chest pain was associated with rest. One week ago he began to experience pain daily, progressively increasing until today.'"

Teach the student how to be comfortable with pauses in the presentation.

"Paul, instead of using the 'uhs' and 'ums,' I want you to try this out. I'm going to have you do the presentation again. When you get to a point that you want to use the 'uh,' just stop and count to three. Just pause and let the silence rule. It will seem weird to you, but believe me, the silence is better than the 'uh.' The silence is like a rest note in music; it will highlight what you said last as people catch up with their writing, and it will add suspense to what you will say next."

Paul nods.

"Now, to make sure that you recognize when you are using the 'uhs' and 'ums', I am going to stop you every time you use one of them. And when I stop you, you will have a 5-second time-out before I will allow you to begin again."

Paul presents again. Although the presentation is choppy with the 3-second silences, it is overall much better. Phaedrus continues: "Okay, Paul. I want you to practice your presentations. As you do so, practice taking planned pauses between sentences. Begin by making yourself stop for 3 seconds after each sentence. Then progress to 2 seconds and then 1 second between sentences." Phaedrus pauses. "And in addition, I want you to take your admission note and highlight the most important parts of the presentation. When you get to one of these items, I want you to highlight its importance by taking a 2-second pause after you have said it. I want you to do so that you come to see 'silence' as a powerful tool in highlighting content, not just a way to get rid of these 'uhs' and 'ums.'"

The Deficit: Lack of Eye Contact or Boring Presentations

A presenter who does not maintain eye contact with the audience has a limited ability to engage the audience. As a result, she loses their attention, and communication is lost. The student should be taught that although the content of the presentation should be sufficient to maintain the audience's attention, it rarely is. People listen to people, not presentations. By engaging the audience using eye contact, the student increases the audience's interest in what she has to say.

The Cause

A primary reason for lack of eye contact is being uncomfortable in front of an audience. Any movement by the audience distracts the student's thought process. Other causes include dependence on index cards or notes, which is another manifestation of the fear of leaving something out.

The Treatment
Encourage the student to practice her presentations in a mirror. Looking someone in the eye is uncomfortable, and the student must become comfortable maintaining eye contact; the mirror is an easy place to practice this skill, but the student must be encouraged to stay focused on the reflection of her own eyes as she presents.

Ask the student to engage in a "note card taper," as explained in the following dialogue.

> *"Paul, I see that you are presenting off of your progress note. There's nothing especially wrong with that, except that you are losing your audience because we can't see you. So here's your challenge ... are you up for it?"*
>
> *Paul nods.*
>
> *"Good. So for your next presentation, I'm going to allow you to use two note cards. You can put whatever you want on the cards, and you can read directly from them. The presentation after that, I'm going to limit you to one note card. And then, Paul ... no more note cards. I want you to present to me, and I want to interact with you. While you are buried behind those note cards, I can't do that. So are you up for it?"*
>
> *"Sure, Dr. Phaedrus. I'll give it a try."*

The Deficit: Nervousness
The first few presentations of the rotation may reflect nervousness, which is understandable; but nervousness that persists after that point should prompt remediation. Symptoms include cracking or shaking of the voice, sweating profusely, or freezing in mid-sentence.

Likely Causes
The student may be afraid of failure or is suffering under the impostor syndrome: the sense that he is masquerading as a physician, that the audience knows much more than he does, and that they are waiting for him to make a mistake that will reveal himself.

The Treatment
Address the impostor syndrome head-on:

> *"Paul, let me tell you that it is true that we are likely to know more about diabetes than you do. We've been doing this much longer than you. But I have to tell you, it is very, very unlikely that we will*

know more about your patient than you do. With regard to your patient's history and condition, you are the expert. You are not expected to know everything about diabetes, so focus on your patient. Before you begin your presentation, tell yourself, 'No one knows more about my patient that I do. I am the expert here.'

The student should be asked to visualize himself presenting successfully, to practice his presentations, to remind himself that everyone has bad presentations, and to understand that no one is "born" knowing how to present a patient on rounds. It is an acquired skill, and one that often requires a bit of coaching.

❖ Conclusion

The Accreditation Council for Graduate Medical Education's core competencies (3), signals to inpatient attendings that the practice of medicine is multidimensional, requiring learners to master competencies much more extensive than just mere medical knowledge. Teaching learners how to master the competencies and "intangibles" of time management, organization, communication, and interpersonal skills has not been a regular feature of the standard attending's job description. Further, the standard job description ends with the end of the rotation, with little time or thought devoted to what happens to the learner after he leaves the rotation. Does the student know how to prioritize tasks, work effectively as a member of a patient care team, and read and study effectively? This chapter provided sample strategies to coach learners in the development of these important skills. The reality is that no attending can ever address all the skills. Residency programs, however, should be taking a coordinated approach to these issues, and encourage attendings to take these skills seriously—they do make an enormous difference, not only in the students' and residents' success on the wards but in their future success as medical professionals.

REFERENCES

1. **Wiese J, Varosy P, Tierney L.** Improving oral presentation skills with a clinical reasoning curriculum: a prospective controlled study. Am J Med. 2002;112:212-8.
2. **Wiese JG, Saint S, Tierney L.** The spoken case presentation: issues and recommendations. Seminars in Medical Practice. 2002;5:29-37.
3. **Accreditation Council for Graduate Medical Education.** Core competencies. Accessed at www.acgme.org/acWebsite/RRC_280/280_coreComp.asp.

Feedback, Evaluation, and Remediation on the Inpatient Service

Jeffrey J. Glasheen, MD
Jeannette Guerrasio, MD
Jeff Wiese, MD, FACP

The practice of medicine requires a commitment to lifelong learning and a commitment to improvement. And while everyone wishes to improve, actively engaging in a process of improvement is no easy task, for it requires taking an inventory of strengths and weaknesses. Emotionally, this can be threatening, and this makes giving and receiving feedback uncomfortable. The unfortunate result is that feedback is either not delivered, or it is delivered in a way that is so generic as to be useless (for example, "Read more," "See as many patients as you can"—as if any learner was previously planning to read less and see fewer patients).

This chapter provides strategies for providing emotionally neutral micro-feedback (feedback in the moment) and macro-feedback (regular midrotation and end-of-rotation evaluations) in the context of an inpatient rotation. These strategies should enhance learner performance and establish a "no-blame" culture of improvement associated with patient safety.

The central tenet to improvement is the acknowledgment of strengths and weakness, and this is at the core of feedback and evaluation. In essence, the goals of feedback and evaluation are fourfold: 1) to encourage learners to emphasize and sustain their strengths; 2) to direct learners to recognize their weaknesses and the need to improve; 3) to empower learners with an action plan for improvement; and

KEY POINTS

- Feedback and evaluation enable learners to appreciate their strengths; recognize their weaknesses; develop an action plan for improvement; and, finally, to instill in learners an internal process of self-reflection, personal inventory, and internally driven advancement toward goals.
- The inpatient attending can establish a culture of improvement that relies on multiple data points and includes both micro-feedback (feedback that occurs daily, as part of clinical teaching) and macro-feedback, which refers to less frequent but more detailed formal sessions for summative assessment.
- For both types of feedback, focus on the performance, not the performer; include as much specific information as possible; and use strategies (and even choice of words) that make the message clear, while maintaining self-esteem.
- Macro-feedback implies a commitment of time and requires special skills to ensure that the session is characterized by accurate diagnosis of the learners' strengths and weaknesses and avoids defensiveness and rejection.
- When dealing with the "problem" student or resident, remediation is beyond the scope of feedback and evaluation as the terms are commonly used. It generally is in the province of the program director, clerkship director, or others in a position of leadership and authority.
- Several behaviors should signal concern about substance abuse or depression, including sudden changes in a resident's performance or appearance, unprovoked outbursts or overreactions to situations, and showing up late for work or leaving the wards at inappropriate times. Inpatient attendings should have an appropriately low threshold for bringing these behaviors to the attention of clerkship and program directors.

4) through this process, to teach students the internal process of self-reflection, personal inventory, and internally driven improvement such that the feedback and evaluation process continues long after the trainee's formal training is complete.

The foundation of feedback and evaluation is built on expectations according to the learner's level of training, and it is important to assess the learner's competence against the backdrop of the level of training (chapter 2). A simple and effective tool to gauge the level of your learner is the mnemonic "RIME": reporter, interpreter, manager, educator (Table 6-1) (1). This tool allows for the standardized assessment of whether learners meet the criteria for proficiency on the basis of their level of training and whether they have the skills needed to progress. Each step in the RIME model is progressive and cannot be achieved until the previous step has been accomplished. In addition, the RIME model should be used across all domains as learners may be progressing differently for different competencies.

❖ Establishing a Culture of Improvement

The attending should recognize that learners may arrive on the wards without the appropriate mindset. Learners may conceptualize rotations just as they did for the preclinical and college courses that they experienced: that each rotation is a challenge to be overcome, a requirement to demonstrate excellence and obtain an "A" or an "Honors" grade. As opposed to the clinical wards, where team-based behavior is required, the preclinical experience

Table 6-1. RIME Education Model*

Level	Description
Reporter	Has consistently good interpersonal skills, reliably obtains and communicates clinical findings; written and spoken presentations are clear and organized
Interpreter	Able to prioritize and analyze patient problems, develop a differential diagnosis and next steps in work up; data are not just data but have clinical significance
Manager	Consistently proposes reasonable diagnostic and therapeutic options, incorporating patient preferences; can take knowledge, integrate it with the findings for a given patient, and form a plan that prioritizes within and among the problem list
Educator	Has sufficient level of knowledge of current medical evidence; demonstrates self-directed leaning and contributes to the education of others

From Pangaro L. A new vocabulary and other innovations for improving descriptive in-training evaluations. Acad Med. 1999;74:1203-7.

*The RIME acronym was developed to provide benchmarks for the progression and evaluation of clinical skills.

socialized learners to be individuals: Only one person takes the exam at a time; only one person gets the grade. The result is that the attending will encounter learners who, through no fault of their own, will be focused on their individual needs ("How will this affect my grade?") and very sensitive to their individual performance ("Did I get an A?"). The deck will be stacked against the attending in getting the learner to take a personal inventory of strengths and weaknesses and to accept constructive feedback necessary for long-term improvement.

Step 1: Establish the New Culture With Expectations
The first step in enabling meaningful feedback and evaluation is to change the culture, which begins with the goals and expectations delivered on the first day. Chapter 2 of this book outlines this process. The key elements with respect to this cultural change are the following: 1) Mistakes are expected (no one will be perfect, and everyone can improve); 2) the "game is won" by team-based play, not individual performance; and 3) the criteria for judging success are based on what helps the patient.

Step 2: Establish a Database of Observation Points
Despite its challenges, the fortunate aspect of the hospital medicine environment is that it allows inspection of each of the core competencies (Table 2-1 in chapter 2). As noted in chapter 3 of this book, the attending should use multiple observation points in assessing a learner's performance. Surrogate evaluation points (attending rounds presentations and admission notes) should be intermittently correlated with direct observations of each trainee to ensure the accuracy of these surrogate evaluation techniques (see chapters 3 and 4 of this book). Through careful attention to observing learners in a variety of settings, performance in each competency can be assessed without excessive time commitments: for example, in the emergency department admitting a patient (professionalism), at the nurses' station interacting with the other members of the health care team (systems-based care), during family meetings (communication), and while accessing the literature to solve a clinical conundrum (practice-based learning). The attending can also create additional opportunities to observe learners by delegating roles and responsibilities. For example, patient care and interpersonal/communication skills can be assessed by asking a learner to lead the bedside patient encounter and describe the plan and goals to the patient. Communication and systems-of-care competencies (such as leadership of a health care team) can be assessed by observing a resident running team rounds.

Step 3: Maintain the Culture With Micro-Feedback

Feedback is the "process by which the teacher provides learners with information about their performance for the purposes of improving their performance" (2). Feedback differs from evaluation. Evaluation is the formal (summary) process of assessing where the learner stands as a whole, occurring at the conclusion of the rotation. Feedback, on the other hand, is the day-to-day assessment of the learner's performance, both in areas of strengths and in areas of improvement.

Micro- Versus Macro-Feedback

It is useful to think of micro-feedback (brief daily doses) and macro-feedback (less frequent but more detailed formal sessions). Micro-feedback provides the learner with short, 1- to 3-minute nuggets of feedback, usually following daily performance of skills (see the dialogue on teaching interpersonal skills in chapter 5). Macro-feedback involves a more formal, 5- to 20-minute, structured feedback session and commonly occurs at the middle of the rotation, at the end of the rotation, or after a significant event (such as a medical error) (2).

The Importance of Feedback to Maintain the Culture of Improvement

Daily micro-feedback sets the stage for the macro-feedback sessions described below. Without regular feedback, the learner may discount or deny the attending's more summative counsel because it will appear to "come as a surprise." But micro-feedback is much more important that just enabling the midrotation feedback sessions.

To appreciate the importance of daily micro-feedback, it is important to understand the psychology of how good students have become "good students" and how bad students have become "bad students." In this discussion, "good" and "bad" refer to the student's performance, not the person's value. The good student enters the clinical environment, and even if she has been given the best of expectations, she will still be forced to learn which behaviors are appropriate and which are not. The student performs a behavior, and the environment, which includes, but is not limited to, the attending or resident, responds to the student with either an approbation ("that behavior was appropriate") or a corrective action ("that behavior was not appropriate"). This "response from the environment," particularly the comments of the attending, is the micro-feedback. Over time, the student builds a set of expectations of what is and what is not appropriate behavior. These expectations make up the student's reality.

> As the team leaves the patient's room, Phaedrus takes a minute to stop rounds.

"Stef, let me stop rounds for a second to comment on the discussion we had with Mr. Tierny's family. It was impressive. He clearly has a diagnosis that is not going to end well, and the easy way out would have been to minimize the prognosis ... but the message delivered to the patient and his family was honest, yet empathetic." Phaedrus pauses. "I just want you know to know that that is exactly the way it needs to be done."

The bad student also formulates a concept of reality, but his reality may not be based on insightful feedback because poor performance often elicits fewer or no comments (3). The difference between the good and the bad student has nothing to do with their initial behaviors: Both will have inappropriate behaviors to start. This leads the bad student to believe that his behaviors are appropriate. This becomes his set of expectations, but unlike the good student, whose concept of reality (what works) is accurate, the bad student's concept of reality is misinformed. In most cases, bad performance results not from fundamental character deficits but from the absence of appropriate re-direction to correctly classify behaviors as appropriate or inappropriate.

As the team rounds on the next patient, it becomes clear to the attending that the team did not come in early enough to collect the necessary information on the patient. The presentation is disorganized, and as the team enters the room, the student's initial presentation—"He is doing fine today ... no acute events overnight"—is juxtaposed against the sight of Mr. Hamm breathing at 30 times per minute with an altered level of consciousness. The attending, although internally frustrated, elects to focus only on the management of the patient, without also addressing the opportunity for micro-feedback to the student.

"Okay." Phaedrus pauses at the sight of the patient. "Moni, can you call a rapid response?"

"Sure, I'll do that right now."

After the rapid response is called, the initial management is complete, and the patient is on the way to the intensive care unit (ICU), the team continues rounds. "All right," Phaedrus say, "Let's move on to the next patient."

In this example, the attending allows his frustration and anger to overcome him. Although he doesn't act on the frustration (which is good), he also misses the opportunity to provide micro-feedback to the team. The correct approach might be something like the following:

As the patient is being moved to the ICU, Phaedrus pauses to give the team feedback. "Let be honest in saying that this is concerning. I know that time is tight, and getting here early enough to see patients before attending rounds can be difficult. I used to be a resident, so I know that is true. I also know that there might have been circumstances that were unusual this morning that kept the team from seeing Mr. Hamm. That said, I want to emphasize the importance of seeing your patients each day, and the importance of taking a personal sign-out from the night-float physician. I am disappointed not in you as people, but I am disappointed in the action of not taking this sign-out and not knowing about the patient's condition." Phaedrus pauses.

"I've communicated my message to you, and now we're done with it. Okay?"

The team nods.

"We have more patients to take care of, so let's keep going on rounds. When we finish, we'll go to the ICU to see how Mr. Hamm is doing. Going forward, remember the lesson that we learned today."

Note that the attending directed his comments to the team, not to any individual team member. This is a deliberate and effective strategy, and one that is recommended for the inpatient service where the learners work as a team. It is easier to criticize a group than an individual. Does this strategy risk not providing a particular learner with feedback necessary to improve future performance? To some extent, it does. But corrective feedback to an individual should not be delivered in public. Having addressed the performance problem of the group, the attending still has the opportunity—and, indeed, the responsibility—to provide private micro-feedback to any individual at a later time, if that is considered helpful. Moreover, in most cases, individuals will "learn" about their own performance when they hear criticism of their group.

Complicating the ward environment is modeling, especially by younger learners who observe and may copy senior-level physicians without fully understanding the circumstances that surrounded the senior physicians' behavior. For example (as noted in chapter 4), a senior-level physician may evoke a diagnostic shortcut by jumping to a diagnosis of *Pneumocystis carinii* pneumonia in an HIV-positive patient who presents with dyspnea. The student may not appreciate that the clinician has the benefit of years of clinical experience that allows him to do this, or that he knows this patient well and has admitted him with this problem before.

The student takes away from the observation that it is "okay to jump to a diagnosis after three or four lines of history." Another example might be a student who observes a resident delivering a cursory presentation to the attending physician, and as a result learns that "cursory presentations are acceptable," even though she did not see that the attending and the resident had discussed the case in detail a couple of hours before.

In both of these examples, the physician's behavior was appropriate, but only because of the physician's level and experience or because of the context. The attending must recognize that the learners are constantly learning and that feedback must be sufficiently frequent to enable the students to adjust their behaviors, and to ensure that the students understand the context or appropriateness of others' behaviors.

As Moni finishes her brief presentation, Phaedrus stops the discussion.

"Paul, I just want you to know that Moni and I discussed this patient at length this morning before we started rounds. Though her presentation is brief, it's only because we had the luxury of talking about it in detail before you arrived. I don't want you to get the wrong idea that we are jumping to conclusions here without all of the information being presented."

Focusing on the Performance, Not the Performer
In both types of feedback, micro and macro, the attending should present information, rather than judgment. The focal point should be on the performance, and not the person. Distinguishing the two will remove much of the emotional overlays that prevent the learner from internalizing the feedback. The distinction can be established by routinely leading with, *"I'm not criticizing you, Paul. I am, however, criticizing the management of Mr. Lawrence's potassium level."*

The attending can mitigate the emotional overtones of judgment by using "I" rather than "you" when giving feedback. The use of the word "I" implies that the feedback is the attending's *perception* of the situation; the use of "you" is perceived as a personal indictment. For example, *"During the interaction with the patient,* **I** began to feel that you were uncomfortable giving her patient bad news" is preferable to "**You** looked uncomfortable giving the patient bad news."

The attending can improve the motivation in feedback by using "and" rather than "but" (4). Learners may tune out positive feedback that precedes constructive feedback because they are waiting for "the other shoe to drop," leaving them only with the areas for improvement, which may make them feel like a failure. The regular use of "and" sends the intended message: Your performance is good in these ways, and this is how you can further improve. For example, *"Your presentations are good,* **but** you need to make it more concise," is not as effective as *"Your presentations are good,* **and** by making them more concise, they will be even better."

Beware the Perils of Praise
Physicians tend to default to positive feedback because it is more comfortable than constructive feedback. The biggest risk is that positive feedback will take the place of important constructive feedback. However, an equally big risk is that positive "feedback" becomes "praise." The former is helpful; the latter turns the focus toward the person, not the performance. For example, "you were great" does not describe the work but rather the learner. The standard of focusing feedback on the performance and not the person has to be consistent, lest the attending set the stage for interpreting subsequent constructive feedback as personal (personal indictments) instead of an assessment of performance. As an example, see the dialogue in the preceding section "The Importance of Feedback to Maintain the Culture of Improvement." In that example, it is tempting for Phaedrus to simply say, *"Stef,* **you** did an impressive job of delivering the bad news to the patient." Instead, the attending keeps the positive feedback focused on the action and not the person by saying, "It [the message] was impressive. ... *The message delivered to the patient and his family was honest, yet empathetic ... I just want you know to know that that is exactly the way it needs to be done."*

Be Specific
The more specific the feedback, the more effective it will be on improving performance. For example, *"The differential diagnosis did not include pulmonary embolism"* is better than *"The differential diagnosis is inadequate."*

Be Conscious of Nonverbal Feedback
Be conscious of nonverbal feedback as well because it may give unintended false confidence. For example, nodding your head to hurry a slow presenter along may be seen as encouragement that she is doing a good job and should keep going.

Function as a Coach
Attendings should see micro-feedback as an extension of their role as the learner's "coach" and should convey from the outset that this is not personal. Using the word "coach" is useful in conveying this sentiment, *"Paul, let me coach you here a bit. Great presentation, and here are some tips on how to make it even better."* The sentiment that this is not personal can be

extended by making micro-feedback a regular part of attending rounds for all learners (so that the learner will think, *"It's not just me that is getting feedback"*).

Step 4: Maintain the Culture of Improvement With Macro-Feedback

The principles of micro-feedback apply to macro-feedback as well. The focal point should be the performance, not the person, and it should be conducted in a manner that is future-oriented, motivational, and not daunting. Comfort with macro-evaluations is contingent on having established the coach–player relationship, which in turn is contingent on frequent micro-feedback leading up to the midrotation and end-of-rotation macro-feedback sessions.

Commitment and Timing
The time pressures and the variability of the attending's day can make finding time to give macro-feedback challenging. The attending must commit to a designated time to provide the feedback, however, because leaving feedback to happenstance will inevitably result in the feedback getting swallowed up by the more "pressing" issues of the day. Clearly setting a time and date for the midmonth feedback during the orientation day (chapter 2) will not only ensure that it occurs but also assuage the fear that can come from being called to a "surprise" feedback session (*"Oh my God, what have I done now!?"*).

> *Phaedrus pauses at the end of rounds. "Okay, today is the midpoint in the rotation. We should discuss how things are going. I want to take some time this afternoon with each of you. Let's do this. I'll start with Moni in the early afternoon before she goes to clinic, and then Stef, I'll send you a page so that we can talk. After that's complete, I'll page Paul."*

Location and Learning Climate
The macro-feedback session should be conducted in a location that is quiet and private and allows both the attending and the learner to sit undisrupted during the discussion. As opposed to micro-feedback, this session should be conducted one learner at a time to allow the learner to confidentially voice any concerns and to reciprocate by giving the attending feedback. It is important that the attending read the situation. Post-call days are not a good time to give feedback, and if the learner is angry, overwhelmed, or hurried, the session should be rescheduled for a better time. From the outset, it is important to communicate to the learner that *"This is feedback"*—if it is not so labeled, learners may not later remember that you gave them feedback.

The rule in teaching students how to take a sexual history is that, *"The patient's discomfort with the discussion will be proportional to the physician's discomfort. The best thing you can do for the patient's comfort is to be comfortable yourself."* The same is true for providing macro-feedback. Attendings must convey that they merely care enough to spend some time reviewing the learner's *performance* and how it could be even better. It is important that the learners perceive that the attending's interest in giving feedback reflects her goal to make them better doctors. Anything short of this will make the learners less open to the suggestions.

Techniques: The Two-Penny Approach
Physicians are keen observers but notoriously poor self-assessors. When asked to rate their performance, weaker residents routinely overestimated their performance, and stronger residents routinely underrated their performance (5). Fortunately, self-assessment skills can be developed with practice, to identify the strengths and weaknesses in learners, if the learners are coached to do so.

The attending should include as part of the macro-feedback session a discussion of how the learner can take charge of his process of self-improvement. This includes a discussion of the method of self-reflection, personal inventory collection, and designing personal strategies to address deficiencies and enhance strengths. In the long run, after the learners have finished their formal training, it will be their skills in self-assessment and self-improvement that will determine their ultimate performance. This is analogous to the learner's use of the medical literature: It is more important to teach the learner how to find a pertinent article in the literature than it is to merely give the learner the article. Likewise, it is important to provide learners with a method for accurately assessing their strengths and weaknesses. For this reason, the method of providing evaluation is as important as what is said.

One method is the "two-penny" approach:

"Paul, thanks for spending a few minutes with me to talk through the rotation thus far. Let me say from the outset that it has been a pleasure being your coach, and it's exciting for me to see you develop as a physician. Everything I say to you is simply because I care enough to see you become a great physician.

"So let me start with this. This session is not for me to tell you how much better or worse you are than other people. This is just about how you can continue to get even better. So, as we talked on the first day, I'll remind you that being a physician requires multiple skills, and since they are all interrelated, the physician can't be

good in only one or two. We have to strive to be better in all of them. But let's do this. I'm going to write out the big skills areas, and I want you to take a few minutes and reflect on the month so far. I want you to think about what is your strongest area, and what is your weakest area. Then I want you to take this penny and put it on the area that you think is your weakest area. I am going to put my penny on what I think is your weakest area. Then we'll talk through strategies to improve both of those." Phaedrus pauses.

"And then, Paul, when we are all done, we are going to do the same process for me ... my strongest and weakest areas, including, of course, my effectiveness as your coach. We'll each put a penny down on the aspect of coaching that I need to work on."

After areas of "greatest improvement potential" are identified, attendings should bring in specific observations as to how they perceived the students' performance in that area and methods or strategies by which performance could be made even better.

The benefit to the "two-penny" approach is that it neutralizes the emotional overtones of the evaluation, and it extinguishes the "how am I compared to my classmates" mentality. Instead, the approach focuses the student on self-reflection, and the attitude that regardless of how good or bad you are, everyone has a "weakest area" and everyone can get better. The method communicates to the student that he has strengths, and the attending can end the session by identifying strengths in other areas as well. Further, the method conveys the message that being strong in one area (such as medical knowledge) does not absolve you from being skilled in other areas (such as interpersonal relations).

The greatest value of this method is that it can be replicated years from now. This is the method that will enable the student to do his own assessment and evaluation years after the formal training is complete, making it a life-long skill. By turning the tables at the end, the attending improves because of the learner's feedback on his coaching performance, but he also models the behavior of self-evaluation, conveying the message that you never outgrow the need to take stock and improve.

Step 5: Consolidate the Culture of Improvement With Evaluation

As noted earlier, "evaluation" is different from "feedback." An evaluation is a final appraisal of performance, determining the extent to which the learner's performance has met the goals and expectations. It is summative, whereas feedback is formative. In essence, the "evaluation" is the coach saying goodbye to his player, preparing her for the next stage of her development, where hopefully she will find a new coach to guide her. There are several crucial elements in constructing meaningful evaluations.

Anticipate What Will Destroy the Effectiveness of the Evaluation

Despite the coach's best efforts at refocusing students toward self-improvement and away from the *"How do I compare to others?"* mentality, students may still slip into the competition-based, me-first mentality. If they do, even constructive criticism on the evaluation may be rebuked instead of being internalized. Even these students will eventually heed the counsel, however, if it is constructive and an alternative "avoidance strategy" isn't an option for them. Thinking of these avoidance strategies ahead of time is important in ensuring that the constructive criticism eventually takes. As it works out, the central elements of preparing evaluations coincide with preventing these avoidance strategies, as noted below.

Synch Expectations With the Evaluation

The avoidance strategy will begin with, *"I reject this evaluation because I wasn't told I was expected to do that."* As chapter 2 noted, it is important to establish expectations from the outset of the rotation. The evaluation should refer only to aspects of performance that were previously directly communicated. It is unfair to judge learners poorly for an aspect of performance of which they were unaware.

Ensure Accuracy

The avoidance strategy will begin with, *"I reject this evaluation because the attending didn't see me do this skill."* To increase the accuracy of an evaluation, the evaluator must have multiple brief observations of performance over a longitudinal period. Try to evaluate as many of the Accreditation Council for Graduate Medical Education (ACGME) competencies as possible, and indicate which areas do not apply because of a lack of opportunity to observe. If the student's time on the rotation is shared by more than one attending, the two attendings should confer with each other and submit one group evaluation. The attending should also evoke the opinions of other team members in constructing a synchronized 360° evaluation, and the evaluation should clearly delineate that all members of the team contributed to the evaluation. This will identify learner behaviors that were masked from the attending because of successful posturing (for example, the student looked great on attending rounds but frequently disappeared during the afternoons, leaving the team stranded). Soliciting opinions from other team members will also insulate the attending from protests about the evaluation; the attending can and should point to the fact that even if he wanted to, he cannot change the evaluation because it is a shared intellectual property of the team.

Make Sure Content Reflects All Relevant Areas
The avoidance strategy will begin with, *"I reject this evaluation because, well, what about my performance with (insert his or her best competency)?"* The attending should provide commentary on the learner's performance in each of the six ACGME competencies. This is a comprehensive and summative report, so it should include all of the attending's observations and judgments regarding the learner's competence. As with feedback, specific examples should be described with unequivocal clarity. The RIME model can also be referenced here to demonstrate whether your learner is at the expected level of performance (1).

Ensure the Evaluation Is Timely
The avoidance strategy will begin with, *"I reject this evaluation because that was a long time ago. I'm different now."* Most evaluations are collected at the end of a series of encounters, such as the end of a month-long rotation. Evaluations that are completed far after the rotation has concluded have an increased probability of being summarily dismissed (on the basis of the preceding rationale), and the content within the evaluation will lose its effectiveness as the details of events become more distant in the learner's memory.

Discuss the Evaluation With the Learner
The avoidance strategy will begin with, *"I reject this evaluation because I would have done something different if only I had been told."* The evaluation should be discussed with the learner, including both positive comments and negative comments. The emotional weight of having this discussion can be offset if the attending uses a synchronized 360° evaluation in which all members of the team have contributed to the evaluation. The learner should be given a chance to process the comments and provide reflections. Turning in evaluations that have not been discussed does not help learners improve; instead, it brews resentment and defensive reactions that are not educationally productive.

Step 6: Overcome Your Own Barriers
Even the thought of a feedback encounter elicits emotional reactions. The common perception is that the learner will be discouraged by negative feedback and that such feedback will do more harm than good, or that it will damage the working relationship between the learner and the teacher. Boehler and colleagues' study on complimentary versus constructive feed-

back showed that constructive feedback improved performance on procedural skills more than complimentary feedback (6). Satisfaction with feedback is a poor marker of the quality of feedback, illustrating that the feedback that makes learners feel great doesn't necessarily make them better.

Another misconception is that giving honest and accurate feedback will negatively affect the attending's own evaluations. The truth is that high-quality feedback is strongly associated with high teacher ratings (7). In fact, Torre and colleagues demonstrated that all feedback activities, on differential diagnosis, oral case presentation, bedside examinations, written history, and daily progress notes, were associated with students' perception of high-quality teaching (7).

❖ Remediation

It is important to appreciate that feedback enables learners to improve only when they are able and willing to do so. Sometimes deficits require remediation, as when a learner proves incapable of achieving an important milestone, or when personal problems, including, unfortunately, substance abuse, preclude satisfactory performance.

Remediation usually warrants intervention by someone of authority, typically the program director or clerkship director (9). The prevalence of residents requiring remediation is 7% to 15% (8). It is important to identify and remediate the struggling trainees because their behaviors and actions affect patient safety and timely care, increase the amount of time faculty spend providing correction, add responsibilities and work for their colleagues, and affect the morale of the entire training program (10). As discussed earlier, a problem learner can also "infect" other learners by way of their bad example, with junior learners modeling bad behavior. It has also been shown that trainees who demonstrate unprofessional behavior during their training are more likely to perpetuate that behavior into their careers (11). But most important, identifying and remediating problem trainees is our professional obligation. A full discussion of remediation is beyond the scope of this book, but there are a few essential points that an attending physician should know.

Identify and Report
The first and most important point is that trainees requiring remediation should be identified and reported to the respective clerkship director or program director. The attending should not be shy about doing this because trainees who have true career-limiting deficits in performance are likely to have had similar events on other rotations. Given the overlapping

schedules between attendings, residents, and students and the "silo" mentality of most medical schools (for example, internal medicine does not review student performances with pediatrics), it is possible, in fact likely, that these trainees have had long-standing problems, including depression and other affective problems, that have not been identified because they were not reported. The program or clerkship director is in a much better position to detect trends in performance. The trainee's personal life during that rotation may have dramatically changed the performance; in that case, this report will probably be a one-time event. Even so, the director will be better able to provide counseling or assistance to the trainee if she knows about the trainee's fall-off in performance as soon as possible.

Suspect Substance Abuse

Accusations of substance abuse should not be made lightly, but clues that might suggest this disorder should be reported immediately so that the resident can receive assistance. Unfortunately, it is rarely as easy as smelling alcohol on a resident's breath or observing pinpoint or dilated pupils. The signs are much more subtle, and are usually identified in the context of trends. A sudden change in a resident's performance or appearance, for example, may suggest impairment. Isolated events of unprovoked outbursts or overreacting to a situation can occur, but if these behaviors become regular occurrences, impairment should be suspected. Routinely showing up late to work or routinely leaving the wards at inappropriate times should also prompt suspicion. The important principle is that *trends are important,* either a deficit in previous good performance or a new set of bad behaviors. As such, it is important to report these events to the program or clerkship director. These individuals have a better perspective on the resident's or student's overall trend of performance and are thus in a better position to detect fall-offs in performance that suggest impairment.

REFERENCES

1. **Pangaro L.** A new vocabulary and other innovations for improving descriptive in-training evaluations. Acad Med. 1999;74:1203-7.
2. **Holmboe E.** American Board of Internal Medicine Faculty Development Conference: Evaluation of Learners, Effective Feedback and Systems Approach. Denver: Univ of Colorado; 2008.
3. **Ginsburg S, Lingard L, Regehr G, Underwood K.** Know when to rock the boat: how faculty rationalize students' behaviors. J Gen Intern Med. 2008;23:942-7.
4. **Weisinger H.** The Power of Positive Criticism. New York: AMACOM; 1999.
5. **Hodges B, Regehr G, Martin D.** Difficulties in recognizing one's own incompetence: novice physicians who are unskilled and unaware of it. Acad Med. 2001;76:S87-9.

6. **Boehler ML, Rogers DA, Schwind CJ, Mayforth R, Quin J, Williams RG, et al.** An investigation of medical student reactions to feedback: a randomised controlled trial. Med Educ. 2006;40:746-9.
7. **Torre DM, Sebastian JL, Simpson DE.** Learning activities and high-quality teaching: perceptions of third-year IM clerkship students. Acad Med. 2003;78:812-4.
8. **Yao DC, Wright SM.** National survey of internal medicine residency program directors regarding problem residents. JAMA. 2000;284:1099-104.
9. **Mitchell M, Srinivasan M, West DC, Franks P, Keenan C, Henderson M, et al.** Factors affecting resident performance: development of a theoretical model and a focused literature review. Acad Med. 2005;80:376-89.
10. **Thomas NK.** Resident burnout. JAMA. 2004;292:2880-9.
11. **Papadakis MA, Arnold GK, Blank LL, Holmboe ES, Lipner RS.** Performance during internal medicine residency training and subsequent disciplinary action by state licensing boards. Ann Intern Med. 2008;148:869-76.

Section II

Clinical Teaching Scripts for Inpatient Medicine

Clinical Teaching Scripts for Inpatient Medicine

Jeff Wiese, MD, FACP

❖ Contents

Print Version

Online Version (www.acponline.org/acp_press/teaching)

❖ What Are Teaching Scripts?

U p until this point, this book has been about process more than content—this is for a reason. The skills required of an attending physician are much more than clinical scientific knowledge. This section, however, is designed to bring the process of teaching in touch with its content. To get into the granularity of all medical knowledge required of the inpatient attending is beyond the scope of this book; indeed, one could argue that given the pace at which clinical medicine is growing and changing, that book could never be written. But that is not to say that clinical teaching, or any teaching for that matter, does not depend greatly on how the content is configured (1, 2).

It is clear that physicians develop patterns that are useful in their care of patients. Illness scripts, for example, are repeatedly used by physicians to identify diagnoses: Fever, cough, and dyspnea are central components to any physician's illness script for pneumonia. Analogous to illness scripts are "teaching scripts": the patterns of teaching that can be used effectively when teaching learners how to address a common clinical problem. This section of the book provides sample teaching scripts for some of the most common clinic problems encountered on the clinical wards.

The value of teaching scripts is twofold. First, because attending physicians routinely evoke the scripts, they find greater and greater proficiency and efficiency in using them. Beginning attendings may find that the first few rotations on the wards bring new teaching challenges each day. As months pass, however, the attendings will find themselves evoking and providing familiar talks, demonstrations, or discussions about the case because the clinical complaints recur; teaching the approach to chest pain becomes more and more familiar. Second, teaching scripts enable attendings to more closely accomplish the goal of clinical education: the ability to extrapolate the lessons learned in the care of one patient to the care of other patients (who may have similar symptoms) in the learner's practice. For example, a teaching script on the approach to dyspnea may be prompted by one patient with pneumonia, but the attending's script empowers the learner with a method that will be equally valuable in identifying the diagnosis in a patient with other causes of dyspnea (such as pneumothorax or congestive heart failure).

It will be tempting to think that this section is the definitive list of teaching scripts— the way that it *has* to be done. It is not. The reality is that *there is no absolute "way that it has to be done."* Each attending can, and should, develop her own teaching scripts. This is part of the artistry that makes clinical education on the wards so fulfilling: the artistic license to develop whatever method the attending finds most useful in approaching clinical problems. The teaching scripts contained here are merely examples, meant to catalyze the creative thought process of readers into developing their own teaching scripts. Analogous to clinical medicine, the details of a method are not nearly important as *having a method*.

That said, there is a rationale behind how the teaching scripts in this section have been constructed. The joy of internal medicine is "figuring things out," and the teaching script (or advanced organizer contained within) should be motivating, not daunting. Students should leave the session saying, *"Wow, this is not as hard as I thought it was going to be."* The reality is that each clinical topic is much more extensive than any advanced organizer could fully capture. But attendings have to be comfortable with the belief that if the method provided in the script empowers students with a sense that competence in the topic can be obtained, the students will be more likely to read about the details of the topic on their own time. Teaching scripts that are mere laundry lists of every possible diagnosis are daunting and will meet with the same results as phase 1 teaching (that is, "look at how much I know") described in chapter 1 of this book.

Further, the teaching script should *anticipate* that students will forget memorized lists—if not now, eventually. The script or method should enable students with a convenient and memorable way of organizing their thoughts such that knowledge can be regenerated at a point distant in time. For example, the causes of chest pain could easily be merely recited to the learners as a script, but this memorized list is unlikely to be recalled at a distant point in time. The method of using the "arrow traveling through the chest, front to back" prompts learners to recall the list later in time and to ensure that their method thoroughly addresses the diagnoses that should at least initially be considered.

Learning clinical medicine should be fun, and the more fun that it is, the greater the engagement on the part of the learners—and the more inspired they will be to read on their own time. Using metaphors and linking examples to areas of interest for the individual learner are features of the teaching script that address this goal, and features that you will find scattered among the teaching scripts below.

Finally, the teaching script should empower understanding of the disease, not merely memorization of associations. Each of the following teaching scripts operates under the Socratic method, the benefits of which are outlined in chapter 1 of this book. By using the Socratic method, the teaching script is designed to move the learner from a baseline "point A" to the wished-for "point B" of understanding. And in doing so, the attending creates a mental road map. Should students become lost in the future (having forgotten what to do), the act of having traveled with that mental map increases the probability that they can re-create the line of questioning that will enable them to find the right conclusion. It is easier to re-create a trip if you drove the car than if you merely rode in the back seat.

In aggregate, all components of the teaching scripts should accomplish the ultimate goal: the improved performance of the learner. The scripts should be targeted at the areas that have the greatest utility to the internal medicine ward team, and they should leave the learner with a greater sense of competence than when they began. The scripts should create an intrinsic vision of how the learner will use the skill, anticipate where learners will forget or struggle with the skill, and motivate the learner to want to practice or use the skill (that is, it shouldn't be daunting). In simple terms, the teaching script should accomplish the fundamental components of clinical coaching outlined in chapter 1 of this book: visualization, motivation, anticipation, and utility.

You will find that the teaching scripts here, with few exceptions, focus on the teaching of diagnostic methods as opposed to management methods. This is merely a feature of space considerations—it is equally likely that attending physicians will (and should) over time develop teaching scripts for management as much as for diagnosis.

You will also find that each teaching script may have exceptions to the rule. Is it possible that there are other causes of dyspnea not captured by the dyspnea pyramid teaching script? Yes, definitely. But each teaching script operates under the principle that "perfection is sometimes the enemy of the good" and that beginning a teaching session on a clinical topic that addresses each possible exception to the rule (for example, a talk that addresses every possible cause of dyspnea) results in 1) a session that never ends and 2) a session that is so daunting that the learner captures nothing from it. The methods in this section operate under the principle that sometimes "understanding is more important that truth," for understanding (having a framework to understand the general rules of a diagnostic method) enables truth (the learner has enough of a grasp to explore and discover the exceptions to the rule). Once a method or teaching script has been delivered, it is the attending's role to supplement the method over the course of the rotation with the exceptions to the rules as they present. But this is the luxury of inpatient attendings, for they will have that opportunity to do so.

The print version of this book features 10 teaching dialogues. For five additional dialogues, go to the companion Web site to this book (www.acponline.org/acp_press/teaching/).

REFERENCES

1. **Shulman LS.** Those who understand: knowledge growth in teaching. Educ Res. 1986; 15:4-14.
2. **Skeff KM, Stratos GA, eds.** Methods for Teaching Medicine. Philadelphia: ACP Pr; 2010.

❖ The 10 Equations

Purpose

Medical students and residents will arrive to the wards with the same psychological frustration: The wards are daunting. Each day learners seemingly fall farther and farther behind, consistently being reminded of more knowledge that they need to learn. Although they will not verbalize it, the sentiment will be there: I might be better off staying at home, at least that way I'll stop falling behind. It is this sentiment that psychologically stands in the way of learners engaging in the discussion of new knowledge, manifest in behavior such as premature closure on diagnoses, failure to address problems two through five on the patient's problem list, and blocking or "turfing" admissions. It is not so much the fear of more work but the fear of revealing greater and greater incompetence that underlies each of these behaviors.

This is especially true for medical students who are coming off a preclinical curriculum that was composed of defined knowledge sets: *"Only the content in the renal block lectures is fair game for the renal block examination," "If you memorize the questions in Q-bank (a finite number) you will pass step 1."* It is this mentality that deters many students away from a career in medicine and toward a career in specialization, captured by the sentiment, *"I feel more comfortable with a small amount of content for which I will be responsible."*

Attending physicians cannot change the reality that there is an infinite amount of knowledge to learn in internal medicine. But they can change the perception of internal medicine by creating a culture of empowerment, and a sentiment that although there will always be an infinite amount of knowledge to learn, each day on the internal medicine service brings greater understanding and competence, moving the learner closer and closer to mastery.

Beginning the month with the "10 Equations" serves several purposes. It demonstrates that despite the complexity of internal medicine, *a few simple principles guide most of what we do as internists*. This addresses the "disempowerment" feeling that learners have with internal medicine. Starting with the "10 Equations" also communicates that despite the breadth of internal medicine (every organ system is in play), these 10 themes recur and apply to most of the new knowledge, regardless of specialty, that will be discussed as the month proceeds. These are the "bones" on which the "flesh" (details of individual diseases) will be hung. And because the "10 Equations" are recurrently used from one disease to the next, the learner starts to get a sense that perhaps there is not an infinite amount of ground to cover after all—*"I've seen this before, it's familiar, it's a repetition"*—lessening the sentiment that the wards are *"a place where I fall farther and farther behind."* Finally, the "10 Equations" send an implicit message that medicine is not about "cookie-cutter protocols," "being the concierge service to direct patients to subspecialists," and "the placement-only service." It sends the message that the joy of internal medicine is figuring things out. The honor lies in not being afraid of all aspects of disease or being afraid of patient presentations that are foreign, unique, or atypical. It sends the message that internal medicine is about reasoning through problems, and with the right methods—the "10 Equations" as the skeleton—even the most atypical, complex, or foreign presentation can be "figured out."

The "10 Equations" is a long dialogue, and the attending can choose to address all equations at one sitting (1 hour) or divide the equations over two or more sessions. The earlier in the rotation the "10 Equations" can be delivered, the better. They will enable efficiency and the benefits of repetition for subsequent teaching scripts because it will set a strong framework ("the bones") on which subsequent teaching can hang. It also saves time going forward, since referencing the equations allows quickly getting to the unique aspects of what is being taught. For example, hypotension, hypertension, congestive heart failure, acute renal failure, hyponatremia, and sepsis talks are all off-shoots of Equations 4, 5, and 6. By having the base knowledge down, the attending can quickly reference the equations to establish the base, and then devote the teaching time to the unique aspects of the disease; this enables teaching during rounds (for example, during non-call, non–post-call days) in a time-efficient manner.

But if time does not allow, the "10 Equations" can be parceled out as four separate sessions. The natural break points are as follows: 1) session 1: Equations 1, 2, and 3 (oxygen from the air to the alveoli, from the alveoli to the blood, and from the blood to the tissues); 2) session 2: Equations 4, 5, 6, and 7 (hemodynamics and ensuring that metabolic needs are matched with oxygen delivery); 3) session 3: Equation 8 (carbon dioxide metabolism); 4) session 4: Equations 9 and 10 (fluid management and understanding chambers in the body). The following dialogues are broken out by these four partitions, although should time allow, one or more of these partitions could be done together.

Setting, Cast of Characters, and Abbreviations

The dialogue begins on the first day of the rotation, in a conference room, in the afternoon. Thus far, the first day has consisted of setting the goals and expectations in the morning (see chapter 2 of this book), and then seeing the patients as a team during the remainder of the morning. The attending, Phaedrus, has been seeing the patients on his own in the afternoon because the team has been doing ward work. The team is on-call, and it is late in the afternoon when most of the work has been finished. Phaedrus has told the team that he would meet with the team one more time on call to do some additional teaching, and to round on any patients who had been admitted during the day. The cast consists of the attending, Phaedrus; the resident, Moni; the intern, Stef; and the medical student, Paul.

The following abbreviations are used in this dialogue: COPD = chronic obstructive pulmonary disease; CT = computed tomography; DO_2 = oxygen delivery; EKG = electrocardiogram; ER = emergency room; FIO_2 = fraction of inspired oxygen; GI = gastrointestinal; ICU = intensive care unit; MI = myocardial infarction; PaO_2 = partial pressure of arterial oxygen.

Dialogue Part 1: Equations 1, 2, and 3

"So Paul, I'm wondering … do you feel overwhelmed by internal medicine? I mean, almost everything is in play … every specialty, every age group—except pediatrics, of course—and every disease."

"Absolutely." Paul looks relieved that his deepest fear has finally been verbalized.

"Hmm …" Phaedrus says. "And Stef, you look afraid that you are going to kill someone because of what you don't know. Is that right?"

"Yes!" Stef shares the look of relief.

"Okay, well, medicine is really not that tough—it's really more simple than you might think. First, let me say this. Stef, Moni has your back. And Moni, I have your back. We have many smart people on this team, and if there is ever a time that you think you have absolutely no idea what to do, or if there is ever a time where you feel that some patient is unsafe, then I want you to let the next person up on the team know. And if that doesn't work, then you call me directly. Here's my cell phone number." Phaedrus writes his cell phone number on the whiteboard. "But all of that said, let me return to how simple medicine really is. Paul, medicine is about one primary task: Getting oxygen from out here in the air …" Phaedrus draws a silhouette of his head on the white board as he speaks. "To the squash—that is, to the brain. And you have to do that without trepanation; no burr holes allowed. If you can do that, Paul, you have done your job as the physician. See how easy this is?"

Getting the "elephant" out of the room will give the learners more focus, and the attending more room to move.

Paul smiles. "Seems simple enough."

"Okay, then. I am going to explain all of internal medicine in 10 simple equations … principles, actually, but you get the point. 10 equations, Paul, that's all you need to know."

"Really?!" Paul looks excited.

There are obviously more than 10 principles needed to understand clinical medicine, but the comment is used to assuage the daunting feel of the first day, and to set a tone of empowerment.

"Well, not really. You'll have to learn about cytokines … let's call that equation 11." Paul smiles.

"There will be many details to learn as the month proceeds, Paul, but these 10 equations are your core. At its simplest, medicine is about ensuring that the brain and vital tissues receive oxygen and can eliminate waste—CO_2—from the body. Disease is your opponent, and it has developed many clever ways of disrupting these two goals. This is your war with disease, Paul, but you have an advantage: You know where disease will go and what it will do. You know this because the 10 equations will tell you. These 10 principles are the axial skeleton of clinical medicine. As clinical problems present, I want you to use one or a combination of these principles to solve the problem. After the general problem has been solved, we'll talk about the specific details of diagnosis and management that we need to know to finish the battle."

Phaedrus pauses to write out Equation 1. "So, Paul, if the brain is not getting enough oxygen, the first step is to determine if the alveoli are getting enough oxygen. Nothing else matters until you know this. What is the driving force that pushes air into the alveoli? And as you answer that, I want you to think about why you can't breathe in outer space."

Paul thinks for a moment and then responds. "Well, the barometric pressure, I guess."

"Right you are, Paul. It's the reason that it's easier to breathe at sea level than it is to breathe at high altitudes like Pikes Peak. Do you run, Paul?"

"Huh?... I mean, yeah, I guess."

"Yeah, I used to run. Got kind of tired of it, though. Did you ever run when it was really humid?"

"Yes, that sucks .... I mean ... uh ... that's not good. It's harder to run when it's humid."

"I agree. It does suck. And the reason that it's harder to run when it's humid, Paul, is that you are getting less air into your lungs. Look at this," Phaedrus points to the first part of Equation 1 (Table 7-1). *"Because the sum of the total pressure of a gas is the sum of all of the pressures of all of the gases in the mixture, you have to subtract out the partial pressure of water vapor—47,*

Table 7-1. The 10 Equations

Equation 1: Alveolar gas equation

$PAO_2 = (760 - 47) FIO_2 - PacO_2(1.25)$

Equation 2: Fick's law of diffusion of a gas across a membrane

$$Diffusion = \frac{Pressure\ gradient \times area}{Wall\ thickness}$$

Equation 3: Delivery of oxygen

$DO_2 = Cardiac\ output\ (hemoglobin \times Sat\%)$

Equation 4: Ohm's law: hemodynamics

Mean arterial pressure = cardiac output × systemic vascular resistance

Equation 5: Cardiac output

Cardiac output = stroke volume × heart rate

Equation 6: Stroke volume

Stroke volume = preload × contractility

Equation 7: How much is enough? Balancing oxygen demand with oxygen supply

Metabolic needs of tissue = CO × (arterial content of O_2 – venous content of O_2)

Equation 8: Excessive CO_2

$PacO_2 = CO_2$ produced – minute ventilation

Minute ventilation = respiratory rate × tidal volume (1 – deadspace %)

Equation 9: How do I approach fluid where fluid should not be? (Starling's law of fluid across a membrane)

Fluid flow = $K[(P_{in} - P_{out}) - (Onc_{in} - Onc_{out})]$

Equation 10: How does the body handle fluid in all of its chambers?

$$Wall\ tension = \frac{Pressure \times radius^4}{Wall\ thickness}$$

FIO_2 = fraction of inspired oxygen; K = permeability of the membrane; Onc = oncotic pressure; P = hydrostatic pressure; $PacO_2$ = partial pressure of arterial carbon dioxide; PAO_2 = partial pressure of oxygen in the alveoli.

typically, but higher when it's humid—that does not contribute to oxygen pressure in the alveoli."

"Hmm .... Hadn't thought of it that way," Stef says.

It would be much more efficient to just write out the equation and fill in the variables, but retention would be lost. The line of questioning one variable at a time is to ensure that the student understands why each variable is in the equation. By using "real-world" examples such as Pikes Peak, the variables are easier to understand and will be recalled with greater ease at a later time (that is, retention).

"Indeed. But the air is not 100% oxygen, is it? It's normally 21% oxygen. So we could say that the total amount of oxygen getting into the alveoli is the barometric pressure, 760 at sea level—minus the water vapor pressure, 47 on a nonhumid day—times the percent of oxygen in the air, 21%." Phaedrus pauses. "Now here's the practical point, Paul. If you take this part of the equation, on room air, it's an even 150, which should make it very easy to do the calculation in our head later."

As the venue in which the content will be used escalates (in this case, the intensive care unit), Phaedrus directs the questions to the learner level (the intern) who will be at that level.

"Now, Stef, here's what I want you to remember. We are eventually going to use this equation to calculate an alveolar-to-arterial gradient. Have you heard of that? The A-a gradient?"

"Yes, I have heard that. I've only done it a time or two so far, though."

"Well, we'll be doing a lot with this calculation, and when we get to it, I want you to remember that we can only use the actual numeric calculation if we know the precise oxygen percentage. If the patient is intubated and we are dialing in the F_{IO_2}, we can use the calculation. If the patient is breathing room air, we can do the calculation with 21%. But if the patient is receiving any additional oxygen and is not intubated, then we can't be sure of what the F_{IO_2} actually is, so the numeric calculation is off. So as a tip to you, I want you to imagine yourself doing night float, responding to a dyspneic patient. Can you see yourself there?" Stef nods.

"Good. If you are going to draw an arterial blood gas to assess the A-a number—and you really need the actual A-a number to make a clinical decision—take the patient off of the supplemental oxy-

gen. Wait a minute; the oxygen will equilibrate, draw the arterial blood gas, and then put the oxygen back on. Got it?"

Visualizing doing the skill consolidates the lesson, and is almost as good as having actually done the skill.

"Got it."

"Great. Paul, back to you. Do you have a roommate?" Phaedrus asks.

"No," Paul replies.

"Ever had a roommate?" Paul looks stunned. Phaedrus continues. "Seen a roommate on TV? Ever lived with your parents?"

Paul laughs. "Uh, sure."

"Okay, so then you know. Even though you drive past your apartment and say, 'Hey, that's my apartment,' it's not fully your apartment, is it? It's partly your apartment, and partly your roommate's apartment. Am I right?"

"Yes, it's partly yours, and partly your roommate's."

"And depending on how much time each of you spends there, the proportion of the apartment that is 'yours' would change. So if your roommate is a 'roommate in name only'—you know—for the family's sake ... if your 'roommate' spends most of his time at the significant other's place?" Stef nods and smiles.

"Then the apartment is, say, 80% yours. But if you are so unlucky as to be the recipient of your roommate's significant other—you know, you pay half the rent, but there are three of you sleeping there every night—then you can say that the apartment is only 33% yours."

"Yeah, I feel that."

"Good. So it is with the alveoli, Paul, and I want you to see it as such. There are two 'roommates': oxygen and carbon dioxide. The more time carbon dioxide spends hanging around the apartment, the less the apartment—in this case the alveoli—belongs to oxygen. So in our equation, we should probably subtract out the amount of 'time' that CO_2 spends around the apartment." Phaedrus points to the second part of the equation.

The "apartment" serves as the advanced organizer to illustrate the point of how the percentages of the two gases can fluctuate. Understanding this principle will be important for the next step, when the A-a gradient is calculated.

"So how do we measure the amount of CO_2 in the alveoli?"

"Great question, Paul." Phaedrus extends a hand for a handshake.

The handshake is the first communication of the message Phaedrus wants Paul to know: Rewards are given not only for providing the right answers but also *asking* the right question. The tone of "open and honest discussions" is beginning to be established.

Phaedrus continues. "So, Paul, here is how I want you to see carbon dioxide—not just here, but throughout the body. CO_2 is nonpolar, so it easily passes through any lipid bilayer ... any cell wall ... and membrane ... it's kind of like Patrick Swayze in that movie Ghost. *Did you see that film, Stef? I know you like movies."*

"Yeah. I saw it with my wife."

"Good answer. I'm not afraid to admit, though, Stef. I liked it. All those scary ghosts and all ... Anyway, as I was saying, CO_2 is Patrick Swayze, passing through walls with ease. So, Paul, we can say with confidence that whatever CO_2 is in the blood," Phaedrus points to the diagram outlining the alveoli-arterial interface and to the pulmonary arteriole, "will be the same amount that diffuses across the membrane to get to the alveoli. But one more question for you, Paul, where does the CO_2 come from?"

The coaching bond can be established only when the two participants, the coach and the player, see each other as people, not roles. Provided that the roles are not eroded, it is beneficial for the coach to show that he is a real person by showing some of his personality, likes, dislikes, et cetera. It also lightens the mood a bit, creating a relaxed atmosphere.

Paul responds, "From the cell—it's the metabolic waste from glycolysis."

"Wow, Moni, I think we lucked out with Paul here. Seems like he knows what he's doing." Moni smiles and nods.

"Indeed, Paul. And the more the metabolism, the more the CO_2. Am I right?"

Being talked about in a positive light is motivational for Paul. A sense of teamsmanship is provided by speaking to the resident, and simply using the word "we."

"Seems correct."

"So the actual formula, Paul, is the CO_2 divided by the respiratory quotient. For a balanced diet of protein, fat, and carbohydrates, that's 0.8. But I have a tough time dividing numbers by decimals in my head. So I prefer to just multiply the CO_2 by 'time and a quarter'—1.25." Phaedrus pauses to let Paul write this down. "Okay, Paul, so the final equation is the amount of oxygen being pushed into the alveoli, minus time and a quarter of the CO_2." Phaedrus points again to the equation. "Paul, this is the one equation of the 10 equations that you are actually going to use to calculate numbers—the others are just principles. I want you to take this equation home tonight and practice plugging in numbers. Because we are going to be using this so frequently, I want you to be able to calculate this in your head. This is important to me, Paul. Will you do that for me?"

"Sure," Paul replies.

"Okay, so Equation 1 will tell us how much oxygen is in the alveoli. That's the first step in getting the oxygen to the squash there." Phaedrus points to the head. "Hey, Paul, have you ever heard of the ABCs ... not the alphabet, but the ABCs like in basic life support?"

"Sure. Airway, breathing, cardiac." Paul answers.

"Yes, indeed. Why is Equation 1 the first equation on our roster?"

"I guess because it's about airway and breathing."

"Good, Paul. Never forget that. Always focus on the airway first."

The sequence of the equations is built to facilitate remembering them by following the natural course of oxygen, but it is also meant to emphasize this key clinical point: airway, then breathing, then circulation.

"So Stef, your turn. Let's say we draw the arterial blood gas on that night-float patient you were imagining earlier, and the CO_2 is 40 and the PaO_2—the arterial oxygen—is 60. What is the amount of oxygen in the alveoli?"

"Well, let's see..." Stef starts to draw out the math.

"Stef, let's see if you can do it in your head. This is important enough that I want you to be able to do this in your head."

"Okay, well, 150 is the first number if he's on room air .... minus 'time-and-a-quarter' of the CO_2 ... that's 50 ... so the alveolar oxygen is 100."

"Well, done Stef. Keep practicing that. And if the arterial oxygen concentration, measured via an arterial blood gas, is 60, then what is the alveolar to arterial gradient? The A-a gradient?"

"Well, that would be 100 minus 60 ... or 40."

"Yes! Fantastic. And as a general rule, Stef, the A-a gradient should be less than a third of the patient's age—with a minimum of 10. We won't hold some 3-year-old responsible for an A-a gradient of 1." Stef laughs. *"So for your 60-year-old patient with dyspnea, what's the cause of his hypoxia? Not enough oxygen in the alveoli, or not enough oxygen getting across the membrane to the blood?"*

"Well, in this case, the gradient is high, so that means that there's probably enough oxygen in the alveoli. It just isn't getting across."

"Fantastic. And that's the focus of Equation 2." (*Figure 7-1*)

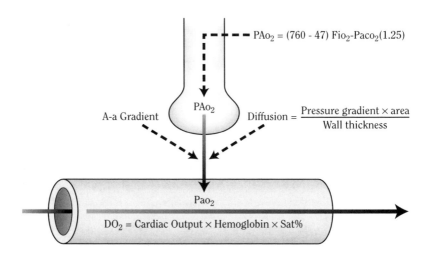

Figure 7-1 The alveoli-capillary interface. DO_2 = oxygen delivery; FIO_2 = fraction of inspired oxygen; PAO_2 = partial pressure of oxygen in the alveoli, $PaCO_2$ = partial pressure of arterial carbon dioxide; PaO_2 = partial pressure of arterial oxygen; Sat% = saturation percentage.

The end of each equation is the end of a "block" (see chapter 1 of this book). As such, it is a time for feedback and evaluation. If the learner cannot demonstrate competence, then the first block has to be repeated. If the student does show competence, and time allows, the discussion will continue to the next block. If time does not allow, this is a clean point at which to break and pick up later.

> *"All right, Paul. I'll draw out Equation 2 for you." Phaedrus writes the equation on the board. "This is a condensed version of Fick's law of diffusion of a gas across a membrane. Now, let me ask you a few questions. Phaedrus points to the diagram of the alveolar-arteriolar interface. "Which would push a gas across a membrane **more**? A high-pressure gradient or a low-pressure gradient?"*
>
> *"A high gradient," Paul answers.*
>
> *"Great. So let's put 'pressure gradient' in the numerator. The higher it is, the more the gas is pushed across. As specific to our discussion about oxygen from the alveoli to the arteries, Paul, what is another name for the pressure gradient?"*
>
> *"Well, that's the A-a gradient," Paul replies.*
>
> *"Great. And let me ask you, would more area or less area increase the diffusion of a gas?"*
>
> *"More area, of course," Paul answers.*
>
> *"Right. So we'll put 'area' in the numerator." Phaedrus writes in 'area' in the numerator of the equation. "And what would be easier for a gas to cross, a really thick membrane, or a very thin, porous membrane?"*
>
> *"A thin, porous membrane," Paul answers.*
>
> *"Correct, Paul. So if the bigger—the thicker—the membrane, the less the diffusion of the gas. So let's put that in the denominator here." Phaedrus writes in "wall thickness" in the denominator of Equation 2. "So there you go, Paul, that's equation 2, the principles that govern a gas—in our case, oxygen—diffusing across a membrane. So Stef, back to your night-float case. If the A-a gradient was … what did you say … 40?" Stef nods. "What two things might be decreasing oxygen in the blood? Look carefully at Equation 2, and remember that the pressure gradient probably isn't the problem, since we know the A-a gradient is elevated."*

"Well, there are only two things left: lung area and the wall thickness."

These two "blocks" will set up the "dyspnea pyramid" dialogue later in the month. (See the online portion of this section for the dyspnea teaching script). At this point, it is worth staying on track with the equations so the team can see how all of the equations relate to each other.

"All right, Paul. Now we have the oxygen in the blood. How does it get to the brain? That is, how is it delivered there?"

"The heart pumps it there, of course."

"Yes. And Paul, let's say that Moni here was a CEO of a grocery delivery business." Phaedrus draws a truck on the board, glancing back and forth at Moni over his shoulder as he draws in the stick figure driving the truck, as if he were creating a depiction of Moni. "Moni, what type of grocery would you like to deliver? This is the art of medicine—you get to choose your 'grocery.'"

Moni smiles. "Bread, I guess."

"The staff of life! Okay, bread." Phaedrus writes in "Moni's Bread" on the side of the truck. "And let's say, Paul, that Moni has 10 trucks in her company to deliver bread. And let's say that five of those trucks get swallowed by potholes—it could happen in New Orleans, you know." Paul smiles. "That's how we fill 'em ... let a car drive into them, put a metal plate over them, fill it with sand and go on ...."

Moni laughs.

"Paul, how could Moni ensure that the same amount of bread was delivered to each of the grocery stores?"

Even if the line of questioning stays with one team member, other team members can be corralled back into the discussion simply by involving them in the analogies.

"Buy more trucks, I guess."

"Good. How else?" Phaedrus waits while Paul thinks. Stef starts to answer, and Phaedrus extends a hand. "I'm sure Paul can come up with this. Let's see what he gets." Phaedrus starts the 5-second clock in his mind.

"Well, I guess the trucks could drive faster."

"Indeed. See, I told you, Stef, Paul would come through." Stef nods.

The line of questioning has to be preserved and held sacred for the learner. This is the first communication of the lesson: Once a person is asked a question, she will be given time to answer it. This is important to ensure that learners engage, especially in response to "think through it" type of questions (see chapter 1 of this book).

"Okay, Paul. But let's say the police are out in force, enforcing the speed limits. How else could the same amount of bread be delivered with fewer trucks?"

"Well, I suppose we could load more bread on each truck."

"Well done, Paul. So here is Equation 3: the delivery of oxygen to the tissues is the number of trucks (the hemoglobin that carries the oxygen) times the speed of the trucks (the cardiac output) times the saturation of each truck (the oxygen saturation of hemoglobin)." Phaedrus draws Equation 3 as he speaks. He then pauses. "Okay, Moni, it's your company, so I'll ask you. At what point do you buy more trucks?"

"Well, I suppose when you can't keep up with the delivery of the bread despite supersaturating the trucks and driving faster."

Phaedrus continues. "So let's make this real. What is the minimum hemoglobin number at which a patient has to be transfused? Assuming that hemoglobin is equivalent to the trucks, and transfusion is equivalent to buying more trucks."

"It depends." Moni looks at the board, and then suddenly her eyes widen a bit and her head moves back slightly. She nods ever so slightly. It is clear now that she has got it.

"Depends on what?" Phaedrus replies.

"It depends on the patient's cardiac and pulmonary function. If the patient has a good heart—that is, good cardiac output—and good lungs … which would be good saturation … then you might be able to hold off transfusing until the hemoglobin got to a lower number."

It would have been easier for the attending to just reveal how the metaphor links to the question of transfusion, but it is much more powerful, and memorable, if the learner makes the connection herself.

"Well done, Moni. Paul, Stef, I think you are in for a great month having Moni as your resident." Phaedrus pauses to let Stef and Paul look at Moni. This is the beginning of the bond between them, and Phaedrus's comment has facilitated it.

"We are going to return to this principle later, but Paul, I want to make sure that you have it. Let's say that Stef has a patient on the wards who has a hemoglobin of 7. She's young, say 30 years old, and otherwise healthy. No heart or lung problems. Does she need to be transfused? And if so, at what number?"

"Well," Paul replies. "It depends."

Phaedrus laughs. "Exactly, Paul. There is no magic number. But as Moni says, the answer to the question can be obtained only by determining when the 'bread' to the 'stores'—in this case, the oxygen to the tissues—is inadequate. I want you to be thinking about how we know that. We'll come back to it in a minute."

This is the finish to block 3, and it ends with feedback and evaluation; Paul demonstrates competence by solving the problem. This will set up Equation 7 that will follow later.

"Okay, Paul we're almost home. We have oxygen to the alveoli, that's Equation 1. Then across the membrane to the blood, that's Equation 2. Then onto the trucks ... the hemoglobin ... and we have it ready to pump to squash ... to mix food metaphors, of course." Phaedrus pauses. "But it sounds like the pagers are going off. Let's stop here, and we'll pick up with what is driving those trucks—Equations 4, 5, and 6 at our next session."

Dialogue Part 2: Equations 4 to 7

"Okay, are you ready for another installment of your 10 Most Important Equations, Paul?"

"Absolutely. I've already had two patients where I used the first three," Paul replies.

"Okay, but first a quick review. You'll remember that Equation 1 was about getting oxygen into the alveoli. What was Equation 2, Paul?"

"Well, let's see. It was getting the oxygen from the alveoli across the membrane to the blood ..." Paul pauses for a second, "and

Equation 3 was about the trucks ... that is, getting the oxygen to the tissues. So we were up to the 'speed of the trucks.'"

"Fantastic, Paul. Glad you have the first part down. In our first session, we said that it was the hemoglobin—the trucks—that was saturated with oxygen. And it was its job to deliver the oxygen to the tissues. And the speed of those trucks was a new variable, the cardiac output."

As subsequent "blocks" or equations continue, it is worth quickly reviewing the previous equations to that point. This consolidates the link between the equations, and is useful for long-term retention in recalling the equations.

Phaedrus underlines "cardiac output" and continues. "And since this appears to be pretty important to our delivery of oxygen to the tissues, perhaps we should determine what goes into it. But first, Paul, let me ask you ... did you have to take physics to get into medical school?"

"Yeah, it's still required."

"Moni, have you ever wondered why you had to take physics? I mean how many pool ball problems have you had to solve in medicine?"

"Well, there is the ER." Moni replies. Stef laughs.

"Okay, that aside, let me reveal the mystery. Paul, the reason you had to take physics was simply that you learned Ohm's law. Remember that? P equals IR. Potential across a circuit is equal to the current times the resistance. Just that principle alone. We were going to tell you that, but then you wouldn't have taken physics." Paul laughs.

"So, Paul, I'm going to put up Equations 4, 5, and 6, and we'll talk about them together. So Ohm's law in medicine is what governs hemodynamics."

Phaedrus writes out equation 4 as he speaks. "The mean arterial pressure, the potential across the hemodynamic circuit, is equal to the cardiac output, the current ... times the systemic vascular resistance, the resistance." Paul writes the question down.

Phaedrus continues. "And there's our friend, 'cardiac output' again. The cardiac output is the stroke volume ... that's what's coming out ... times the number of 'strokes per minute' ... or the heart rate." Phaedrus writes out Equation 5. "And the stroke volume is the volume in the heart to start with—we'll call that the preload—times the amount of heart squeeze per pump, the ejection fraction."

Speaking only in scientific terms (such as "ejection fraction") sounds impressive, but it prompts learners to memorize the terms. Combining the vernacular ("the amount of heart squeeze per pump") with the scientific term "ejection fraction" promotes understanding.

Phaedrus pauses while Paul writes it down. "Okay, Paul, let me ask you a few questions. And Stef, you get ready, 'cause I'm coming for you next." Stef smiles. "And Moni, if they can't get them right, you'll have a chance to steal … in a 'Family Feud' sort of way." Moni smiles as well.

"All right Paul, let's say you go down to Frankie and Johnnie's and have a big bowl of crawfish … it's salty … really salty … so you go throw back three or four Cokes. Have you done that?"

"No, not yet. I just moved to New Orleans."

"You are missing out, my friend. It's a delight. But okay, imagine all of that salt and fluid going to your gut. Where does it go then?"

"Well, it's absorbed into the veins … then past the liver … and then to the heart."

"Great. So if the volume in the veins was higher, what would happen to the preload to the heart?" Phaedrus asks.

"It would increase."

"Correct. And with increased volume to the heart—preload— what would happen to the stroke volume?"

"It would increase," Paul replies.

"Correct again. And if the stroke volume increased, what would happen to the cardiac output?"

"It would increase as well," Paul says.

"Correct again! Wow! Moni, things don't look good for your chance of stealing, here—Paul's on a roll." Moni smiles. It almost looks as if she is proud of Paul, even though it is their first day on the service. "And Paul, if the cardiac output increases, what would happen to the mean arterial pressure?"

"It would increases as well … hey, is that why you get hypertension from eating a lot of salt?"

"Indeed. Well done, Paul. Do you see how easy this is?"

This is a true Socratic method, taking the student from point A (consuming salt) to point B (hypertension). It is useful to further consolidate the links ("the neurons"; see chapter 1 of this book) by beginning with the conclusion of the previous link (that is, "if the cardiac output increases") and then asking the next question ("What would *happen to the mean arterial pressure?*").

"You know, it's not like I didn't know that salt causes hypertension. I guess I just never thought it through. I'm kind of dumb, huh?"

"To the contrary, Paul. You are like most of us. We 'learn' things without taking the time to fully understand it. This month is going to have a lot of those moments if you let me coach you." Paul looks at Phaedrus with a new appreciation. The coach–player bond is forming. *"Okay, Stef, you're up."*

Stef sits up in his chair. "Okay. I'm ready."

"Let's say, Stef, that your patient has a huge GI bleed. What will happen to his venous volume?"

"It will go down."

"Right. And if his venous volume goes down, what will happen to the preload?"

"It will go down," Stef replies.

"Indeed. And if there is less preload, what will happen to his stroke volume?"

"It will also go down."

"Nice. And if the stroke volume goes down, what will happen to the cardiac output?"

"The cardiac output will go down."

"Yes. And if the cardiac output goes down, what will happen to his blood pressure?"

"It will drop," Stef says.

"So put yourself in the vision, Stef. I know you are nervous about being the night-float tonight, so let's just address that. You're on call tonight and the pager goes off. One of the patients you are cross-covering has a large bloody bowel movement. The nurse wants to know what to do. What do you do?" Stef looks frozen. It is clear that he is deeply in the vision, which has struck to the core of his fears. "Don't panic, now. Think through it just like you did with me. He's had a big GI bleed … What happens to his preload?"

The measure of performance is not what happens in a conference room. The attending paints a very scary vision to test the intern's ability to perform under duress. Anticipating that performance will drop under crisis, the attending teaches the intern how to use his method to work his way out of the problem and identify the right things to do.

"Okay, I would go see the patient and …" Stef pauses to think. Phaedrus waits and Stef begins to talk out loud. Phaedrus is thinking, "Exactly, Stef. Exactly what I want you to do. Talk it out now … just like you will when it actually happens."'

Stef continues, "So if the preload dropped, the stroke volume would drop, and the cardiac output would drop, and his blood pressure would drop … Okay, I would check the vital signs and see how much his blood pressure had dropped."

"Fantastic. And look at Equation 5 carefully now. If the preload and thus the stroke volume had both dropped, how would the body compensate to keep the cardiac output the same?"

"Well … oh, I would check the heart rate as well. If preload and stroke volume dropped, the heart rate would go up."

"Excellent. So you'll check the blood pressure and the heart rate to see how much preload he had lost. If the blood pressure is low, and the heart rate is high, then you know there's been a pretty big bleed. That will give you an idea of how serious this is. Let's say it's the worst case … pretty serious. What are you going to do then?"

"Well, I would call Moni."

"Perfect. And Moni, let's say you are on your way." Phaedrus looks to Moni, who looks equally nervous. "Stef, what can you do in the meantime while you are waiting for Moni to arrive? Look at your

equations and work backwards. The mean arterial pressure is low; how could you fix that? Start with Equation 4."

The best way to absolve the nervousness that goes with fear is to acknowledge it outright: "We have nothing to fear but fear itself."

"Well, I could increase the systemic vascular resistance."

"Yes. We would use pressers to do that, but that will mean transferring him to the ICU. And it is good of you to start thinking that way. It might be worth a call to the ICU resident as well, just so that she is aware. But is there anything else you could do? Look at Equations 5 and 6."

"Well, the heart rate is already high. I guess pressors would do that too. Hmm … and we could increase the contractility…. That would be pressors again."

"Anything you could do without the ICU, Stef." Phaedrus waits patiently.

"Oh, I could increase the preload. I would start two large-bore IVs and start normal saline. I could also transfuse him, so I would draw some blood to type and cross."

"See, Stef, it's not that hard. Well done. Moni, anything else to add?"

"It would be worth getting some coags to make sure we didn't need to fix that. And of course to stop any of his blood pressure medications that might make the blood pressure lower."

"Nice. Stef, that feeling you just had … you know, where you thought you might have a patient with a large bloody bowel movement?"

"Yeah."

"You are going to have that feeling again when it happens in real life. Probably even more intense. And when that day does come, and you have that feeling, I want you to remember what you did here to get out of it. You talked out loud, systematically working through your method. And your method took you to the right answers, even after you had forgotten what to do in the panic of the moment."

"Thanks, Dr. Phaedrus."

This ends block four: Equations 4, 5, and 6. Other disease dialogues could be used to test the learner's competence, and this sequence of equations will set up quick "on the wards" talks about the diagnosis and rational management of hypotension, hypertension, myocardial infarction, congestive heart failure, sepsis, and the effect of other fluid-loss diseases (such as ascites, pancreatitis, and dehydration) and other fluid-gain conditions (such as renal failure and pregnancy) on hemodynamics.

"Okay, Paul, let's review. Equation 1 got the oxygen into the alveoli. Equation 2 took the oxygen to the blood. Equation 3 told us we would need trucks (hemoglobin), saturation of the trucks (oxygen saturation), and speed of the trucks (cardiac output) to get the oxygen to the tissues. And Equations 4, 5, and 6 gave us a method for figuring out what went wrong if the cardiac output wasn't sufficient—that is, if our trucks weren't moving fast enough—and 4, 5, and 6 also gave us a method for dealing with hypertension and hypotension. So, now let me ask you. How much is enough? I mean, Paul, how much oxygen delivery to the tissues do we need? Put another way, how much bread does Moni have to deliver to the grocery stores?"

"Hmm. I don't know. As much as they need, I guess?"

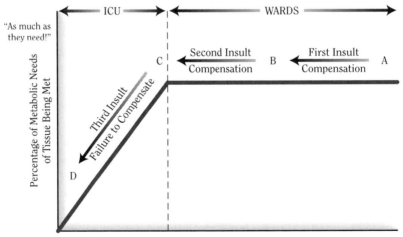

Figure 7-2 Metabolic needs vs. oxygen delivery. DO_2 = oxygen delivery; ICU = intensive care unit.

"Correct! Well done, Paul." Phaedrus draws the graph in Figure 7-2 as he speaks. "Listen, I'm going to draw you this graph … I'm going to label the y-axis as 'as much as they need'—that is the 'metabolic needs of the tissue'—and I'm going to label the x-axis as the 'delivery of oxygen to the tissues.' One of the rare times in medicine that the x- axis is something other than time. Okay?"

Phaedrus turns from the board. "I've labeled four points on the graph: A, B, C, and D. Moni, are you still thinking about that GI bleed patient that Stef was dealing with on night float?"

"Actually, yes. It's kind of nerve-wracking. I mean, I've done both the ICU and the wards as an intern, but I still don't have a good idea of who goes to the ICU, when, and why."

"Well, I have something special for you then. So help me out with these questions, Moni. At point A, here," Phaedrus points to point A on the graph, "we'll say that the delivery of oxygen, or the 'DO$_2$,' is normal, and the metabolic needs of the tissues are being met." Phaedrus points to the corresponding part of the y-axis. "So, Moni, name me a disease that might take us from point A to point B—remember your Equation 3."

"Well, it looks like the DO$_2$ has decreased as you go from point A to point B. And Equation 3 is the DO$_2$ … the number of trucks, the speed of the trucks, and the saturation. So that would be something like, well, the GI bleed we just talked about. Both the hemoglobin and the preload would go down, so the DO$_2$ would decrease."

Phaedrus turns to Paul. "Paul, do you follow that?"

"Sure."

Higher-level questions are best directed to higher-level learners, both to maintain clarity for the group (the answers are likely to be correct and more clear) and to involve the higher-level learners in the discussion. To ensure that lower-level learners are not getting lost, it is worth intermittently asking them to confirm their understanding.

"But Moni, what happened to the metabolic needs of the tissues being met as you moved from point A to point B?" Phaedrus points to the same point on the y-axis.

"It stayed the same?"

"Well, how is that possible?" Phaedrus asks.

Paul interjects. "Is that because of the compensation you talked about before ... you know, the heart rate going up?"

"No. Remember all of that compensation is to keep the cardiac output—and thus the DO_2—at the same level. In this case, we are past that compensation point. The body has raised its heart rate as much as it can, and the DO_2 has still decreased. But again, how is it possible that the 'grocery stores' are still getting the same amount of bread as they did before, even with less delivery?"

Moni thinks for a while. Phaedrus waits, counting down on the internal 5-second clock. Then she speaks. "I got it. They are taking more bread off of the truck with each pass."

"I was told you were a superstar, Moni. I'm starting to see why." Moni smiles. She is proud, and has the look of someone who is starting to have fun again. "Yes, I won't get into the details, but you remember that when the tissue beds become hypoxic, the elevated CO_2, the 2,3-diphosphoglycerate, and the acid environment will shift the oxygen dissociation curve such that more oxygen is removed from each hemoglobin molecule. That is, more bread is removed from each truck."

A fundamental principle of "winning friends and influencing people" is that people like to hear that they are talked about in a favorable way. The "superstar" comment is motivating for the resident; it's the first day on call as a resident, and boosting her confidence will improve her performance.

"Now, Moni. Stef's patient is having a GI bleed ... he's lost preload and he's lost hemoglobin. The heart rate is high, and the increased work of the heart has caused him to have chest pain. In fact, he's now had an MI, and he's lost some contractility of the left ventricle. The stroke volume decreases because of that, and the cardiac output decreases. The DO_2 decreases even more, and we move from point B to point C ... and still the metabolic needs are being met, extracting even more oxygen from the hemoglobin."

"I think at this point I would take him to the ICU," Moni says.

"But tell me why. And as you formulate your answer, I want you to think about what happens to the cells for every increment the DO_2 moves to the left of point C."

"Well, as the DO_2 starts to drop—that is, as we move to the left of point C—well, the metabolic needs of the tissues stop being met,

probably because the tissues have reached their max in compensating by extracting more oxygen."

"Exactly, Moni. And past point C—we'll just call point C the 'critical care point' if that's all right with you—the point where the body has done all that it can to compensate for the insult … for every increment to the left, some cells die."

Phaedrus follows the graph with his pen right down to point D and then turns to the team. "And that will continue down to point D— D for disability." Phaedrus pauses. "So Moni, which, why, and when do patients go to the ICU? Think about what defined point C."

"Well, at the point that the body has done all that it can in compensating for the insult."

"Indeed. And that's where the body needs you to step in to compensate for it. And I'm sure Stef knows … Stef, have you done the ICU yet?"

"No, not yet. I'm not looking forward to it."

"Well, don't sweat it. The only difference between the ICU and floors is that you have a lot of nurses … one for every one to two patients in the ICU. There's really nothing different about the place. Let me ask you, Stef—and Moni, you correct me if I'm wrong with this—what are the things that we can do in the ICU to fix this problem? Start with the basis of the problem: The DO_2 is below the level it needs to be to maintain the needs of the tissues."

"Well, we have to increase the DO_2. That's the problem."

"Okay, Equation 3. How would you do it?" Phaedrus waits for the response.

"Well … ventilate the patient … that would increase the oxygen saturation."

"Great. That would be Equations 1 and 2. Right?" All three nod. "And what else?"

"And … transfuse the patient … that would increase the hemoglobin … and give fluids and pressers … that would increase the cardiac output by increasing the preload, contractility, and heart rate." Stef has learned the method.

"Correct. That would be Equations 3, 4, 5, and 6 if I'm not mistaken." Phaedrus pauses to let the connection between the equations

sink in. "See, Stef, nothing to be afraid of in the ICU. That's about all that we do there. Am I right, Moni?"

"Yeah, that's basically it. I guess I had never really thought of it that way."

Linking the equations reinforces each of them. This serves to demystify the ICU, which novice learners will see as a "magic car wash" where really sick patients go for awhile, and then they come back all fixed. This also enables the learners to see the key elements in this area of transition of care.

"So you see, you know the answer to that question ... who goes to the ICU ... People who have maxed out their compensation and need our help to do it for them."

"Yeah, I guess so. I feel better about that. Is there anything we can do to decrease the metabolic needs of the tissues? That might rematch the metabolic needs with the DO_2."

"A few things ... we'll talk about managing sepsis, seizures, and euthyroid sick later. For now, it sounds like the ER is calling you. Let's take a break there and we'll pick up with Equation 8 later."

The importance of Equation 7 is that it illustrates that no physiologic variable can be considered in isolation. The case in this dialogue focused on the extreme example (the patient with a GI bleed going to the unit). This will serve as a foundation for "on the wards" discussions about interpreting variables such as ejection fraction, hemoglobin, and saturation in the context of the patient's illness (metabolic needs) and the patient's other organ dysfunctions that might limit compensation.

Dialogue Part 3: Equations 8, 9, and 10

"All right, Paul, where were we with our equations? Seems like we only had two or three to go."

"We got through Equations 1 to 7 ... you said we start with Equation 8," Paul says.

"Indeed," Phaedrus replies. "Paul, let me ask you: What happens to the oxygen once we deliver it to the tissues?"

"Well, it's used to make adenosine triphosphate, with glucose, of course. Glycolysis."

"Absolutely right. It's metabolized. That's the 'metabolic rate.' And what is the byproduct of that metabolism?"

"Carbon dioxide … CO_2."

"Indeed. So our last problem in this circuit is how to get the waste—the CO_2—out of the system. And to help us with that is Equation 8." Phaedrus begins to draw a picture of a bathtub and then writes out Equation 8. *"Do you have a bathtub, Paul?"*

"Umm … no, I have a shower."

"Okay, have you seen a bathtub? Maybe on TV?"

Paul laughs. *"Yes. I know what a bathtub is."*

"Okay. So here's the problem to pose to you. If the bathtub has too much water in it, there are only two explanations. What are those explanations?"

"Well, there's too much faucet, or not enough drain."

"Great. And if the bathtub has too little water in it, what are the explanations?"

"Well, there's too little faucet or too much drain."

The bathtub "advanced organizer" will be used throughout the month to explain anemia, thrombocytopenia, calcium, or any any topic where the problem is "too much" or "too little."

"Excellent. Let's say your patient has too much CO_2—that is, too much water in his bathtub. What are the only two causes?"

"Well, too much being made … that would be the faucet. Or, not enough elimination of the CO_2 … that would be the drain."

"Indeed, Paul. And for most patients, we'll assume that the cause of their increased CO_2 is not because they had just finished doing 100 one-armed pushups."

Moni laughs. *"I think that's safe to say."*

"Well, you never know," Phaedrus replies. *"I can do 100 one-armed pushups—as far as you know."* All three laugh. *"Okay, Paul. What's the drain? How does the body get rid of CO_2?"*

"The lungs."

"Indeed." Phaedrus writes in the back half of Equation 8. *"The drain for CO_2 is the 'minute ventilation,' or the 'ventilations per*

minute.' That is, the respiratory rate times the volume of respiration per breath—otherwise known as the tidal volume. But remember that you don't get credit for the whole tidal volume. Some of this is deadspace."

Paul interjects, "I remember that. That's the part of the tidal volume that doesn't get to the alveoli."

"Correct, you are, Paul, and since CO_2 can make its way only into alveoli that have blood flow to them, that is, the non-deadspace areas of the lung, only non-deadspace ventilation contributes to removing the CO_2." Phaedrus pauses." Let me draw this figure, and don't have a post-traumatic stress disorder attack—I'm taking you back to first year of medical school." Phaedrus draws out the West zones (Figure 7-3).

"Now look at this. There are two variables on the board: pulmonary artery pressure and pulmonary alveolar pressure ... only

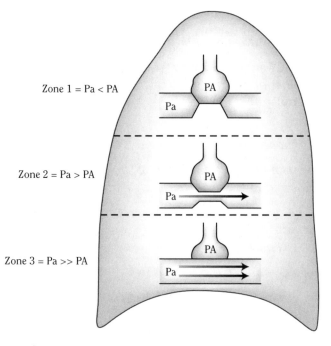

Figure 7-3 Pulmonary lung zones. Pa = pulmonary artery pressure; PA = pulmonary alveolar pressure.

two variables. What is the difference between zone 1 and zone 3, and why?"

Paul jumps on the chance to answer something that he knows. "Well, in zone 1, there is less pulmonary artery pressure, so the alveolar pressure overcomes the pulmonary artery and squishes it. That makes it deadspace—ventilation put no perfusion."

"Indeed. And why is that not the case in zone 3?"

"Gravity."

"Well done, Paul. Now tell me. How could I make zone 2 look like zone 1? That is, how could I make zone 2 deadspace? Remember, there are only two variables on the board, and for zone 1, the definition of deadspace, the pulmonary alveolar pressure was much greater than the pulmonary arterial pressure."

The attending more or less gives the answer to the question even as he is asking it. For tougher questions, leading the audience with the answer allows them to get the information while still interacting with the content (answering the question themselves). With respect to retention, a question that a learner answers correctly, even if spoon-fed, is 10 times as valuable as a piece of knowledge that is merely provided.

Stef interjects, "Can I do this one?"

"Sure. Have at it."

"Well, either the pulmonary alveolar pressure is increased … or the pulmonary artery pressure is decreased."

"Great. And can you think of a disease that would, say, degrade the collagenous support of the bronchial walls such that on inspiration they popped open, but on exhalation they flopped closed, trapping air and pressure in the alveoli?" Phaedrus draws the picture of a floppy bronchiole to illustrate the point.

"Uh, yeah. That's chronic obstructive pulmonary disease. The floppy bronchioles result from the oxidative damage from long-term smoking."

"Fantastic. We'll spend some time later this month talking about COPD. But before we leave this topic, I want to remind you that there are two variables up there. Moni, this is probably at your level, but later on I want to talk about how biventricular heart failure, especially if you overdiurese it, can lead to very low pul-

monary artery pressures and resulting deadspace. Can you see how that might happen?"

"Sure."

"Can you see how that patient might be dyspneic because of the elevated CO_2 because of the increased deadspace?"

"Yeah."

"Can you see how a patient with biventricular heart failure who is dyspneic might be given even more diuretics under the erroneous belief that she had pulmonary edema?"

"I can," Moni replies.

"And can you see how you could kill that patient by diuresing them more?"

"Yes," Moni responds.

"Okay, we'll talk more about this when we address heart failure and the dyspnea pyramid. But this is a quick reminder to you all: When dyspnea is present, you need to get an arterial blood gas. Be disciplined in your method. It will ensure that you never make that mistake."

"Got it." Moni makes a mental note.

"Paul, will you keep a list of the topics we want to talk about?" Paul nods. "Okay, write that one down—dyspnea pyramid and congestive heart failure."

The attending gives just enough of the biventricular heart failure talk to consolidate the point at hand, but remains disciplined in not going on a tangent. When tempted to digress, use the learners as the "scorekeepers," keeping track of the agenda of topics to be discussed later.

"Okay, Stef, let's see if learning took place here. You are called to see a patient tonight who is short of breath. In addition to a history and physical examination, what do you do first?"

"Well, based on what you just said, I would get an arterial blood gas?"

"Learning did take place. How about that? And let's say the CO_2 is elevated. Talk me through your method ... look at Equation 8 now."

"I would first exclude one-armed pushups." Phaedrus smiles. "Okay, then I would look at the respiratory rate to make sure that was adequate."

"And let's say that his breathing was appropriate for the elevated CO_2 was normal or high, Stef. What next?" Phaedrus crosses out "respiratory rate" on the board.

"Then I would look at depth of the respirations."

"And let's say that was normal—big deep breaths—that can't be the problem." Phaedrus crosses out "tidal volume." "What's left?"

"Well, the only thing left would be deadspace. I guess I would listen to his lungs to see if there was wheezing—that might suggest COPD or asthma."

"Fantastic. And what could you do to decrease the deadspace?"

"Well, bronchodilators … and steroids."

"Nice. And maybe some noninvasive ventilation … we'll talk about that later. Paul, you got that?" Paul nods as he writes it down.

The attending has clearly found the intern's hook: He's deathly afraid of night float, and each successive example couched in night float is not only increasing attention and thus motivation to learn it but also creating a series of visions in which the intern succeeds in each scenario. Success begins with visualizing success.

"All right, Paul. That completes the circuit. We have successfully taken oxygen from the lungs, to the tissues, made some adenosine triphosphate, and eliminated the CO_2. This is the skeleton of internal medicine—almost everything else we talk about this month will just be 'flesh' that you can hang on this skeleton. But there are two important details we need to discuss. You see, this whole discussion has presumed that the chambers in the body— the alveoli, the heart, the arteries, the veins—all of that was intact. So to really ensure that this system works, we have to know a little something about the chambers in the body. Can you see how a disruption in the chambers—leaky chambers—would cause chaos in this system?"

"Yeah, I can see that." Paul replies.

The dialogue continues here, but this is another natural break point. Equations 9 and 10 can be done separately if time does not allow.

"Okay, then, Equation 9 … This is Starling's law of fluid flow across a membrane." Phaedrus writes the equation on the board. "Do you remember this, Paul?"

"I do. But I always forget the equation."

"Indeed. Let's talk through it, and then I'll give you a simple way to remember it. Okay, to start, what would fluid flow across easier, a very permeable membrane, or a not-so-permeable membrane?"

"Permeable, of course."

"Okay, so we'll put the letter 'K' first—that will be the permeability of the membrane. Now, I think we can agree that a higher pressure gradient pushing the fluid across the membrane will result in more fluid going across the membrane. Is that safe to say?"

"Sure."

"Okay, hold that in your left hand; keep your right hand free to work with the next concept. I think we can also agree that osmotic molecules inside a chamber will hold on to more fluid, and osmotic molecules outside of the chamber will draw more fluid out of the chamber. Is that safe to say?"

Paul thinks for a moment. "Um, yes … that's right."

"Okay, so let me rearrange the terms here a bit, and I'll give you an easy way to remember it." Phaedrus writes as he speaks. "The fluid flow across a membrane is the permeability of the membrane—K—times the following. There are two sets of parentheses in the brackets. We'll put the 'Ps' first, and the 'Os' second." He writes a P in the first parentheses and an O in the second, then repeats the act as he says, "Post office box, post office box—do you see, 'P's' in the first parentheses and 'Os' in the second." Paul nods. "Okay, Paul, it's minuses all the way across: Minus, minus, minus." Phaedrus writes in the minuses in the equation. "Now, Stef, you're from California, right?"

"That's right."

"So the quintessential fast-food restaurant is …?"

"In-N-Out Burger."

"Indeed." In each set of parentheses, Phaedrus fills in the subscripts for each letter as he speaks, "In-N-Out Burger … In-N-Out

Burger." He pauses. "Not Out-N-In Burger, Paul … that would be gross." The three team members laugh. "So in sum, Paul, it's the permeability constant times the difference in the hydrostatic pressures—the 'Ps'—minus the difference in the oncotic pressure— the 'Os.'"

"Wow, I think I can remember that," Paul says.

It is important for the attending to ensure that the mnemonics used to simply complex problems, or in this case, Equation 9, are not more difficult to remember than the actual problem being solved. An added layer of teaching (the instruction booklet for how to use the tool) may be required.

"All right, Paul, so here is where we are going to use this equation. Whenever there is 'fluid where fluid should not be', we are going to use this equation. Stef, can you think of a patient who might have 'fluid where fluid should not be'?"

"Sure. Heart failure. Those patients have fluid in their lungs, peripheral edema, and sometimes ascites."

"Well done." Phaedrus pauses, "Okay, Paul, this is going to be your method. We will always start with the 'Ps.' Now I'll tell you, 'fluid where fluid shouldn't be' is almost always due to too much pressure inside the chamber—it is almost always not due to too little pressure outside of the chamber. Do you understand that?" Paul nods. "Okay then, here is your method. Look at my chest. Can you visualize where my aorta would be?" Paul nods again.

"All right, then, we are going to start at the aortic valve and work our way all the way back to where the fluid is; knowing, of course, that a valve stenosis or incompetence, or any obstruction to fluid along the way, will put increased back pressure all the way down the system. So, Paul, let's say Stef gets called tonight for a patient who has peripheral edema. And you are still around to go see the patient with him. You are starting at the aortic valve—what are the causes of the increased pressure?"

"Well, as you said, aortic stenosis … and aortic insufficiency."

"Good, so can you see yourself listening for a murmur?" Paul nods. Stef nods. The mere mention of night float has reengaged him. "Great, what's next?"

"Well, the left ventricle … so left ventricular failure."

"Good, so that might result from a new myocardial infarction. Can you see yourself getting an EKG? Maybe even ordering an echo?" Stef nods. "There are other causes of left ventricular failure to consider, and we'll talk about that as well as it comes up this month. Write that down, Paul." Paul obliges. "So, then, what's next?"

The attending not only walks through the method but also links the physical examination and laboratory tests that would be useful in evaluating each diagnosis. In essence, the diagnostic strategy is being laid down simultaneously with the method. This is the way the attending wants the learner to think: Let your differential diagnosis drive the diagnostic testing strategy.

"Well, mitral stenosis or mitral insufficiency."

"Good. You would listen to the heart for that murmur as well. Then maybe left atrial obstruction—it's an academic institution, Paul—atrial myxomas can happen." Stef laughs. Phaedrus continues. "Okay, then pulmonary hypertension … we'll talk about that later as well. But let me stop here. Paul, for any of the abnormalities we have just mentioned, will the pressure in the pulmonary capillaries be increased or decreased?"

"It will be increased, of course."

"And if there is increased pressure in the vessels, what will be the fluid flow from the vessels into the pulmonary interstitium? Look at Equation 9 carefully."

"It will be increased," Paul replies.

"Pulmonary edema," Stef adds.

"Exactly, so that's the first clue as you work through this method. Look not only for where the 'fluid is that it shouldn't be'"— Phaedrus made the quotes sign as he says this—"But also where else there is 'fluid where fluid shouldn't be.' That will tell you where the obstruction or incompetence in the chamber exists. So for all of these causes, we could listen for crackles or get a chest x-ray to see if fluid was there as well. Am I right?"

"Sure," says Stef.

Teaching the pathophysiology of a disease allows learners to link multiple symptoms into one disease state. It moves the phase 1 clinical reasoning to phase 2 (see chapter 4).

"Okay, let's keep going. Then pulmonary stenosis and pulmonary insufficiency—also very rare, you understand, but it could happen, especially here. Now your turn, Stef, what's next?"

Even as the method is taught, it is worth calling out the prevalence of the diseases on the method. This helps the learner move from phase 2 to phase 3 clinical reasoning (see chapter 4).

"Well, right ventricular failure and tricuspid disease."

"Good, and remember that right ventricular failure is usually due to right ventricle infarcts, or compression around the right ventricle like you might see with tamponade or constrictive pericarditis. Hey, Paul, if the obstruction was at this level, would we see pulmonary edema?"

"No, the obstruction would be before the lungs."

"Remember that. It will be important. Okay, so we have tricuspid stenosis, tricuspid insufficiency, right atrial myxoma … rare … Hey, Paul, what will the jugular venous distension be with all of the causes up to this point? Increased distension or decreased?"

"Well, it would be increased."

"Indeed it would. So continuing on … Paul, are you following the anatomy on my body as we move through this system?" Paul nods. *"Good, that's what I want you to do it. If you ever forget this information, just look at your patient's aortic valve, and start moving backwards, chamber by chamber."* Phaedrus pauses. *"But when we get down to my ileac veins, look away."* Paul laughs. *"All right, so inferior vena cava obstruction, like you might see with a thrombus, or compression on the vessel from a tumor or a baby— cirrhosis or hepatic vein thrombosis if we are headed to ascites— and if we are headed to peripheral edema, then a deep venous thrombosis or venous incompetence in the legs. You can add on lymphatic incompetence as well, I suppose. Same principle. How would you diagnose these, Stef?"*

"Well, I guess a CT for the obstruction in the abdomen, or for the legs, and ultrasound—all of these wouldn't have jugular venous pressure or pulmonary edema either."

"Wow. Fantastic thinking, Stef." Phaedrus extends a handshake. *"But we're not done, are we? What else is on the equation, Paul?"*

"Oncotic pressure."

"Right. Oncotic pressure is mostly due to albumin in the blood—that is, protein. So imagine yourself eating a large porterhouse steak ... lots of protein in that. Follow the steak into your gut, and then to the liver, where it's turned into albumin. So first, it's not having the porterhouse steak ... that is, not eating enough protein. Kwashiorkor, I believe. Then it's not being able to absorb the steak ... protein-losing enteropathy. Then it's liver failure. And we can talk about liver failure later. Paul, write that down for us." Paul obliges. *"And then, Paul, think about ways that the body loses protein ... so pancreatitis, burns, and the nephrotic syndrome. How would you diagnose these, Stef? Would the edema with these causes be just in one spot, or would it be all over? That is to say, would you have lots of protein in one part of the body, and no protein in other parts?"*

"I would guess that it would be all over—we could also measure the albumin level and ask about the dietary history."

"Indeed, Stef. Well done. So one small point: As opposed to hydrostatic pressure, where the 'outside' pressure didn't play much of a role, the 'outside oncotic pressure' can actually play a role here. Imagine, for example, that you had a bacterial infection in your pleural space or in your abdomen—the protein in the bacteria might pull some fluid toward it. We'll talk about that more when we talk about ascites. Wow, Paul, we're building a pretty good list, huh?

"Yes, we are."

"Well okay, the last part of the equation is the permeability constant. And it's a short list, but here goes: sepsis, anaphylaxis, hypothyroidism, inflammation and, let's see, yes, pit viper bites. But that's pretty rare." Paul laughs. *"Seriously, though, think of inflammation as disrupting the permeability constant. Have you ever sprained your ankle, Paul?"*

"Sure," Paul answers.

"Did it swell?"

"Yes."

"Well, that's 'fluid where fluid shouldn't be'—actually the swelling is a good thing since it stabilizes the joint. But we can agree that 'normal' ankles aren't swollen."

"That's pretty cool—you sure know a lot."

"No, not really, Paul. I just have very good methods. And after this month, you'll have most of those methods, too. The rest is just because I have more experience. But remember, practice doesn't make perfect ... perfect practice makes perfect. Experience without methods is just making the same mistakes over and over again."

Attendings often worry about not looking smart enough. What they should worry about is looking too smart because this image is daunting to learners who can't imagine ever knowing that much. Learners should be redirected to the methods that enable the perception of "knowing a lot."

At the end of the method, Phaedrus takes the time to ask Stef to go through how he would approach a patient who presented with new-onset ascites. Feeling confident that Stef has mastered the method, he asks Moni to do the same for a pleural effusion. Feeling confident that the team has mastered the concept of 'fluid where fluid shouldn't be,' he moves on to Equation 10.

"So, Moni, one quick last method—and I'll make it quick, because I see that your pager is going off. Equation 10 is Laplace's law. It defines how chambers handle pressure. This is less about diagnosis and more about understanding what happens to chambers with too much pressure if we don't do something about it. It's about understanding the natural history of disease, and how complications develop will help you recognize the relative importance and urgency of treating disease. This is especially true for silent diseases like hypertension and diabetes."

Novice physicians see all disease as more or less the same: It needs to be cured. Providing an understanding how a disease causes the complications it does can give insight into why we manage different diseases the way we do.

"I think we have a few minutes. This is 7 West telling me that Mrs. Roberts has arrived on the floor," says Moni.

"Okay, I'll make it fast. Real patients are better than conference rooms. So Laplace's law defines wall tension in a chamber, Paul. And that's important to us because wall tension is proportional to popping ... and in medicine, Paul, just like in surgery, letting things pop is very poor form." The three laugh. Phaedrus contin-

ues. *"Paul, have you ever blown up a balloon? You know, like a clown does."*

"Umm, sure."

"Did you ever blow up a balloon … and blow so hard that it made your cheeks tingle and hurt … you know, like when you first start blowing up the balloon?"

"Yeah."

"I hate that." Phaedrus replies. "Do you like clowns?"

"No, not really"

"Me either … in fact, they creep me out." Paul waits in silence. Phaedrus continues, "Okay, well, that's not the point, but here is. When did the balloon pop? When you first started blowing it up, or when it got really big?"

"When it got big."

"Indeed, and the reason is because that is when the wall tension was the greatest …. Because at that point, Paul, you had put a lot of pressure into the balloon—am I right?" Paul nods. "And the balloon had a very big radius—am I right?" Paul nods again. "And the wall of the balloon had been stretched very thin—am I right about that?"

"Yes. Right on all three accounts."

"So here it is, Paul." Phaedrus writes out Equation 10 as he speaks. "The wall tension of a chamber—its risk for popping—is proportional to the pressure in the chamber times the radius of the chamber to the fourth power, divided by the wall thickness." Phaedrus pauses. "This is simply to say that the bigger a chamber gets, the greater the risk for popping. Kind of like a pulmonary bleb in a COPD patient, or an aortic aneurysm, or a bowel obstruction … right, Moni?"

"That's right."

"Confirm this for me, Moni. What is the indication for operating on an abdominal aortic aneurysm?"

"When it gets to be 5 centimeters in diameter."

"Five centimeters ... not the appearance, not even the pressure ... but the size of the aneurysm. How about that. Why do you suppose that is, Stef?"

"Well, because wall tension is proportional to the radius to the fourth power ... that makes it the critical variable."

"Indeed. And Stef, let me ask you ... what does the left ventricle look like in a patient who has aortic stenosis or long-standing hypertension?"

"It's thick."

"That's right. But why do you suppose that is?" Stef pauses. Phaedrus waits for 5 seconds and then brings him along in the method.

Once a student stalls at 5 seconds, he should be brought along in the method.

"What's the pressure in the ventricle for a patient with aortic stenosis or a very high afterload resistance ... that is, hypertension? Will it be higher or lower than a normal left ventricle?"

"It will be higher."

"Right. And what will the wall tension be? Look at Equation 10."

"It will be higher."

"So the ventricle will blow apart unless the body does something to correct the problem. It can't do much about the radius, but it could do something about the ..."

Stef has it. He jumps back in: "It will increase its wall thickness."

"Indeed it will. So the left ventricle will be thick, huh?" Stef nods. "We'll spend some time with the cardiac exam later. Write that down, Paul." Phaedrus pauses. "I'll show you how to feel the point of maximum impulse to get a gestalt of how long your patient has had hypertension." Phaedrus pauses again. "Hey, Stef, what do you suppose the pressure in the vessels will be for someone who has had hypertension for a long time?"

"Increased, I suppose," Stef replies.

"And what would be the wall thickness of those vessels?"

"They would be thicker."

"And wouldn't it be cool if you could take out a few of those vessels and just look at them—and then you'd know, right? Just how long this patient had had hypertension. Because it's always the question for the patient who presents with hypertension, you wonder, 'Wow, I wonder just how long this patient has had hypertension?' Because you know that the longer she's had it, the greater the risk to the heart and other organs. Well, if you could just look at those vessels, you would know. Wouldn't that be cool?"

"Yeah, it sure would be."

"Do you have an ophthalmoscope, Stef?"

There was silence. Stef finally replies, "So you're saying that I could look at the retinal vessels and know how long someone has had hypertension. And that could tell me how much damage there might have been to the other organs ... like the heart and the kidneys."

"That's exactly what I'm saying." Phaedrus puts his lab coat back on as he speaks. "You see Stef ... and Paul ... and Moni ... internal medicine is not a game of checkers where you just wait for your opponent to move and then you respond. This is a strategy game like chess. You have to think several moves ahead before you move your piece ... and in a Sun Tzu sort of way, the more you know about how your opponent will behave—what your opponent will do—the greater your chance of heading off your opponent and winning the game. We're fighting disease here, and we have the advantage—we have a mind; disease does not. It has to do what it was destined to do. But you have to learn about those destinies. Equation 10 is an example of thinking about how the disease ends up, which enables you to prevent it from happening in the first place."

"Wow. That's deep," Stef replies.

"I'll just pretend that you mean that in a complimentary way," says Phaedrus, smiling. "But wait and see if I'm not right. Okay, go get at that patient. Moni, call me if you need me. Anytime for anything." Phaedrus pauses at the door. "And Paul ... tell me tomorrow: Which do you take to the operating room first, a small bowel obstruction or a large bowel obstruction? I've been wondering about that. By Equation 10, I'm sure you'll figure it out."

There are two rules for student assignments. First, students must always be given time to show their work whenever it was scheduled to be reported, lest they learn that there is a probability with every future assignment that they might not actually have to do it. Second, assignments that are creative and not drudgery, like the riddle in this dialogue, inspire the student to think and to read. The goal is not in finding the answer. The goal is inspiring thinking and reading: life-long habits.

❖ Congestive Heart Failure

Purpose
Of all diagnoses seen on the internal medicine wards, congestive heart failure has one of the highest mortalities and one of the highest rates of re-admission. As such, coaching students and resident in the management of heart failure is an opportunity for the attending to teach the principles of heart failure management to ensure successful clinical outcomes, and to teach the principles of transitions of care.

The second part of this dialogue illustrates an important teaching principle of hospital medicine: selectively choosing which topics will be taught in detail. Although the management of all issues has been addressed as part of the clinical discussion, the attending in this dialogue adeptly recognizes that time will not permit detailed teaching of all topics. But the multiple-day stay that is typical of inpatient admissions is the luxury of hospital medicine: the luxury of choosing which teaching topics will be taught in detail on one day, and choosing teaching topics that will be deferred to subsequent days.

Setting, Cast of Characters, and Abbreviations
The team is rounding post-call and consists of the attending, Phaedrus; the resident, Moni; the intern, Stef; and the medical student, Paul. The attending has read his team and sees that they have had a difficult first night. Although there were not that many admissions, the work intensity was clearly high, and the team looks fatigued. The attending has elected to start the 7 a.m. post-call rounds in a conference room, where the team can have some coffee, followed by on-the-ward work rounds. This dialogue takes place in the conference room.

The following abbreviations are used in this dialogue: ACE = angiotensin-converting enzyme inhibitors; ATPase = adenosine triphosphatase; BNP = brain natriuretic peptide; CHF = congestive heart failure; DIG = Digitalis Investigation Group; EKG = electrocardiogram; ER = emergency room; ICU = intensive care unit; JG = juxtaglomerular; JVP = jugular venous pressure; SVR = systemic vascular resistance.

The attending's investment in the "10 Equations" on the previous on-call day will afford him the great luxury of referring to the equations to quickly teach the principles of diagnosing and managing congestive heart failure. The reiteration of the principles on the post-call day is also valuable in consolidating the lessons. It is also motivating in that the familiarity of the 10 equations provides a sense of psychological security: *"I learned something yesterday, and now I'm using it. Maybe I'll eventually get my arms around this task."*

Dialogue

Paul begins rounds by presenting his first patient.

"Our first patient is Mr. Lawrence. He is a 55-year-old man who presented with 3 days of progressive shortness of breath. He noted associated leg swelling and the inability to sleep while lying flat..." *Paul continues his presentation through the physical examination and laboratory values. He stops as he approaches the assessment and plan. "So that's Mr. Lawrence."*

"Well done, Paul. What is your assessment?"

"Umm, I don't really know. We started him on Lasix, and I guess our plan was to discuss him with you."

"A good plan ... that's what I'm here for. But it could be made even better if you told me what you thought was causing his symptoms, and what we should do for him."

"Me?" says Paul with a frightened face.

"That's okay, Paul. I know it's the first post-call day. Going forward, here's what I want you to do." Phaedrus looks at the team. "It's very important to me that you invest in your patients ... I want you to be their doctors. Take your best shot at making the diagnosis, and then have the courage to present what you decided, and what you decided to do. I'm not going to get mad at you or belittle you if you get a diagnosis or management decision wrong. That's part of learning how to do this ... so 'discussing with me' is a fine idea, but I never want that to be all that there is to your 'plan.'"

Even after expectations have been laid out for the team (see chapter 2), the attending should anticipate that the team will initially revert to what they have seen in their past experience. It may take additional "doses" of the expectations, especially for getting learners to engage in active decision-making.

> *The team nods in agreement. Paul begins again. "Well, we did think that it was congestive heart failure. His BNP was 860, so I guess our plan was to try to make that normal."*

> *Phaedrus chokes back the impulse to explode at hearing the physical examination reduced to the BNP, and instead spends some time talking through the differential diagnosis with the team, outlining the clinical reasoning that they had done but not clearly elucidated. Then he turns to Paul, "Paul, how have you seen congestive heart failure managed?"*

The student is demonstrating that he sees all lab values as the same: "They must all be made normal." The underlying motivation, however, is to remain within his world of "security." It is much safer to treat a number than it is to engage in assessing and managing the patient. The attending redirects the discussion to the physical examination, which brings the focus back to managing the patient, not the laboratory value.

> *"Well, I haven't really. I guess Lasix is the treatment," Paul says.*

> *"Or furosemide …" Paul looks confused, but he would get the point later when he looks up furosemide. "Well … let's talk through it. Do you remember Equations 4, 5, and 6?"*

> *"Kind of … I'm not sure I remember the numbers," says Paul.*

> *Phaedrus laughs. "That's okay, it's the principles I care about. Let me ask you this, Paul. What do you suppose caused Mr. Lawrence's heart failure?"*

> *"Well, he did have a heart attack a few years ago … probably that."*

> *"A myocardial infarction, you mean?"*

> *"Yes, a myocardial infarction." Paul feels the gentle readjustment. "That would have impaired his heart's contractility."*

> *"Indeed, Paul. And if the contractility went down, what would happen to the stroke volume? Remember Equation 6—contractility times preload equals stroke volume?"*

The attending quickly reads the phase 2 clinical reasoning: The student has memorized that "if congestive heart failure, then Lasix," without understanding the rationale for its use. The goal of this dialogue is to get the student to see CHF as a hemodynamic problem. This will enable him to understand why the medications used in the management of CHF are prescribed (preload- and afterload-reducing agents), and will enable him to anticipate the side effects and consequences.

> *"Well, if the contractility went down, the stroke volume would go down," says Paul.*

> *"Yes, and if the stroke volume went down, what would happen to the cardiac output? Remember Equation 5 ... stroke volume times heart rate is cardiac output?"*

> *"It would go down, of course," replies Paul.*

> *"Good, Paul. And what would happen to the mean arterial pressure if the cardiac output went down? Do you remember Equation 4, Ohm's law?"*

> *"If the cardiac output went down, then the pressure would go down?"*

> *"What was his blood pressure again, Paul?"*

> *"It was 110 over 70 .... Is that why he was a little on the low side?"*

> *"Indeed, Paul, and that is going to be important in our management, as you will soon see." Phaedrus pauses. "But let me ask you, Paul, as the mean arterial pressure goes down, what happens to the perfusion of the kidney?"*

> *"I suppose it would go down as well." Paul replies.*

> *"Nice," Phaedrus says as he draws out a nephron. "What's this Paul?"*

> *"That's a nephron."*

> *"Oh, so close Paul ... this is that scary worm from the movie* Tremors. *Here, let me draw Kevin Bacon in for you." The team laughs and Phaedrus continues. "I'm just kidding, Paul. It's a nephron. So let me ask you, if I drew a box around Kevin Bacon and the glomerulus here, what would the pressure in that box be if the perfusion pressure to the kidney was decreased?"*

The attending is making good use of yesterday's investment in the "10 Equations," which is making the dialogue go quickly. The risk, however, is that the audience may get bored. The *Tremors*/Kevin Bacon reference is inserted to lighten the mood and turn up the "energy dial" a bit.

"It would be less, of course."

"Yes. And what would be the amount of glomerular filtration if the pressure was less?"

"It would go down."

"Right, and this part you may not remember, but I'll lay it out for you. This part of the nephron is called the JG apparatus—the juxtaglomerular apparatus—because it's "juxta" to the glomerulus." Paul smiles. *"And when the JG apparatus senses no sodium being delivered to it..."* Phaedrus points to the tubule next to the JG apparatus, *"... it releases renin. And renin converts angiotensinogen to angiotensin I, which is later converted in the lungs to angiotensin II."* Phaedrus pauses. *"Okay, so Paul, let me ask you ... if the GFR is less, what happens to the total amount of sodium delivered to the JG apparatus ... not the concentration, now ... just the total amount of sodium?"*

"Well if the GFR was less, then the total sodium delivered to the tubule would be less."

"Good, Paul, and what would happen to the JG apparatus' production of renin?"

"It would increase," Paul replies.

"And what would happen to the amount of angiotensinogen, angiotensin I, and angiotensin II?"

It would have been more time efficient to just tell the team about the renin-angiotensin axis, but this is the first part of the rotation. The attending is setting himself up for success in teaching other topics, such as hyponatremia and renal failure, by investing the time here.

"All of them would increase as well."

"Correct. And Stef," Phaedrus turns his attention to the intern. He *knows that Stef knows this one.* "What does angiotensin do? Do you remember?"*

From the outset, discussions about angiotensin should be linked to both its SVR properties and its aldosterone properties. This will enable teaching about uses and complications of ACE inhibitors, particularly hyperkalemia and hypotension.

"Well, it increases the aldosterone, which in turn brings more sodium into the body."

"Fantastic, Stef. And one other thing it does ..." Phaedrus pauses for effect, "...it 'tenses the angios' ... that is, it increases the systemic vascular resistance." Paul smiles. "Paul, return to Equation 4 for me... Ohm's law. What would be the purpose of 'tensing the angios' in the setting of very low preload, very low stroke volume, and thus very low cardiac output?" Phaedrus emphasizes the words "very low cardiac output."

"Oh, I see. The increased 'tensing of the angios' ... that is, the increased SVR, would balance out the very low cardiac output."

"Indeed, and the only downside to that, Paul, is that the arterioles—the controllers of SVR—are the gateways to the tissues. So if the SVR increases too much, the tissues aren't perfused. As an aside, Paul, what was the temperature of his skin, like on his legs?"

The attending uses the physiology of CHF to explain the physical findings, thereby moving the student from phase 1 to phase 2 clinical reasoning (seeing all symptoms as a syndrome as opposed to separate problems). The management of CHF is an exercise in "balancing on the tightrope": too little preload reduction (diuresis) and the patient is dyspneic, too much preload reduction and the patient is weak or syncopal. The attending's focus on the explanation on the physical examination abnormalities brings the learner's focus back to the patient's symptoms and examination as the focal point for assessing success or failure of management.

"It was cool ... I do remember that."

"Right, so you get the point. Okay, so Paul, hold all of that in your left hand ... we'll come back to it. But I want to come back to Stef's point about the increased angio II causing increased aldosterone. What is the purpose of the increased aldosterone? Stef?"

"Well, it increases sodium reabsorption."

"Indeed it does, and that in turn increases water reabsorption. So Paul, with all of that salt and water coming into the body ... what happens to the preload?"

"Oh, I get it. The preload increases, and that, too, is the body trying to correct for the decreased stroke volume."

"Absolutely. So we can say that when a patient like Mr. Lawrence has a myocardial infarction, he loses contractility, which decreases stroke volume, which decreases cardiac output, which decreases mean arterial pressure ..." Phaedrus writes out the equations as he speaks, pointing to each variable as he comes to it. *"... and the body uses the renin-angiotensin axis to fix the problem by increasing SVR and preload."* At that end, Phaedrus writes out Equation 9. *"So that sounds fine. There's only one downside to this. Paul, what was Mr. Lawrence's primary complaint?"*

"Shortness of breath."

"Indeed. Let's think about that. If the contractility is less, what happens to the pressure behind the left ventricle ... say in the left atrium and the pulmonary veins?"

"It increases," replies Paul.

"And do you remember Equation 9 ... Starling's law of fluid flow across a membrane? Remember, 'In-N-Out Burger, In-N-Out Burger?'"

"Yeah, I remember that one," Stef jumps in.

"Okay, so what would the pressure be at the alveolar-capillary interface if the pulmonary vein pressure were higher?"

"It would be higher," says Paul.

"And if it were higher, what would be the amount of fluid pushed across the membrane?"

"It would increase ... uh ... I mean, there would be fluid that would move across the membrane." Paul pauses. *"Oh, so that's the pulmonary edema ... and thus the pulmonary edema."*

"Correct. And what would be the pressure in the right ventricle?"

"It would be increased."

"Right. And as an aside, remember that BNP is released when the pressures in the ventricles increase. So the BNP would be...?"

"Ah, that's the cause of the increased BNP."

The attending does not negate the purpose of the BNP, but he does link the BNP to the physiology, allowing the student to see why trying to "normalize" this number in a patient who will be perpetually preload-dependent is not rational.

"Yes. And what would the pressure in the jugular vein be if the pressure in the right ventricle was increased?"

"It would increase as well."

"And how about the pressure in the inferior vena cava?"

"It would increase as well."

"And based on Starling's law again—Equation 9—what would be the symptom we might expect if the pressure in the, say, feet, was increased?"

"Peripheral edema. He has that, you know," Paul says.

"I'm not surprised," replies Phaedrus. "Hey, let me ask you … this guy with elevated JVP, peripheral edema, crackles in his lungs— Did you need that BNP level?" Phaedrus pauses. "Let me put it another way, if the BNP had been in the normal range, would it have changed your diagnosis?"

"I guess not," says Moni. "But we didn't order it, the ER did."

The discussion of BNP in diagnosis and management of CHF will set up a talk later in the rotation on the evidence-based use of BNP.

"Okay, that's fine. So long as you know." Phaedrus pauses. "So Paul, how about management? How are we going to decrease his shortness of breath?"

"Well, we started Lasix."

"And what does furosemide do?" Paul looks stunned. It is clear that he had memorized 'if heart failure, then Lasix.' Phaedrus continues. "Well, remember, Paul, furosemide blocks the reabsorption of sodium from the nephron, and with more sodium in the urine, more water is lost into the urine. So look at these equations … 4, 5, and 6. Which of these variables are we changing with furosemide?"

"Well, the preload … it is reducing the preload."

"Absolutely, Paul, and that's how I want you to see it. Furosemide and all of the diuretics are preload reducers." Phaedrus pauses. "And as we reduce the preload, what happens to the fluid in his left ventricle?"

As explained at the end of this dialogue, shifting learners away from "drug names and disease indications" to "active classes" such as preload, afterload, and contractility reducers or augmenters not only enables them to choose the next most appropriate medication when the standard drug does not work but also enables them to identify corrective actions when management is excessive.

"It goes down," says Paul.

"Correct, and as it goes down, what happens to the pressure in the pulmonary veins?"

"It goes down ... and the fluid into the lungs would go down as well."

"Correct, Paul. And his dyspnea would improve." Phaedrus pauses. "But remember, Paul, we are accountable for both the intended and unintended consequences of our interventions. With less pre-load in the left ventricle, what happens to the stroke volume?"

"It would go down ... so the cardiac output would go down as well, wouldn't it?" Paul asks.

"Yes, indeed. And what would happen to the mean arterial pressure? Look at Equation 4."

"It would go down as well ... so there would be less perfusion pressure." Paul pauses. "Hmm, maybe that explains why his blood pressure went down this morning."

"I suspect so," says Phaedrus. "Paul, here's a term you might not have heard because I made it up. The term is 'blood pressure currency.' And as you manipulate this hemodynamic system, I want you to think of this term. Our goal with Mr. Lawrence is to reduce his preload such that his pulmonary edema improves. But for a man like Mr. Lawrence," Phaedrus points to Equation 6, "His whole life depends on more than normal preload .... because he has less than normal contractility. So we are only going to have so much blood pressure currency to work with. The more we reduce the preload, the better he will breathe, but the more we reduce his preload, the less his cardiac output will be ... and thus the less his mean arterial pressure ... and the less his perfusion of his vital organs." Phaedrus pauses.

"Paul, let's say we overdid it. Let's say we took off too much pre-load. His BNP number would normalize, right?" Paul nods, realizing that normalizing the BNP number was no longer the goal. "And his cardiac output and thus his mean arterial pressure—and

thus his perfusion of the organs—would drop. What symptoms might tell us that we had gone too far?"

"Blood pressure currency" is the attending's own concept, illustrating the infusion of style into the instruction. The attending does the right thing by calling it out as his own, so as not to confuse it with the standard terms. It is a useful concept, however, that enables the learners to conceptualize the limiting variables on their hemodynamic management.

"I guess he would pass out … and maybe his kidneys would shut down."

"Right, and that's an important lesson not only for management of heart failure but for all of internal medicine. So in this case, we are thinking about the potential complications even as we start his therapy."

"That sounds good." Paul pauses. "Can't we just make his contractility stronger?"

"Well, good question, Paul. Unfortunately, no. We can use pressors such as dobutamine in the ICU, but as far as long-term management, your only option is digoxin. Digoxin works by binding up the sodium-potassium ATPase pump, and that increases the intracellular calcium concentration, which does increase contractility. The downside is that it also increases the cells' membrane potential, bringing the cells closer to their arrhythmia threshold. Later, when we talk about EKGs and arrhythmias, I'm going to make the case to you that while digoxin is a good thing in increasing contractility, it is also a not-so-good thing in increasing arrhythmias—which might explain why the DIG trial showed decreased hospital admissions for patients taking digoxin, but no change in their overall mortality. You'll see when we talk about it, Paul, but for now, I want you to remember this very, very important point in managing congestive heart failure." Phaedrus pauses for effect. "These patients die of arrhythmias. Moni, this is probably at your level, but remember this is the reason that very-low-dose beta-blockers, despite their negative effect on an already low contractility, save patient's lives."

The attending should anticipate that a hemodynamic discussion about heart failure will eventually turn to digoxin. In the preclinical years, on paper, it looks too good to be true. The attending in this case gives just enough rationale for the use and limitations of digoxin. This will set up the lecture on electrocardiography that will follow later in the rotation. The attending also infuses evidence-based medicine (the DIG trial) by linking it to the pathophysiology.

> *"Is there anything else we can do?"*

> *"Well, let's talk about it, Paul. The big problem was not having enough contractility. It would be really cool if we could give a drug that would allow the heart to pump against less resistance, huh? Since this would allow whatever contractile function that he had to pump more blood forward."*

> *"Yeah, that would be cool. What drug is that?"*

> *"You tell me. What is the resistance that is opposing the cardiac output ... I mean, what is the systemic vascular resistance that does that?"*

> *Paul smiles. "Oh, the SVR. So we need a drug that reduces the SVR."*

> *"Right. And what drug would un-tense the angios?"*

> *"Ah, an ACE inhibitor!"*

> *"Exactly, Paul. Just remember that angiotensin also stimulates aldosterone, which means if you block the production of angiotensin II, you are both afterload reducing—that is, decreasing the SVR—and preload reducing—that is, shutting off the aldosterone that is bringing in the salt and water. Just be careful, as you already have him on a preload reducer. I believe you called it ... Lasix."*

Learners will often consider one drug at a time (for example, furosemide is good, nitrates are good, ACE inhibitors are good), failing to see the potential for excessive management when more than one drug per class is added. Having switched their focus to "active classes" and having discussed the concept of blood pressure currency, the attending has set up the learners to come to the correct conclusion on their own.

> *"Right. And we have to be careful with our blood pressure currency ... especially since we are now reducing his SVR as well."*

> *"Well, done, Paul. Moni, a mighty fine team you have." Phaedrus pauses. "For all of you, I want you to remember these lessons. From now on, when we talk about hemodynamics, I want us to start with the action they have: preload-reducing agents, which might include nitrates, opiates, diuretics, ACE inhibitors; after-*

load-reducing agents, which might include ACE inhibitors, cloni-dine, hydralazine; and contractility agents, like beta-blockers, calcium-channel blockers, and digoxin.

"It is important to me that you think in this manner. If you do so, then when we meet the patient, Paul, and we can't give the stan-dard drug that goes with the problem—say, a patient with heart failure AND renal failure—we can look in the 'action class' and say, 'Well, if I can't use an ACE inhibitor, what other tools do I have in this afterload-reducing box?' Then, we just might find our-selves using something such as hydralazine and nitrates." *Phaedrus pauses again. "Okay, Paul, what other problems did Mr. Lawrence have that we need to address? Remember the 'solvency issues' talk we had? What other solvency issues do we need to address today?"*

Essential Components of Teaching Heart Failure
1. Anticipate that learners will be stuck in the "if CHF, then Lasix" mode.
2. Use a pathophysiologic line of questions to get students to think in terms of preload, afterload, and contractility. Diuretics, nitrates, and opiates are preload reducers; fluids are preload increasers. ACE inhibitors and hydralazine are after-load reducers. This level of understanding will prevent learn-ers from doing two opposing interventions at the same time (fluids and diuretics), and will enable them to choose the next-best intervention within a category if one is prohibited (hydralazine as an afterload-reducing agent if renal failure prevents using an ACE inhibitor).
3. Get students to understand the concept of "blood pressure currency" (how much blood pressure the patient has). Each heart failure agent will "cost" some currency (reduce the blood pressure), and agents may have to be prioritized accord-ing to what currency is available.
4. Use a pathophysiologic line of questions to get students to understand that increased preload is a natural compensation for decreased contractility.
5. Get students to see that there is an optimal preload for patients with heart failure and that because of the poor con-tractility, this preload will be higher than normal.
6. Refocus students to use patient symptoms, and not BNP levels, as the measure of success: enough preload to maintain func-

tion (no syncope, no renal failure, no weakness) but a low enough preload to avoid congestion or dyspnea.

7. Should time allow, emphasize that arrhythmia is the largest single mortality risk among patients with heart failure; low-dose beta-blockers are indicated for their arrhythmia protection, despite their negative contractility features.

❖ Anemia

Purpose

Anemia is one of the most commonly encountered problems on the inpatient medical service. Anemia is so common, in fact, that the attending should be comfortable prioritizing other teaching sessions above anemia if the choice has to be made, deferring a detailed teaching session on anemia until time allows: You can be confident that there will be a patient with anemia next week. Nonetheless, anemia does need to be taught, and no learner on the inpatient medical service should leave the rotation without a strong method of approaching anemia.

The attending should anticipate that learners are likely to arrive with a preset, nonmethodical method for approaching anemia. They will either have memorized a list of causes of anemia or default to a method with two diagnoses: 1) iron deficiency or 2) all other causes of anemia collectively lumped together as "anemia of chronic disease." Although anemia of chronic *inflammatory* disease does exist, the category is unfortunately used as a "wastebasket diagnosis" for all anemias the learner couldn't or didn't want to figure out.

The "bathtub" advanced organizer outlined in this dialogue will move students to a more organized way of understanding the diagnostic evaluation of anemia, beginning with a central question: "Is it too little faucet (production) or too much drain (loss)?" The method is designed to get students to see that too much drain (hemorrhage or lysis) should be excluded first (an assessment to discover hidden blood loss, and a peripheral smear to exclude hemolysis). A pathophysiologic discussion of how erythrocytes are formed will help the student understand (as oppose to memorize) the microcytic, normocytic, and macrocytic causes of anemia. It will also enable the student to understand the other values on the complete blood count (such as mean corpuscular volume and red blood cell distribution width) that are useful in the assessment of "too little faucet" causes of anemia. The faucet method directs students, should they get to the end of the method without an answer, with a bone marrow biopsy, which should be the standard for all undiagnosed anemias. The "bathtub" analogy is also useful in approaching platelet disorders, which, although not presented in this book, is a teaching script that the attendings should have in their repertoire.

Setting, Cast of Characters, and Abbreviations

The team is rounding on one of the patients admitted the day before. It is the post-post-call day, and with the acute issues of the post-call day addressed, the attending has the luxury of addressing anemia in greater depth. The cast of characters is the same: Phaedrus, the attending; Moni, the resident; Stef, the intern; and Paul, the student.

The following abbreviations are used in this dialogue: GI = gastrointestinal; MCV = mean corpuscular volume; RES = reticuloendothelial system; TSH = thyroid-stimulating hormone; TTP = thrombotic thromocytopenic purpura.

Dialogue

"So problem number two is anemia. This is probably anemia of chronic disease because he is in the hospital. We ordered some iron studies and we'll check on the results of those later. Problem number three is ... "

"Paul, let me stop you there. Moni, do we have some time to talk through this?"

On a post-call day, the resident will know better than the attending how much time expenditure and intensity remain because she knows the patients the attending has not yet met. The attending here uses the resident to guide his time management for the rounds.

"Sure, Dr. Phaedrus. I think we have only one other new patient to discuss, and then a consult."

"Okay, Paul. What is your approach to anemia?"

"Well, I'm not sure I have one. In the past, we've just scheduled the patient for an outpatient work-up in the hematology clinic."

"Hmmm. Can I give you a method? You can try it on for size, and if it doesn't fit, you can come up with your own."

Telling learners that they "have to use this method" is not effective. The better approach is to provide a sample method, emphasize the principles that should be incorporated into whatever method they choose, and then encourage learners to develop their own methods. Methods that are forced on learners will lead to them dismissing the methods as merely a "style preferences," reverting back to bad habits they have seen before. Encouraging learners to develop their own methods also encourages free thought and discussion, which are important to establishing the "no-blame" culture, and the creativity that makes medicine fun. Further, it emphasizes "method development" as its own skill, which is important for the learners in their life-long learning, enabling them to construct new methods in the future as new problems present.

"Sure."

"Do you have a bathtub, Paul?"

"Umm … no, I have a shower."

"Okay, have you seen a bathtub? Maybe on TV?"

Paul laughs, *"Yes. I know what a bathtub is."*

"Okay. So here's the problem to pose to you. If a bathtub has too much water in it, there are only two explanations. What are those explanations?"

"Well, there's too much faucet, or not enough drain."

"Great. And if the bathtub has too little water in it, what are the explanations?"

"Well, there's too little faucet or too much drain."

"Excellent. Your patient has too little water in his bathtub … or in this case, too few blood cells in his bathtub. Do you get the metaphor?"

"Sure."

"Okay. So what are the two causes of not having enough blood in the 'bathtub'?"

"Well, I guess too little production or too much removal of the red cells."

"Fantastic. Let's start with too much drain, since I want that to be the starting point for your method. How are blood cells removed from the body?"

"Bleeding, I guess."

The first step in approaching anemia is "to stop the bleeding." The attending emphasizes this point by starting with a discussion of "drain" causes of anemia. Remember, how it is laid down in the learner's mind is how it will be recalled.

> *"Double fantastic, Paul. The first step in approaching anemia is to 'STOP THE BLEEDING!'" Paul smiles. "Seriously, the first step is to make sure that the cause of the patient's anemia is not due to hemorrhage. Most external hemorrhage is pretty obvious … I'm assuming there was no blood squirting out of his arm, or anything?"*

> *"No, nothing like that."*

> *"Okay, so we are left with the five causes of hidden bleeding. Are you ready?"*

> *Paul pulls out his notebook and readies his pen. "Sure."*

> *"By far and away, the most common is gastrointestinal bleeding. It's the reason that a guaiac examination of the stool is an important first step in all causes of anemia, especially given the prevalence of colon cancer and ulcer disease. The second most common cause is menstrual loss, as might occur with menometrorrhagia from fibroids, or just heavy periods. The third most common cause is excessive phlebotomy. That's probably not the case in this patient who was just admitted to the hospital, but it is worth thinking about for all patients when you go to order labs each day. Ask yourself if you really need those labs. The other two causes are rare, but worth remembering. The thighs and the retroperitoneum can hide a lot of blood. Usually this follows some procedure, such as a cardiac catheterization or a central line placement where the artery has been punctured. Okay, Paul, assuming that the cause of the anemia is hemorrhage, what would the red cells that remain in the body look like? Assuming that everything was NORMAL before the hemorrhage?"*

The novice physician waits for the signs to respond. Hemorrhage in internal medicine is unique in that the hidden causes of bleeding, unless a method directs the physician to exclude them, present with few or no signs until it is too late. The importance of the method is to direct the learner to these diagnoses, even in the absence of obvious signs.

> *"Well, I suppose they would look normal."*

> *"Excellent. The initial appearance on the smear, and their mean corpuscular volume—the MCV—will be normal. Now, if the bleeding goes on for awhile, iron is lost from the body, and the*

hemorrhage causes of anemia can turn to an iron-deficient cause of anemia. But see this as a lesson we've learned before, Paul: Let your method drive your tests, not the other way around. So tell me, assuming you will take a history to address the pretest probabilities of all of the diagnoses we talk about on this method, what will be the first tests you will order?"

"Well, I guess a physical exam to exclude the causes of bleeding you noted, then a peripheral smear and an MCV."

"Fantastic, Paul. Good of you to do the physical exam before the labs. Relative to laboratory testing, the physical examination is cheap, quick, and noninvasive, and that is why it is important that it precede the laboratory testing. Further, it can help us choose the best laboratory tests by advancing our pretest probabilities established in the history. All right ... now how else could blood cells be lost from the body?"

From a clinical reasoning perspective, physical examination maneuvers should be considered the same as diagnostic tests, with their own likelihood ratios unique to each disease. The attending seizes the opportunity to emphasize why the physical examination is complementary to the laboratory testing, and why it should precede laboratory testing. The rationale is contained in the dialogue.

"Well, I guess they could be destroyed. Like in hemolysis."

"Excellent, Paul, and how would you make that diagnosis?"

"By the peripheral smear."

"Nice. Should you find the schistocytes on peripheral smear, use the following micro-method to think through causes of hemolysis. Start at the inside of the cell and work outward. First, is it due to abnormal hemoglobin? That is sickle cell or sickle-beta thalassemia. A hemoglobin electrophoresis will help evaluate both types. Next, think about the cell structure: Is it a spectrin or ankyrin deficit? Both will have unusual appearances on the peripheral smear, and the hematologist can help in diagnosing both. Third, think about infections to the red cells. Is this bartonella, babesiosis, or malaria? You'll see the intracellular inclusions in the red cells. Fourth, think about external damage to the cell. This comes in two flavors: mechanical damage to the cells as might be seen with abnormal heart valves, aggressive dialysis, or

TTP—and immune damage to the cells as you might see with autoimmune hemolytic anemia.

"We can get into the details of all of these if that works out to be the case, but for now, I want you to remember that the 'drain' approach to anemia begins with excluding external bleeding, and then obtaining a peripheral smear to exclude internal cell loss due to hemolysis. Are you ready for the faucet, Paul?"

The quick micro-method based on the red cell anatomy gives the student a way to rationally consider each diagnosis in this subset. This is much superior to merely listing a random list of causes. The attending defers the details of each diagnosis of hemolysis so as to not burden the overall method, and to not overwhelm the learner.

"Sure."

"Okay. Red cells are made in the marrow. I'll walk you through the life of a red cell, and then we'll go back to the beginning and you can take me through the causes of anemia due to an inadequate faucet."

"I haven't read about this, you know."

"I know. I'm after the method here. This will guide your reading tonight. So the life of a red cell begins with a stem cell that differentiates into a red cell. The red cell initially has a nucleus and a cytoplasm like every other cell. The cell will continue to enlarge until the nucleus has completed its job of building the RNA necessary for the cytoplasm. Once it has completed its task, the nucleus is expelled. The red cell is then ready for release into the body. Through all of this, Paul, the red cell has to have the following nutrients. It has to have DNA/RNA, which means that it has to have B_{12} and folate to do the single-carbon transfers necessary to build the DNA/RNA. It also has to have hemoglobin to fill the sack, and like all cells, it has to have thyroid hormone to drive its metabolism. And finally, it's nice if there isn't anything else in the bone marrow that's toxic to the red cell." Phaedrus pauses. "Okay, Paul, you're up. I'll walk through it with you. What might be the causes of inadequate red cell development? That is, the causes of not enough faucet?"

The student demonstrates the typical mindset of the early learner on the clinical wards: *"If I haven't read about it, I'm not responsible for it."*

The attending redirects him to a new way of thinking: *"See and learn things on the wards, and then use this to guide your reading."*

"Well, if there were no stem cells, then there would be no red cells."

"Fantastic. So diseases that destroyed the stem cells ... like, say, other blood tumors such as leukemia, lymphoma, myeloma, or the myelodysplastic and myeloproliferative disorders. If any of these tumors occupied the bone marrow to the point that they squeezed out the red cell progenitors ... anemia would result. And remember, too, it's good not to have toxins or other infections sitting in the bone marrow. Namely, alcohol, drugs, and mycobacterial disease. How would you look into the bone marrow to establish this diagnosis?"

"I guess a bone marrow biopsy."

"Indeed. It's kind of invasive, so we'll hold that to the end of the method if we can't find another cause, but good of you to have it in your method. By the way, what would the peripheral smear look like? Would the red cells that escape be abnormal?"

The attending emphasizes that while the method is sequential in building the differential diagnoses, the diagnostic plan may not be. Alerting the student to the invasiveness of the bone marrow biopsy emphasizes the testing threshold concept discussed in chapter 4 of this book.

"I don't know. It seems that if they made it out, they should be normal."

"Indeed, that is usually the case. The red cells look normal, there are just fewer of them. If the bone marrow becomes packed with one of these other diseases, the red cells might be squeezed out of the bone marrow. The squeezing out results in a tear-drop appearance to the cell. Either way, it's good that you have the peripheral smear early in your method." Phaedrus pauses. *"Okay, let's say the stem cells were normal. What happens next? Think about how the red cell develops."*

"Well, you said the cell had to make its DNA/RNA, and needed the vitamins to do so. So I guess B_{12} and folate deficiency would be a cause ... Oh, and thyroid ... You said it needed thyroid to drive the metabolism."

"Excellent, Paul. And remember for all three causes, the cell cytoplasm will continue to grow and grow until the nucleus has completed its job of DNA/RNA synthesis and then is expelled from the cell. So let me ask you: If we didn't have B_{12}, or folate, or thyroid, would the nucleus take a longer or shorter time to finish its job?"

"Longer, of course."

"Indeed. And would the cytoplasm have a longer time to grow bigger and bigger, or a shorter time?"

"A longer time, of course."

"So what would be the size of the red cells when you looked at them on the peripheral smear?"

"They would be big ... the MCV would be big."

Understanding what goes into causing macrocytic cells enables the learner to recall this list at a later time, even after he has forgotten a memorized list.

"Indeed, Paul. They would be big. So, what else does the red cell need to do in its development?"

"Well, it needs to put the iron, that is, the hemoglobin, into the 'sack.'"

"Excellent. And let me ask you. If you had two of those stretchable garbage bags ... you know, the ones that stretch as you put more garbage in it?" Paul nods. *"Which would be bigger, the bag where you put a lot of garbage in it, or the bag where you put just a little garbage in it?"*

"Well, the 'lot of garbage' bag would be bigger."

"So if you have a red cell with not that much hemoglobin in it— either because the hemoglobin was abnormal ... say thalassemia ... or because there wasn't much iron because of iron deficiency— would the cell be larger or smaller than normal?"

"Smaller ... the MCV would be smaller."

"Indeed. We're almost done, Paul. One other thing you should know, one thing that is very, very cool. Did you know that most bacteria cannot make their own ferrous iron that is necessary for their survival? They have to rely on the body's ferrous iron to survive?"

"I didn't know that."

"Wouldn't it be cool if our ancestors evolved such that they had a way of sensing when there were bacteria in the body—or something like it—and then could move all of the iron out of the blood stream and sequester it away from the bacteria? Like, store it in the RES or something, away from the bacteria or whatever the inflammation cause was?"

"I'm guessing they came up with that."

"Indeed, Paul. So easy, even a caveman can do it ... Any chronic inflammation to the body will sequester away iron. The result is that very little iron gets put into the 'stretchable garbage bags' so they look smaller. It's almost exactly the same as iron deficiency anemia, except that there is more than enough iron in the body. Indeed, it can grow to be too much total iron in the body ... just not enough in the red cells." Phaedrus pauses. *"In that case, what will the red cells look like?"* Phaedrus looks to Paul.

"Small .... Hey, is this anemia of chronic disease?"

*"Yes, Paul. But to capture the physiology, I would rather you refer to it as anemia of chronic **inflammatory** disease ... since we really do have to have a disease that is inflammatory in nature, and it has to be present long enough—that is, chronic—to make this happen."* Paul nods. *"Okay, Paul, so let's review the method. Talk me through it. But when you get to the faucet part, I want you to start with the small cells, then the big cells, and then the normal cells."*

This is the end of the first block. The attending is asking the student to recall the method to this point to ensure that he has it down (feedback and evaluation) before moving to the next block.

"Well, first I make sure there is no bleeding ... thinking about in the GI tract, the uterus, phlebotomy, the thighs, and the retroperitoneum." Paul pauses to think. *"Then I'll look at the peripheral smear to make sure that it is internal cell death ... that is, hemolysis. That would be the drain."*

"Good. And how about the faucet?"

"Then I would look at the MCV. Starting with the small cells. This would have to be not enough hemoglobin in the 'stretchable garbage bags.'" So the MCV would be small for iron deficiency,

anemia of chronic disease, and abnormal hemoglobins like tha-
lassemia."

"Nice. How about the big cells?"

"Well, if the MCV was big, I would think about something that
slowed the development of the nucleus so that the cytoplasm
would grow very big. So B_{12}, folate, and thyroid disease."

"Excellent. And how about normal-sized ... that is, a normal
MCV?"

"That would be something in the bone marrow that was either a
cancer, an infection, or a toxin ... so I would probably get a bone
marrow biopsy."

"Well, done, Paul. The one last step to the method is distinguish-
ing between the diseases in each of the three 'faucet' categories.
For the small cell category, how would you distinguish iron defi-
ciency, anemia of chronic disease, and abnormal hemoglobins?"

"For the abnormal hemoglobins, I guess an electrophoresis. For
the other two, iron studies, I guess."

"Hmm. What do you mean by 'iron studies'?"

"I don't know. I don't really write orders. I think you just write
'iron studies.' I guess, a serum iron then."

Phrases that the expert speaks (such as "rheumatology panels," "iron
studies," "broad-spectrum antibiotics") are often copied by learners without them fully knowing what the phrase means. If in doubt, it is worth asking the learner what she means by these terms to ensure that there is
understanding, and not just mimicking of behavior.

"Okay. Two words of caution. Be careful when you find yourself
ordering "panels" of tests ... you may end up with test results that
you don't want or need. Second, regarding serum iron, think
through this with me. For iron deficiency, the serum will natural-
ly be low, correct?"

"Correct."

"Now, regarding anemia of chronic inflammatory disease ....
remember what we talked about regarding the pathophysiology:
What will the serum iron be for that disease?"

"Well, since the iron is being sequestered, it could be low as well."

"Correct. So what you would really like to see is a measure of the total-body iron. Right?"

"Yes. The total-body iron should be high with anemia of chronic inflammatory disease, but it would be low with iron deficiency. That would be a great test."

"And the ferritin is the test that does that for you, Paul."

"Wow. Okay, ferritin as the test for the small MCV causes. I'm guessing that a B_{12}, folate and TSH would be the best tests for the big MCV causes."

"Yes, though actually, it is the red blood cell folate that you want to know, and the methylmalonic acid level to assess the B_{12} deficiency. We'll talk more about that later. The TSH is the right test for thyroid disease. How about the normal-size anemias?"

"Well, I guess a bone marrow biopsy if there is no definitive cause by this point in the method."

"Exactly, Paul. Leave no anemia undiagnosed. Not everything has to be done in the hospital, but I also want you to pay attention to the transition of care from the inpatient hospital to the outpatient clinic. What we can't do is just hope that someone out there in the clinic world will work all of this up. We can do our part in starting the evaluation for the problem, doing those tests that are more easily accomplished in the inpatient arena, and then, importantly, Paul, communicating what we have done and what still needs to be done to the clinic physicians who will assume the patient's care." Phaedrus pauses. *"Well, there are some finer points to discuss later, but for now, that is an excellent general method. Let's hear about that last patient."*

Essential Components of Teaching Anemia

1. Good methods prompt learners to remember components of a diagnostic evaluation that would have otherwise been forgotten (in this case, the peripheral smear, the MCV, and so forth).
2. Get students to see the two causes of anemia: too little production (faucet) and too much loss (drain). This model will be useful for other teaching topics (for example, electrolytes). Start with the drain to emphasize the need to exclude active hemorrhage and to ensure that the peripheral smear is ordered early (before transfusion negates its accuracy).

3. When addressing production, use pathophysiology to ensure that students understand why microcytic, normocytic, and macrocytic anemia develop. This will help them recall the differential for each (What factors would impair the erythrocyte's nucleus development? These are the causes for macrocytic anemias), and will emphasize the importance of using the MCV to guide the diagnostic method.

4. If the evaluation ends without a diagnosis (usually normocytic anemias unexplained), the method should direct the team to the bone marrow biopsy. While ambulatory evaluation of many problems is appropriate, the attending should ensure that learners know which problems require inpatient evaluation and which problems are appropriate for ambulatory evaluation. Many learners will have blindly acquired the phrase "it can be worked up as an outpatient" as code for "problems we do not want to address." Even for problems reserved for ambulatory evaluation, the attending should teach the learners what portion of that evaluation can be done as an inpatient, and emphasize the team's responsibility to ensure that the evaluation actually occurs (transitions of care).

❖ Hyponatremia

Purpose

Like anemia, hyponatremia is encountered frequently enough that the attending can pick and choose when he wants to get into the teaching session. Also like anemia, sodium disorders are common enough that the ward team should not leave the rotation without understanding the pathophysiology that causes the disorders, and the method for diagnosing the problem.

The central component of sodium disorders is that they are not disorders of sodium at all; they are disorders of water. All teaching of sodium disorders should begin with that principle. The attending should anticipate that many learners will see these disorders as separate from renal pathophysiology. Teaching the method using renal pathophysiology will not only enable the attending to make the link between renal function and sodium but also will enable the learner to understand (as oppose to memorize) the pathophysiology that underlies the diagnostic testing.

Setting, Cast of Characters, and Abbreviations

The team is on their pre-call day. With all of the acute management issues addressed, and the service size at its nadir, Phaedrus, the attending, has the luxury of spending some time on sodium disorders. Paul, the student, is accompanied by Moni, the resident, and Stef, the intern. Paul is presenting a patient with a low sodium, and as the dialogue notes, the team has elected to defer addressing the problem by reflexively ordering a renal consultation.

The following abbreviations are used in this dialogue: ADH = antidiuretic hormone; GFR = glomerular filtration rate; JG = juxtaglomerular; JVP = jugular venous pressure; SIADH = syndrome of inappropriate antidiuretic hormone hypersecretion; SVR = systemic vascular resistance; T3 = triiodothyronine.

Dialogue

"So problem number three is hyponatremia. He has a sodium of 128. We will call renal for evaluation. Problem number four is ... "

"Paul, let me stop you there. Calling renal sounds like it might be a good option, but talk me through what we have done to evaluate his hyponatremia."

Learners may consult needlessly to avoid adequately addressing a clinical problem. The attending in this case validates the potential value of consultation but redirects the team to try to deal with the problem first. This emphasizes active clinical management (as opposed to passive consultation), cost, and time efficiency (length of stay increases while the team awaits needless consultation results), and ensures that the consults that are obtained are meaningful, and have been worked up to the point of a critical question.

"Well, truthfully, we haven't really done much of an evaluation. We focused most of our efforts on his heart failure."

Phaedrus looks over his glasses at Moni, the resident. She returns the look, exhales, and drops her head. "Yeah, I'm sorry about that. We were hit pretty hard last night on call. All we had time for was the heart failure, but I know that we have to work this up."

"No worries. I understand. You did take care of the big issue, but let's talk a bit about how we are going to evaluate his low sodium. Paul, are you okay with that?" Paul nods. "Moni, is that okay?"

"Sure. We do need to do it."

"Okay. Paul, what was his sodium concentration, again?"

"128," Paul replies.

"No. What was the concentration? You know, there are some labels that come after that number."

"Oh, I'm sorry. The sodium concentration was 128 mEq/L."

"Great. I understand the milli-equivalents. A liter of what?"

"Water, I guess."

"There you go, Paul. That is perhaps the most important part of the whole method. Sodium disorders are not disorders of sodium, they are disorders of water." Paul nods. *"Okay, Paul what is your method for low sodium?"*

The attending is not being nit-picky. Emphasizing the "concentration" redirects the learner away from the numerator (the sodium) and emphasizes the importance of the denominator (the water).

"Well, I know to start with the patient's fluid status ... either hypovolemia, hypervolemia, or euvolemia."

"And how do you do that, Paul?"

"Honestly, I don't know. Look for JVP, I guess ... or skin turgor."

"Okay, let me evoke some experience, here." Phaedrus pauses. *"Moni, how many patients—excluding the elderly, of course— have you seen that have had noticeable decreased skin turgor?"*

"Honestly, excluding the elderly—none."

"So while that's the right answer for the boards, it is important that we be honest about the strengths and limitations of the physical examination. You know me, Paul, I'm a big advocate of using the physical examination. It brings you closer to your patient, and it's a good way to choose the right diagnostic test, if not to obviate doing some of them. But I promised you at the outset of the month that I would be honest as to which maneuvers were not useful and which were useful ... Useful, of course, being defined by maneuvers that have big positive likelihood ratios and low negative likelihood ratios." Phaedrus pauses. *"Skin turgor is one of those maneuvers that is not that useful. So that said, let me talk you through the physiology of this, and maybe we can come up with a better method."*

Emphasizing the physical examination is a good thing; it saves cost and brings learners closer to their patients. Blindly endorsing the physical examination, however, will lead to a backlash. As students learn that one physical finding doesn't work, they are prone to dismissing the entire physical examination. A better approach is to endorse physical examination maneuvers that do work (as judged by their likelihood ratios), and be honest about the efficacy or lack of efficacy for the remainder.

"Sounds good," says Moni.

"Okay, Paul. Do you remember when we talked about diagnosing renal failure last week?"

"Yeah … I think I do."

"Alright, well, let's walk through it again, but with a focus on sodium. One of the categories of low sodium that you evoked was hypovolemia. I assume you mean dehydration, is that right?"

"Yes. That's what I was thinking about."

"Okay. So let's say you get sick, like with the flu. You don't feel like eating or drinking anything. What happens to the volume in your veins as you get dehydrated?" As he says this, Phaedrus draws out the diagram in Figure 7-4 and points to point A on the diagram.

"It goes down, of course."

"And as the volume in the veins goes down, what happens to the preload to the heart?" Phaedrus points to point B on the diagram (see Figure 7-4).

"It goes down as well."

"And with lower preload, what happens to the stroke volume? Remember Equation 6."

"It goes down."

"And as the stroke volume goes down, what happens to the cardiac output?" Phaedrus points to point C on Figure 7-4.

"It goes down."

"And as that goes down, what happens to the renal filtration across the glomerulus?"

"It goes down."

*"And remember that the JG apparatus responds to decreased **total** sodium being filtered by increasing renin. So if the filtration decreases, and the sodium to the JG apparatus goes down, what happens to the renin level?" Phaedrus points to point E on Figure 7-4.*

"It goes up."

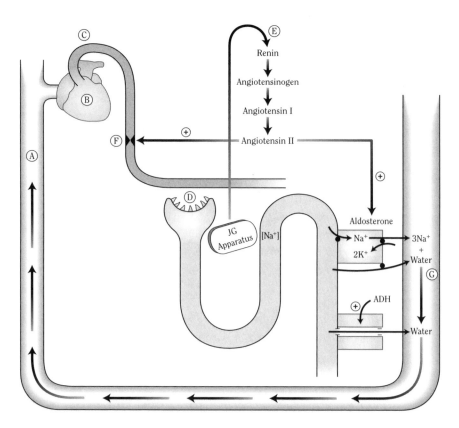

Figure 7-4 The renin-angiotensin axis. ADH = antidiuretic hypersecretion; JG = juxtaglomerular. A = decreased preload volume returns to the heart; B = decreased preload volume returning to the heart decreases stroke volume; C = decreased stroke volume from the heart decreases cardiac output; D = decreased cardiac output from the heart decreases volume, and thus pressure, at the glomerulus—the glomerular filtration rate decreases; E = decreased volume across the glomerulus results in less sodium delivery to the juxtaglomerular apparatus, and this apparatus responds by producing increased renin; F = the increased renin eventually increases angiotensin, which increases vascular resistance, and the increased vascular resistance balances the decreased cardiac output to keep the mean arterial pressure momentarily normal; G = the increased renin eventually increases angiotensin, which stimulates the production of aldosterone; aldosterone increases reabsorption of sodium, and thus preload, into the veins.

"Great, Paul. I think you remember this next part, so I'll go quickly. If the renin goes up, what happens to the angiotensin I, and the angiotensin II?"

"They both go up," says Paul.

"And remember that angiotensin II does two things. First, it 'tenses the angios'—that is, it increases the SVR to offset the drop in cardiac output. Remember Equation 4?" Paul nods. Phaedrus draws a slight stenosis in the artery in the figure (point F) "And it increases aldosterone. Paul, I think you know this, so I'm going to give you a chance to shine. What does aldosterone do and why?" Phaedrus draws out the diagram of the tubular cell, point G in Figure 7-4, as he speaks.

"Aldosterone increases sodium reabsorption. It does that to increase fluid retention to correct the deficit in preload." Phaedrus draws a line from point G to point A to close the loop.

"Well done, Paul. I see that you've learned."

"Well, I've been practicing visualizing myself using it … just like you said."

"Fantastic, but there is one problem, isn't there? If the aldosterone is elevated, why is the sodium concentration low and not high? I mean if I put you in the desert somewhere, your sodium concentration would go through the roof. Why does the patient with flu, who is dehydrated, have a low sodium concentration?"

The attending *anticipates* the question that the student has not yet thought of, but someday will. When the student studies hypernatremia, he'll discover that the primary cause is dehydration. This will be a source of confusion: "Both hypo- and hyper-natremia are caused by dehydration?"

Paul cocks his head. "I don't know."

Phaedrus waits and then says, "Think about it." He waits some more. "Think about what is the common denominator of sodium disorders. If the sodium concentration is low, yet the sodium being reabsorbed back into the body via the kidneys is as avid as it can be, there is only one possibility."

"Hmm … water … Oh, I got it. He's drinking a lot of water."

"Yes, Paul. What do you eat and drink when you have the flu?"

"Popsicles … Sprite … " Paul replies.

"Indeed. All things that have a lot of free water, but no salt. And what did your mother tell you to eat when you are sick?"

"Chicken soup."

"Indeed …. Lots of sodium in chicken soup to balance out the free water you're taking in. Mothers are smarter than you think." Paul nods. "So call her and tell her so. The upshot is this, Paul. The only way a dehydrated patient can get a low sodium concentration is if he consumes an excess amount of free water. But before we leave this category … what will the urine sodium concentration be if the aldosterone is high? I mean, if all of the sodium is being reabsorbed out of the urine, into the body?"

"It will be low."

"Indeed. Hold that in your left hand—keep your right hand free to deal with what comes next. Now let's move to the 'hypervolemia' category. Moni, what are the common diseases that cause this?"

"Well, cardosis, nephrosis, cirrhosis," Moni replies. Phaedrus waits, looking over his glasses. Moni continues: "Okay, congestive heart failure, nephritic syndrome, and cirrhosis."

"Good. And all of these have what in common?"

"Fluid leaks out into the third space."

"So Paul, with fluid leaking out into the third space, what happens to the volume in the veins?" Phaedrus points to point A on the diagram (Figure 7-4).

"It goes down."

"Okay. So talk me through it again. I want to hear you do it. Take it all the way to the aldosterone."

"Well, with less venous volume, preload will go down … so stroke volume and thus cardiac output will go down." As Paul speaks, Phaedrus follows along by pointing at the letters on the diagram; first A, then B, then C. "And with decreased cardiac output, the GFR will go down …" Phaedrus points to letter D. Paul continues, "…and with that, the renin, angio I, and angio II will go up. So eventually, the aldosterone will go up."

"Indeed. So how is it that these patients have a low sodium concentration?"

"I would guess the same way—they have to be consuming a lot of free water."

"Yes, Paul, well done. It's just like the hypovolemia category. What will the urine sodium be?"

"Well, the aldosterone will be high, so the urine sodium will be lower as well."

*"So here is where the physical exam is useful. If the urine sodium is low, you are between the hypovolemia and the hypervolemia categories, the exam will be telling. So that leads to the euvolemia category. Paul, here's the quick mnemonic: RATS. **R**enal tubular damage, **A**ddison's, hypo**T**hyroid, and **S**IADH."*

"Yeah, I know SIADH," Stef says. "But I've never understood how SIADH causes euvolemia."

Most learners will have blindly learned that "euvolemic hyponatremia is SIADH," although few will have learned why. With this understanding, the learner has a better sense of how the laboratory tests (the urine sodium) can be useful in diagnosing the disease, and the other diagnoses that share the pathophysiology (renal tubular damage, hypothyroidism, and Addison's disease).

"It's interesting, isn't it, Stef? Everything else in medicine got to be excessive or deficient, but not ADH. It's 'inappropriate.' " Phaedrus pauses. "I mean, I like ADH … good guy, dresses well …but sometimes, just … 'inappropriate.'" Paul laughs. Phaedrus continues. "I'm just joking … okay, let's walk through it. I'll start you out." Phaedrus points to the distal tubule on the diagram of the nephron in Figure 7-4. "ADH opens up canals in the distal tubules, and the high osmolarity in the medulla of the kidney draws free water into the body. Do you remember that, Paul?"

"Sure."

"Okay, so if more volume is coming into the body, there is more volume in the veins." Phaedrus pauses to point at point A in Figure 7-4. "Paul, take it from here all the way back to aldosterone."

"Okay … well, the preload will go up because of the increased venous volume. The increased preload will increase stroke volume, which will increase the cardiac output … which will in turn increase perfusion to the kidney." Phaedrus's pen follows the letters, point A, then B, then C, as Paul speaks. "That will increase the

total amount of sodium to the JG apparatus, which will …" Paul pauses. Phaedrus waits with his pen on point E in the diagram. Paul studies it, then continues, "Decrease renin production."

"Well done, Paul. And what will that eventually do to the aldosterone?"

"Well, the angiotensin I and II will go down, so the aldosterone will go down."

"Good, and with aldosterone shut off, what will happen to the sodium reabsorption?"

"It will decrease."

"So what will happen to the urine sodium?"

"It will be elevated."

"Quite a difference from the other two categories, huh? Both of those had a decreased urine sodium."

"Yes indeed. So I guess we should check a urine sodium, huh?"

"Sounds like a plan. But Paul, why is the patient euvolemic? I mean, there is increased free water coming into the body by way of the kidneys, so that explains the hyponatremia. But why wouldn't the patient be hypervolemic?"

"I was wondering that myself."

"Think about the aldosterone and the sodium reabsorption." Phaedrus waits.

"Okay … because the aldosterone is shut off … Oh, we lose as much volume because of the low aldosterone as we gain from bringing more water into the body."

"Indeed, Paul. And just to finish off the category. Remember that cortisol and T3 both negatively feed back to the brain to shut off ADH release. So if you are deficient in either—that is, Addison's or hypothyroidism—you functionally have SIADH. And why would renal tubular damage at the distal tubule cause a SIADH-like syndrome? Think of how ADH works."

"I would guess that the breaks in the cells cause similar sort of aqua-pores."

"Correct. Paul. Okay, see what his urine sodium is. I'm guessing it's going to be high. You might also read up on causes of SIADH, especially as it relates to the lung. I think you will find it interesting."

Essential Components of Teaching Hyponatremia

1. Get students to see that sodium disorders are disorders of free water. Hyponatremia is due to excessive free water, either from the kidney retaining free water or from the patient overly consuming free water.

2. Teaching hyponatremia is a game of anticipation. The attending must be prepared to anticipate where the points of confusion will reside. Only very self-confident learners (rare) will have the courage to ask the question to resolve the confusion, so the attending must be prepared to ask the questions they are afraid to voice.

3. Anticipate that students will get stuck or confused on why dehydration causes hyponatremia (when dehydration also causes hypernatremia). Emphasizing the "free water intake greater than solute intake" using the "chicken soup when you are sick" example will resolve the confusion.

4. Anticipate that students will get stuck on why "SIADH," which is effectively pulling in *more* free water from the kidney, would cause "normovolemia" as opposed to hypervolemia. By using the pathophysiology-based Socratic method, the attending can make the case that SIADH does increase free water volume but also decreases aldosterone (and thus less sodium and water retention), which offsets the total-body volume increase from the ADH.

5. Anticipate that students will get stuck on why heart failure and all other causes of third spacing (such as ascites) would continue to produce ADH (and thus the hyponatremia) when the low serum osmolarity should shut off ADH production. A critical point in the teaching is to emphasize that the production of ADH is regulated by both osmolarity and volume perfusion. When the two conflict, as in the case of heart failure, volume perfusion wins. Thus, ADH production continues to be high in heart failure, despite the low osmolarity, because of the low perfusion.

6. The method for teaching hypernatremia is the mirror image of that for hyponatremia, again with emphasis on the renal pathophysiology.

❖ Diabetes

Purpose

The long-term management of diabetes is best suited for the ambulatory environment because glucose levels can be adjusted with patients in their natural environment. Diabetes, however, is the most common comorbid condition in most inpatient services, and it is perhaps the one responsible for many of the transitions-of-care fallouts, both on the receiving end as the patient is admitted (home doses of insulin are maintained despite the illness-induced decreased oral intake) and upon discharge (inpatient doses of insulin are not increased as the patient's oral intake increases upon discharge). In between are multiple pitfalls of which the inpatient team must be aware. Diabetes renal morbidity, and the interaction of insulin levels with renal filtration, create a great risk for hypoglycemia during the hospital admission.

Teaching about diabetes, then, hinges upon the pathophysiology of insulin production and insulin clearance. In the context of that discussion, the attending has the opportunity to show the learners why diabetes induces the organ disease that it does, and in doing so, enabling the team to become familiar with the pitfalls they must avoid. This dialogue focuses on diabetes as a comorbid condition; a separate dialogue on management of diabetic ketoacidosis and hyperosmolar nonketotic coma should also be in the attending's repertoire. Because of space considerations, however, it is not included here.

Setting, Cast of Characters, and Abbreviations

The team is post-call, and because the number of patients admitted was less than usual, the attending has the luxury of addressing diabetes. It is early in the rotation, and the attending, Phaedrus, has wisely targeted this discussion to start the rotation because the team will frequently encounter diabetes as a comorbid condition as the rotation ensues. Paul, the medical student, is presenting the patient he admitted last night. With the primary problem addressed, he is moving on to address other "solvency issues," one of which is the patient's diabetes. Moni, the resident, and Stef, the intern, look on, as Paul defers the diabetes management to another consultation.

The following abbreviations are used in this dialogue: ACE = angiotensin-converting enzyme; AGE = advanced glycosylation end product; DCCT = Diabetes Control and Complications Trial; LDL = low-density lipoprotein.

Dialogue

"So problem number four is diabetes. We will start a sliding scale and consult endocrine. Problem number five is ... "

"Paul, let me stop you there. What is our plan for her diabetes?"

"Well, I'm not sure. We restarted her home regimen for diabetes, but that's about all. What else should we be doing?"

"Moni, do we have time to talk through diabetes quickly?"

"Sure. We have two patients who will probably take 20 minutes each, so we have 5 or so minutes."

"Great. That's all it will take. So, Paul, here is what you need to know first. Your proteins come with three essential characteristics." Phaedrus draws a small curved line as he speaks. *"First, the proteins are small. Second, they are negatively charged—and that's important, Paul. I want you to think of all proteins in the body as negatively charged ... all except antibodies, that is, which I want you to think of as positively charged."* Phaedrus pauses to draw small minus signs around the curved "protein" line. *And finally, the proteins do not have large, sticky carbon chains attached to them. And all of this, Paul, prevents your proteins from sticking to-gether ... to keep them from plugging up your vessels."*

"Okay," Paul replies, wondering where this might be going.

"So, Paul, what happens when you put sugar in a glass of water?" Phaedrus draws a glass of water.

"You get sugar water."

"Yep. Just like that soda you are drinking. And what happens when you add in even more sugar?"

"The sugar crystallizes out."

"Correct. Which was the whole point of eating unsweetened cere-al, wasn't it? So you could add sugar to it, and then eat the sugar at the bottom of the bowl."

Paul laughs. *"I suppose."*

"And when you put excess sugar in the bloodstream, the same thing happens ... it crystallizes out. The difference is that there is no bottom to the glass in the body. The sugar crystallizes onto those proteins." Phaedrus draws wavy lines coming off of the ini-

tial protein line. "And this does three things. First, it makes the proteins bigger. Second, it insulates the negative charge such that the proteins no longer repel each other. And third, it puts large, sticky carbon chains on the proteins, which makes them even stickier. And these Paul, are what we call advanced glycosylated end products: AGEs."

Learners memorize the complications of diabetes as if they were a grocery list. Beginning with the pathophysiology will link them together with their common origin, and refocus the student on the important key issue: glucose control.

"Hmmm." Paul is following along but is still trying to figure out where this is going.

"So all of the complication of diabetes, Paul, you can understand and prevent if you just stay focused on this one simple principle: prevent the development of AGEs."

"Wow. Tell me how."

"Well, by the end of this, I think you'll be able to tell me." Phaedrus turns to Stef to keep him involved in the discussion. "Stef, what are the complications of diabetes?"

"Peripheral neuropathy, kidney failure, retinopathy, and vascular and heart disease."

"That's a nice list. Let me also add diabetes as being an immune-compromised state."

"Really? Why is that?" asks Stef.

"Stay tuned, since I'm going to take you to that answer," replies Phaedrus. "But first ... Paul, back to you ... which of the vessels in the body will these AGEs most likely plug up? The really big ones, or the smallest of the smallest ones?"

"The smallest ones, of course."

"Indeed, and as you know, we start with a really big artery in the middle—the aorta—and then the arteries arborize, becoming progressively smaller as they go to the periphery. So where would the smallest vessels be? Close to the center, or out in the periphery?"

"Out in the periphery."

"Indeed. And we could with good reason suspect that the smallest vessels to the smallest nerves—the vasonervosum—might be affected first. Does that sound reasonable?"

"Sure."

"So what's the longest nerve in the body? Since that nerve by definition would be the farthest from the center of the body—the one most likely to be affected by plugging of the vasonervosum by these AGEs."

"Well, the sural nerve ... the one to the feet," says Paul.

"Yes. And what would be the second longest nerve?" Phaedrus holds out his arms.

"The nerves to the hand?" Paul replies.

"Indeed, and the third longest nerve ... that wandering 'vagrant' of a nerve ... "

Stef smiles. Paul answers, "The vagus."

"So where might we first expect the neuropathy of diabetes? Paul?"

"Oh, the hands and the feet ... the sock and glove. Hmm, I hadn't thought of it being due to that reason. I had just memorized that pattern."

"And then the vagus nerve," inserts Stef. "The vagal neuropathy causes the gastroparesis and the inability to sense myocardial infarction."

"Well said, Stef." Phaedrus nods with approval. "Stef, you seem on top of your game." Phaedrus draws a picture of a nephron, with the afferent arteriole tapering down to the efferent arteriole (Figure 7-5). "Stef, this is a nephron, not that evil worm from Tremors." Stef likes the movie reference and smiles. "Here, I'll draw in Kevin Bacon for you." Phaedrus draws in a stick figure sitting on top of the glomerulus. "Stef, which of these two arterioles will be preferentially plugged by these AGEs? The bigger afferent arteriole, or the smaller efferent arteriole?"

Obviously the *Tremors* and Kevin Bacon references have nothing to do with learning diabetes and renal disease, but they lighten the mood, allowing the learners to loosen up just enough to stay focused on the principles, and not the details.

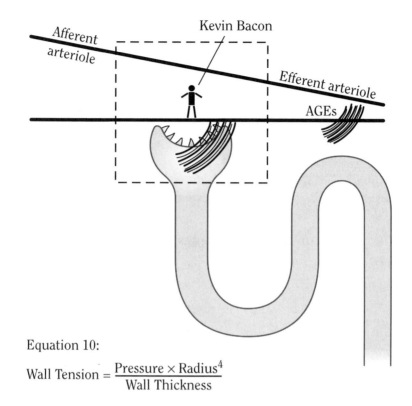

Equation 10:

$$\text{Wall Tension} = \frac{\text{Pressure} \times \text{Radius}^4}{\text{Wall Thickness}}$$

Figure 7-5 The diabetic kidney. AGE = advanced glycosylated end products.

"The small one ... uh ... the efferent arteriole."

"Yes. And what will happen to the pressure at the glomerulus here?" Phaedrus points to Kevin Bacon in the diagram.

"It increases," Stef replies.

"Yes. And based on Equation 10, remember that? Laplace's law of how a chamber handles pressure?" Phaedrus can see that this is a little vague. It is in there, but it is a little dusty. "No? Okay, remember that wall tension in a chamber is proportional to the risk for the chamber popping, which in medicine is very poor form. And wall tension is proportional to the pressure in a chamber times the radius to the fourth ... all of that divided by the wall thickness." Phaedrus pauses to draw a dotted box around the glomerulus, inclusive of Kevin Bacon. "So Stef, let's imagine the glomerulus as inside a box. As the AGEs plug up the efferent arte-

*rioles, what happens to the pressure inside this chamber?"
Phaedrus points to the middle of the dotted box.*

"It increases."

"And what happens to the wall tension?"

"It increases, too," Stef replies.

*"And since the nephron can't really decrease its radius, it has only
two choices: either it pops as the wall tension increases or it offsets the wall tension by …" Phaedrus points to the denominator
of Equation 10.*

"Increasing its wall thickness!" says Stef.

*"Well done, Stef. For simplicity's sake, we'll call that 'increasing
wall thickness'—crescentic glomerular sclerosis—the glomerular
pathology you see with diabetes." Phaedrus draws lines through
the "teeth" of the glomerulus. The reference to a preclinical term
raises Paul's interest. Not that he has any interest in pathology: It
is just that the preclinical years seemed to be worth it now. "And
while in the short term this is a good thing, since it's better than
the glomeruli popping, in the long term it leaves glomeruli that
are overrun with sclerosis and thus no filtration. Renal failure
results. Okay, Moni, here's one at your level. What could you do
to offset the glomerular damage due to diabetes?"*

The pathophysiologic link between diabetes and glomerular renal disease enables understanding of why ACE inhibitors are beneficial.

*"Well, tight control of the diabetes for one … that would prevent
the AGEs … but also ACE inhibitors. That would preferentially
dilate the efferent arterioles, thereby unloading the pressure in
the glomeruli and preventing the renal damage," says Moni.*

*"Hey, that's something we could do. We could start an ACE
inhibitor!" Paul exclaims.*

*"How about that?" Phaedrus replies. "Moni?" Moni nods. "And
now about that vascular disease. Paul, how does your body get rid
of cholesterol?"*

*"Well, the LDL molecules bring it to the liver, and the liver gets rid
of it."*

*"And the LDL molecules dock on LDL receptors at the liver, right?
And what are those LDL receptors composed of?"*

"Proteins ... oh, are you saying that there is glycosylation of those proteins as well?" Paul has clued in.

"Indeed. And if those receptors don't work, the LDL dumps the cholesterol elsewhere."

"Like on the arterial walls," notes Stef. "That's the coronary artery disease. Wow. But I still don't understand the immunocompromised state."

The pathophysiologic link between diabetes and hypercholesterolemia enables an understanding of why diabetes is its own cardiovascular risk factor, and in a transitions-of-care perspective, why aggressive lipid-lowering therapy should be started before discharge.

"Well, what sits on the outside of the polys? That is, how do the polys recognize the antigens they engulf?"

"Oh ... " Stef notes, then continues, "Glycosylation of the proteins on the polys as well ... impairing their ability to function. I get it."

"So Paul, can you think of a protein that turns over ... oh, say, every couple of months ... that we could measure to see how much glycosylation there is? Like something that rhymes with 'hemoglobin A_{1c}'?"

Paul smiles. "So that's why we follow the hemoglobin A_{1c}? Hmm, I knew that was the thing to do, but didn't really know why."

"Indeed, Paul. And now you know what the DCCT told us—control the AGEs and you control the complications. But for now, let's cancel the sliding scale. Start her on half of her home regimen, because I don't think she will be eating that much in the next day or so. Then just check the glucose levels three or four times a day. We'll adjust her NPH and regular insulin on the basis of the glucose levels we observe. Sound like a plan?"

"And the ACE inhibitor?"

"Sounds like a plan. Before she leaves, Paul, we need to make sure that we set her up for podiatry and ophthalmology appointments. Knowing what you now know, I'm sure you know why."

The pathophysiologic understanding of diabetes enables the transitions-of-care issues: arranging for podiatry and ophthalmology appointments.

Essential Components of Teaching Diabetes
1. Understanding diabetes (and its complications) begins with making the link between high glucose and glycosylation of proteins (AGEs).
2. Once students can link high glycosylated proteins (for example, a high hemoglobin A_{1c} value), then the principles of glucose control become easier to teach.
3. As with many things in hospital medicine, learners will be tempted to treat themselves (make the numbers look better) instead of treating the patient. Overdoing glucose control can lead to hypoglycemia, which is the largest risk in the hospitalized patient. Learners should be encouraged to "hold on loosely" with respect to glucose control, and keep the focus on a transition-of-care plan that enables tighter control in the outpatient setting.
4. Attendings should anticipate that learners do not see diabetes as an immune-compromising state, and should be prepared to link the "glycosylation of neutrophils" to "immune compromise" as part of the diabetes instruction.

❖ Renal Failure

Purpose
Renal failure is one of the most common diagnoses seen on the hospital medicine ward. This dialogue emphasizes two primary goals: to establish the diagnostic approach in distinguishing between prerenal, renal, and postrenal causes, and to understand the physiology-based treatments for each. Because of space limitations, the dialogue focuses solely on the two most common causes of renal failure in the inpatient setting: prerenal failure and postrenal failure. The attending should acquire over time a teaching script for intrinsic renal failure as well.

Setting, Cast of Characters, and Abbreviations
This dialogue takes place on daily attending rounds. The intern, Stef, has the day off. Participating in rounds are the attending, Phaedrus; the resident, Moni; and the student, Paul.

The following abbreviations are used in this dialogue: ACE = angiotensin-converting enzyme inhibitor; BUN = blood urea nitrogen; FENA = fractional excretion of sodium; FEUA = fractional excretion of uric acid; FEUrea = fractional excretion of urea; SVR = systemic vascular resistance.

Dialogue

"Phaedrus, our first patient is Mr. Wellikson. You'll remember he's the 62-year-old man who presented with lower abdominal pain and renal failure."

After hearing the events overnight and the most recent physical examination and laboratory values, Phaedrus realizes that the renal failure has still not been adequately addressed. He inquires, "Paul, do have a plan for Mr. Wellikson's renal failure?"

"Well, not really. I know we talked about this yesterday, but this is Stef's patient, and I don't remember what was said."

One of the skills in attending is patience. You have to get over your anger at the relative incompetence of students and residents—they are not at the attending level; otherwise they would not be trainees. Despite the anger the attending is feeling for violating one of the expectations (the team rounds as a whole, with each member responsible for knowing each other's patients), he does not show it. Instead, he reiterates the expectation, taking advantage of the fallout to illustrate the rationale that underlies the expectation. He then continues with the management of the patient.

"Okay, Paul. I'll help you through this. But remember, I want all of you to know about each other's patients. That was one of the expectations we laid out at the beginning of the month. The importance is illustrated here. Without that knowledge, patient care slows or falls apart when one member of the team is off."

"I know," Paul says. "I'm sorry."

"It's okay, Paul. Remember that it's okay to make mistakes—just not okay to continue to make the same mistake. But don't sweat it. Let's focus on Mr. Wellikson. How have you seen renal failure approached?"

"Well, that's the real problem. I haven't seen a really good approach. We usually just call renal. Is that what you want me to do?"

"Okay. Nothing wrong with getting a consultation. But let's see how far we can get before calling renal. If we can get this down to a concise question, we'll get more from our consult." Phaedrus pauses. "Paul, do you have a stereo?"

"Umm ... sure."

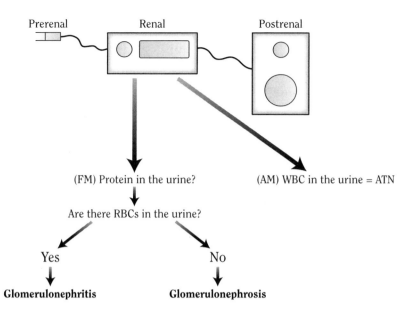

Figure 7-6 The "stereo" advanced organizer for renal failure. ATN = acute tubular necrosis; RBC = red blood cell; WBC = white blood cell.

"A kind with speakers you plug in and all?"

"Yeah," Paul replies.

"Well, let me ask you. If your stereo wasn't making any sound, what's the first thing you would do?"

"I would make sure it was plugged in."

Phaedrus begins to draw the diagram in Figure 7-6. "Fantastic, so you are one third of the way home. If there's no 'juice' to the stereo, there's no sound. If there's no blood flow to the kidneys, there is no sound of urine hitting the bowl."

"Oh, I get it now."

"All right, what would you do next if the stereo still didn't make sound?"

"Buy a new stereo, or call the help line, I guess."

Phaedrus laughs. "Okay ... the equivalents of a renal transplant and a renal consult. But even before that, what would you do? Think carefully now about all of the wires."

Paul thinks for awhile. "Oh, I would make sure the speakers were plugged in."

"Fantastic. The sound has to leave the stereo to get out. The same is true with the urine. Once the kidneys have made it, it has to get out. We'll call that postrenal." (See Figure 7-6.) Phaedrus pauses as he writes. "Systematically, Paul, I want you to think about each step of the way from the renal calyx, to the ureters, to the bladder, past the prostate, and through the urethra. And if the stereo, after you plug it into the outlet and plug in the speakers, still didn't make any sound?"

"Well, I guess I would focus on the stereo itself."

"Right, and that's the time to crack the case on the receiver and see what's wrong inside."

"That's a good approach. But how to do you tell one from the other?" Paul asks.

"Great question, Paul. And that's where your mind comes in."

"What? My mind?"

"Yes, Paul. This is internal medicine; the mind is our 'intellectual scalpel.' Which you do first is based on your pretest probability. I think we've established that starting with 'intrinsic renal caus-es'—the stereo itself—doesn't make much sense. But here are some general guidelines. Presuming that it is prerenal makes the most sense for patients who are currently in the hospital, or for those who have obviously not been eating or drinking before coming into the hospital. It also makes sense to presume postrenal if the patient is an older man, or has a history of renal stones, or has any trauma to the lower urinary tract." Phaedrus pauses. "For all patients, I'll give you a good approach. But first, let me walk you through this, such that you understand the method and not just memorize it. That's important to me, you know."

The attending illustrates that pretest probability can also be important in choosing the sequence of evaluation, as much as it is in arriving at the correct diagnosis.

"Oh, I know." Paul replies.

"I'm going to draw you a picture." Phaedrus draws Figure 7-7 while he speaks. "Now, what is this?"

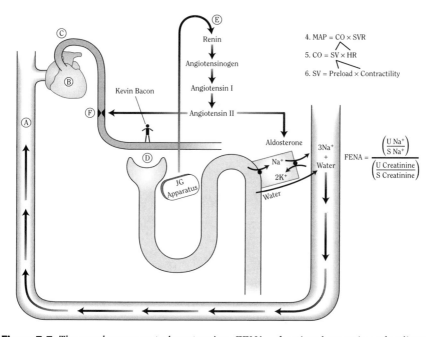

Figure 7-7 The renal response to hypotension. FENA = fractional excretion of sodium; HR = heart rate; JG = juxtaglomerular; MAP = mean arterial blood pressure; S = serum; SV = stroke volume; SVR = systemic vascular resistance; U = urine. A = decreased preload volume returns to the heart; B = decreased preload volume returning to the heart decreases stroke volume; C = decreased stroke volume from the heart decreases cardiac output; D = decreased cardiac output from the heart decreases volume, and thus pressure, at the glomerulus—the glomerular filtration rate decreases; E = decreased volume across the glomerulus results in less sodium delivery to the juxtaglomerular apparatus, and this apparatus responds by producing increased renin; F = the increased renin eventually increases angiotensin, which increases vascular resistance, and the increased vascular resistance balances the decreased cardiac output to keep the mean arterial pressure momentarily normal; G = the increased renin eventually increases angiotensin, which stimulates the production of aldosterone; aldosterone increases reabsorption of sodium, and thus preload, into the veins.

"It's a nephron."

"Ohhh … close, Paul. This is that worm from the movie Tremors. *Here, I'll draw Kevin Bacon in here for you." Phaedrus draws in the stick figure. Paul laughs, as Phaedrus continues. "Okay, we'll call it a nephron … if you insist. Now let me complete the diagram." Phaedrus connects the veins to the heart and the arteries from the heart to the kidneys, and then continues. "This is not drawn to scale, Paul … unless you are a nephrologist, of course." Paul laughs again. "I'm just kidding, Paul. Okay, here's how pre-*

renal starts. Let's say the patient has a gastrointestinal bleed … or diarrhea … or persistent vomiting … or just doesn't consume enough fluids. With respect to the amount of intravascular volume in the veins, what do all of these causes have in common?" Phaedrus points to point A in Figure 7-7.

"The intravascular volume would be less."

"Correct. Can you think of other causes of not enough intravascular volume?"

Paul is motionless, thinking. After 5 seconds, Phaedrus intervenes.

"It's a tough one. Moni, any thoughts?"

"I guess volume leaking out of the vasculature …. like in ascites or peripheral edema."

"Fantastic. Good team play. All of those would be the same with respect to having too little volume in the veins. But how would those latter causes be different from the first ones I laid out? In particular, how would the patient appear?"

"Well, in the latter causes, the patient would look puffy or bloated. He wouldn't look that way with the former causes."

Linking the physical examination to the method will help prompt the learner to look for this examination information when he finds himself in the diagnostic dilemma in the future.

"Great. I'm going to come back to that on a later day." Phaedrus makes a mental note to return to hyponatremia at a later point as it comes up. "For now, though, we can agree that all of the above causes would have less volume in the veins. So how much volume would return to the heart?" Phaedrus points to point B in Figure 7-7.

"Less would return."

"And based on what you know about Equation 6 … remember that? Preload times contractility equals stroke volume?" Paul nods as Phaedrus writes out Equations 4, 5, and 6. "Good. So with less volume coming to the heart, what would happen to the stroke volume?"

"It would go down."

"Great, and based on Equation 5—stroke volume times heart rate equals cardiac output—what would happen to the cardiac output?" Phaedrus points to point C in Figure 7-7.

"It would go down."

The student clearly knows the sequence of Equations 5 and 6, but it is a time-inexpensive way to consolidate the importance of the physiologic method of thinking.

"Excellent. And with a lower cardiac output, what would happen to the amount of volume to Kevin Bacon here?" Phaedrus points to the stick figure at the glomerulus.

"It would go down."

"Correct. And imagine the glomerulus as a box with Kevin Bacon inside." Phaedrus draws a dotted line around the glomerulus. "If less volume was delivered to the box, what would be the pressure at Kevin Bacon?"

"It would be less."

"And with less pressure, how much fluid would be pushed across the glomerulus?" Phaedrus points to point D in Figure 7-7.

"Less fluid would be pushed across." Paul pauses. "Okay, I get it … that's the cause of the lower urine output."

"Indeed. But a few more questions to make sure you understand the method. What would be the total amount of volume delivered to this part of the nephron?" Phaedrus points to the distal convoluted tubule, point E in Figure 7-7.

"It would be less, of course."

"All right, Paul, here's something that you probably remember, but I'm going to review it for you. If less total sodium is delivered to this part of the nephron, the juxtaglomerular apparatus—so named because it's 'juxta' to the glomerulus—makes a hormone. And that hormone is renin." Phaedrus pauses to let the first part sink in. "Do you have that, Paul?" Paul nods. "Okay, the renin then converts angiotensinogen to angiotensin I … and if there is a 'one,' then you know there must be a 'two.' So angiotensin I turns into angiotensin II … and angiotensin II does two things."

Paul jumps in. "It increases aldosterone."

"Indeed, it increases aldosterone, and it also 'tenses' the 'angios'—that is, it increases your systemic vascular resistance." Phaedrus draws a stenosis at point F in Figure 7-7 to emphasize the contraction of systemic vascular resistance, and then continues. "I want to come back to the aldosterone in a second, but a brief time out here. Do you remember Equation 4? Ohm's law?" Phaedrus points to point F again, and then to the SVR in Equation 4 at the top of the figure.

"Sure. That's P equals IR. Or for us—the mean arterial pressure is equal to the current (the cardiac output) times the resistance (the systemic vascular resistance)."

"Well done, and again, Paul, just to ensure that learning took place here, walk me through what happens when fluid is lost from the body. Start with the venous volume."

The attending is asking for a review of the physiology to bring the student back to the systemic vascular resistance, just to make the link that there is a physiologic purpose to the renin-angiotensin pathway. This will be important later when the use of ACE inhibitors is discussed, particularly in identifying hypotension as a potential complication.

"Well, the venous volume goes down … the preload goes down … which makes the stroke volume go down … which in turn makes the cardiac output go down … which … "

"Okay. Stop there. If the cardiac output goes down, what happens to the mean arterial pressure? Use Equation 4, Ohm's law."

"The mean arterial pressure goes down."

"Great. Now use what you know about the renin-angiotensin axis. How does the body compensate for this drop in the mean arterial pressure?"

"Oh, I get it. The angiotensin II increases the SVR to balance out the drop in the cardiac output."

"Exactly the way I want you to see it. Later on we'll talk about hypotension and hypertension, but for both, I want you to remember this axis. Instead of thinking about drug names, I want you to start thinking about hemodynamic classes—that is, pre-load agents, contractility agents, and after-load agents. Got it?"

"Yes." Paul replies.

Getting students to think of antihypertensive agents in hemodynamic classes allows greater flexibility in their future management of hypertensive patients, especially those with complicating conditions. Because many teaching physicians do not explain why they do what they do, students may memorize the use of a particular antihypertensive agent, usually by drug name, for a particular indication. When patients become complex, the student is left with no recourse in choosing the next most appropriate agent to address the physiologic need of the patient.

"Okay, back to the increased aldosterone. You'll remember that aldosterone increases the absorption of sodium." As Phaedrus speaks, he draws out the aldosterone pathway to the right of Figure 7-7. *"So if the aldosterone is increased, what happens to the amount of sodium being reabsorbed into the body?"*

"It increases," Paul replies.

"Right. And that's good, huh? Because the increase in sodium reabsorption leads to increased fluid retention, and that helps to balance out the decrease in preload due to the hemorrhage, or whatever disease kicked it off."

"Nice. But how we know that this is happening, or, uh, how do we diagnose it?"

"Great question, Paul. Let's look at it. If the pressure at Kevin Bacon is less, and the filtration across the glomerulus is less, what will happen to the rate of filtration of creatinine?"

"It will be increased."

"Right. That's the core component to diagnosing renal failure. But now for distinguishing prerenal from renal or postrenal." Phaedrus pauses. *"If the aldosterone is increased, and the sodium absorption into the body is increased, what will be the amount of sodium in the urine? Increased or decreased?"*

"Decreased."

"Right again. So let me draw out this formula." Phaedrus writes out the formula for the fractional excretion of sodium (FENA) (see Figure 7-7). *"The operative variable in this formula, Paul, is the urine sodium."* Phaedrus pauses to emphasize the point. *"So if the urine sodium is decreased in prerenal failure, which it will be because of the high aldosterone, the FENA will be very low. We use 'less than 1%' as the diagnostic cutoff for pre-renal failure."*

"Wow, that makes sense now. I've heard people refer to that, and I had memorized that formula, but I didn't really understand it."

"There are other clues that you can use as well, Paul. Remember that aldosterone also induces hyperreabsorption of BUN and uric acid."

"Is that why the BUN goes up?"

"Yes, out of proportion to the creatinine because not only is it not filtered as a result of the decreased pressure at Kevin Bacon, but it is also hyperreabsorbed by the aldosterone." Phaedrus pauses. "Moni, I'm sure you know this, but as a reminder we can also do equations similar to FENA, with uric acid and urea. We call them the FEUA and FEUrea. You just have to remember that there are different cutoff points for making the prerenal diagnosis. Less than 35% for FEUA, and less than 10% for FEUrea."

Teaching higher-level learners in the context of lower learners can be complex. The attending avoids the risk for insulting the upper-level resident, especially in front of her student, by leading with "I'm sure you already know this, but as a reminder ..."

"Why use these if you have the FENA?" Paul asks.

"We usually don't. But there are times when a patient is on a diuretic such as furosemide, which of course is going to artificially elevate the amount of sodium in the tubule because it is blocking sodium reabsorption, and that makes interpreting a FENA impossible if it is above 1%. In these cases, the FEUA and FEUrea can be useful."

"Hmm. That's pretty helpful," says Moni.

"One last question, Paul, just to see if learning took place here. In patients with gout, we instruct them to eat a diet low in uric acid, but we also tell them it is very important that they stay well hydrated. Based on what you know here, why is that?"

"I haven't read about gout yet."

"That's okay. See if you can figure this one out. I'll give you a clue that gout attacks occur when uric acid crystallizes out of solution into the joint—and of course, the higher the concentration of uric acid, the higher the probability that the crystals will fall out of solution."

"Hmmm. Well, if a patient became dehydrated, their preload would go down … their cardiac output to the kidney would go down … the angiotensin II and thus the aldosterone would go up …. Oh, I got it! If the aldosterone was high, then the uric acid would be hyperreabsorbed into the body."

The gout is not a tangent. It is a method to see whether the student can apply the same physiology to a related disease by using the same method of thought.

"Well done, Paul." Phaedrus extends a hand for a handshake. "Now, how would you fix someone who was in prerenal failure?"

"Fluids …. that would fix the preload, which would fix the cardiac output, which would fix the perfusion to the kidneys."

"Spot on, Paul. I think you have it. We'll talk about fluids later, but remember the cardinal rule. If fluids are being used for preload, normal saline is the answer. Do you have that?"

"Normal saline equals preload. Got it."

There is no teaching dialogue for fluids in this book because it really is that simple. Provided learners make the connection between normal saline and preload, 90% of the teaching topic is complete.

"That was the hard one. Postrenal is pretty easy. You simply need to ensure that there is no obstruction. The easiest way to exclude an obstruction of the lower tract … that is, the bladder and the urethra, is to place a Foley catheter. If a lot of urine returns, you know that you have simultaneously made the diagnosis and solved the problem. For the upper urinary tract, you will probably need an ultrasound. Just remember that both ureters have to be obstructed to cause renal failure. And by the way … why does the creatinine rise with postrenal failure?"

Paul thinks. "I don't know."

Moni interjects, "I would guess that it's because of the back pressure on the kidneys."

"Absolutely right, Moni. The filtration across the glomerulus will be less if there is increased pressure from below. Paul, what do you suppose will happen to the cells along the nephron as the pressure inside of the tubule increases from below?"

"It will be increased … I don't suppose that's good."

"No, not at all." Phaedrus says. "Remember that the kidney, like the heart, is an oxygen-requiring organ, and the blood supply (Equation 3) is from the outside in. So doubling the pressure on the inside—the pressure pushing from inside out—is the equivalent of halving the perfusion pressure from the outside-in. The cells become ischemic and die." Phaedrus pauses for effect. "Here is the lesson. And Moni, I want you to help me out by teaching all of your students this. If you let 'postrenal' or 'prerenal' go uncorrected, both will become 'intrinsic renal' failure because of ischemia to the kidneys. For postrenal, it's the pressure inside the kidney opposing perfusion pressure; for prerenal, it's the failure to perfuse the kidney that causes the ischemia."

The learning material is below the level of the resident, although this is a point that many residents miss. The attending involves the resident by including her as a teaching colleague.

"Wow, I hadn't thought of it that way," says Paul.

"Well, now you will. And that makes me happy. So, we'll talk about causes of intrinsic renal failure on a different day. For now, you have a couple of kidneys to save. Go get it ...." Phaedrus pats Paul on the shoulder and reaches for the Purell dispenser. "Let's go in and talk with Mr. Wellikson."

Essential Components of Teaching Renal Failure

1. "The stereo" advanced organizer is a useful way to organize and prioritize the learner's thought process in approaching renal failure: prerenal (current to the stereo), postrenal (the speakers), and renal (the stereo itself). This will keep the learner's focus on prerenal first, then postrenal, then renal.

2. Using Equations 4, 5, and 6, the attending can link "preload augmentation" to "prerenal blood flow." This will enable the student to see a central lesson: Preload augmentation (fluids) is the corrective action for prerenal failure and prevent them from erroneously concluding that preload reduction (diuresis) is indicated for renal failure (that is, the temporary increase in urine due to diuresis is not a corrective action for renal failure; it will eventually make matters worse).

❖ Asthma/Chronic Obstructive Pulmonary Disease

Purpose

Asthma and chronic obstructive pulmonary disease (COPD) are common admitting diagnoses for the inpatient service. Although the two are different diseases, they are clustered together in the dialogue as an example of the importance of empowering learners to see the unique features of each (that is, to distinguish the two as different diseases even though both involve the bronchioles).

The first step in teaching this dialogue is to distinguish asthma from COPD, then to distinguish intrinsic asthma from precipitant asthma (that is, reflux or sinus drainage). Understanding the pathophysiology of the natural progression of asthma will enable the learner to identify levels of risk for the asthmatic patient (a critical presentation vs. a mild exacerbation) and to use physical examination and laboratory data to assign this risk assessment. Understanding the pathophysiology also enables the learner to remember the appropriate level of treatment for each presentation.

Setting, Cast of Characters, and Abbreviations

The team is on-call, and an asthmatic patient has presented to the emergency department. The attending, Phaedrus, is making afternoon "solo" rounds when he learns of the admission from his resident, Moni, who is asking whether the patient should be admitted to the floor or to the ICU. Phaedrus makes his way to the emergency department, where he finds the team. Paul, the medical student, is presenting what he knows of the case thus far; Moni and Stef, the intern, are looking on.

The following abbreviations are used in this dialogue: ABG = arterial blood gas; COPD = chronic obstructive pulmonary disease; ICU = intensive care unit; OB = obstetrics; Po_2 = pressure of oxygen.

Dialogue

"So, Paul, tell me about your patient." Phaedrus joins the team at the patient's bedside.

"Well, she is a 28-year-old woman who presented with the sudden onset of shortness of breath. She says that she was sleeping last night, when she suddenly awoke at 4 a.m. with the onset of shortness of breath. She took her inhaler—albuterol, I think ..." Paul pauses and looks to the patient, who in return nods but does not speak. Paul continues, "So she took albuterol and it didn't get any better. In fact, over the next 6 hours the dyspnea worsened, prompting her to call 911. She arrived here about 2 hours ago."

"Paul, this is a great presentation, and you know that I don't like to interrupt, but since we are managing this case together in real time, do you mind if I ask a few questions as we go?"

"No, that would be fine. I'm only part of the way through the history and examination anyway. She's having a hard time answering the questions, and we still don't have any laboratory tests back yet."

Phaedrus turns his attention to the patient. "Mrs. Eggerding, would you mind if we have a conversation back and forth here? I just want to make sure that we have all of the right information."

The patient nods, and after a couple of seconds, manages to say, "That ... would be ... okay."

"Okay, great. Listen, we are going to take care of you. You've had these attacks before, haven't you?" She nods. "Okay. It's going to be okay." Phaedrus pauses and turns to Moni, and in a softer voice says, "Moni, I think your assessment was correct. While Paul and Stef and I continue talking, why don't you call the ICU team and ask them to join us here in evaluating her." Moni nods and leaves the room. Phaedrus continues, "Mrs. Eggerding, we are going to step out for a second to talk. When is the last time you had one of the nebulized treatments?"

"Umm ... about an hour ... ago," the patient replies.

"Okay. I'm going to ask the nurse to come in. We'll be right back."

As the team exits the room, Phaedrus turns to Stef. "Stef, can you touch base with the nurse taking care of Mrs. Eggerding? We need to make sure that we have a repeat arterial blood gas, and she probably needs another albuterol treatment. Also, has she received steroids yet?"

"I think they gave her 60 milligrams of prednisone when she came in, but I'll check." Stef replies.

"Okay, great. Listen, if she hasn't received 125 milligrams of methylprednisolone intravenously, can you make sure that she receives that? And the albuterol nebulizer, of course."

"Sure," Stef replies, "I'll be right back."

The attending prioritizes the clinical need, and then uses the downtime between the order entry and order execution to set the stage for teaching the asthma management.

Phaedrus continues, "Okay, Paul. Tell me what you know about asthma."

"Well, not much," Paul replies. "I've only done the surgery and OB rotations so far."

"Okay," Phaedrus replies. He pauses for a second. "Hey, Paul. Have you ever worked with chemicals?" Paul looks confused. Phaedrus continues. "You know, things like house cleaners and the like ... the stuff that smells really pungent."

"Yeah, I guess so. Things like ammonia, you mean?"

"Yes, exactly. Have you ever had the misfortune of catching a strong whiff of the chemical?"

"Yeah, I know what you are talking about ... for me, it's followed by a coughing fit." Paul replies.

"And why, Paul, do you think you cough?"

"To get it out of my system, I guess."

"Exactly, Paul. The body is responding with the cough to eliminate whatever noxious chemicals where inhaled. And as uncomfortable as that is, it's a good evolutionary advantage. Because as the body senses the insult, it immediately tries to remove it." Phaedrus pauses. "But that's not all. The body also has the ability to constrict the bronchioles to resist inhaling any additional fumes."

"Well, I hadn't really thought of it like that, but that makes sense."

"So here's my point to you, Paul. The body has the ability to bronchoconstrict ... and for most people, that's a valuable adaptation. But for a select few, the bronchoconstriction is out of control, occurring either excessively in response to relatively mild insults or, even more frighteningly, spontaneously constricting with no precipitant at all."

The attending establishes that bronchoconstriction is a normal physiologic feature. This helps establish that bronchoconstriction exists on a spectrum: For those on the far left of the spectrum (most people), the bronchoconstriction occurs only in response to severely noxious fumes; those on the far right have spontaneous bronchoconstriction to no stimulus at all. This will help the learner understand that even among asthmatic patients, some patients have more severe bronchoconstriction than others.

The attending sets the stage for using prior events (such as previous intubations) and nocturnal asthma as markers of patients who are far to the right on this spectrum. The student volunteers the cough, which is fortuitous, because this will also set the stage for discussing "asthma variants" such as cough.

> *"I see where you are going. That's COPD and asthma."*
>
> *"Partly correct, Paul. What we have just described—the excessive or spontaneous bronchoconstriction—is definitely asthma. But let's take a moment and distinguish asthma from COPD. By 'COPD,' I think you mean chronic bronchitis and emphysema. Is that correct?"*
>
> *"Yeah, that's right. But in class, they put all three together. Is there a difference?"*
>
> *"Indeed, Paul. A very important difference. Let's talk through COPD—that is, chronic bronchitis and emphysema—first."*
>
> *"Sounds good." Paul replies.*

Asthma is an obstructive pulmonary disease, but unfortunately its grouping with emphysema and chronic bronchitis in preclinical years leaves students believing that they are all the same disease. The attending anticipates the error, and begins by comparing and contrasting the two disease types to define the clinical presentation of asthma.

> *"All right. I'm going to start by talking through what causes COPD, then we'll return to asthma so that you can see the difference. Here's how COPD starts ..." Phaedrus pauses. "It begins with the chronic inhalation of a toxin, most commonly tobacco smoke, but it could also be other inflammatory agents, such as coal dust or other occupational hazards. The terminal bronchioles trap the toxins, and the body responds by trying to eliminate the toxins. At first, there is ciliary clearance via coughing the impurities out. Then comes the neutrophil response to the toxins. While this is good—the neutrophils ingest the toxins and remove them—there is eventually a price to pay. Namely, the enzymes released by the neutrophils, the myeloperoxidase and the like, start to digest not only the toxins but also the normal collagenous support of the terminal bronchioles. The result is that the terminal bronchioles, over time, become floppy."*
>
> *Paul replies, "Yeah, I remember that now. The floppy bronchioles then cause air trapping in the lungs."*

"Right," Phaedrus replies. "During inspiration, when the pressure in the chest is negative, the floppy bronchioles of a patient with COPD are pulled apart, easily allowing air into the alveoli. But during exhalation, when the pressure in the chest is positive, the floppy bronchioles collapse, trapping air in the alveoli."

"And that's what causes the wheezing of COPD," Paul replies.

The student does the work here, but had the attending not been so lucky, this is the time to link the physical examination as a diagnostic tool in COPD and asthma, as well as a marker of severity. Although not addressed in this dialogue, it is worth indicating that the absence of wheezing, especially when it had been present before, might be a harbinger of worsening airway constriction.

"Indeed. And you'll remember Equation 8, right? The one that governed CO_2 elimination from the body?"

"Sure. The CO_2 in the blood is the CO_2 being produced, minus the CO_2 being eliminated."

"Correct. And remember that the CO_2 being eliminated was the 'minute ventilation.' That is, the respiratory rate—the number of ventilations per minute—times the tidal volume in the ventilation." Phaedrus pauses as Paul nods. "And remember, Paul, you don't get full credit for the tidal volume. Do you?"

"No, you have to subtract out the deadspace ventilation."

"Right. So let's take a moment and review those 'West zones' that defined deadspace. Do you remember those?" Phaedrus takes a minute to draw out Figure 7-3. Paul nods, showing the pain that he recalled from his first-year medical school curriculum. Phaedrus continues. "Okay, Paul. It's not that bad. You'll remember that the top zone was representative of deadspace. There was elevated alveolar pressure, but the pulmonary artery pressure was much less, allowing the alveoli to compress the pulmonary capillaries. That's what defined deadspace: ventilation with no perfusion." Phaedrus pauses to ensure that Paul remembers, and seeing that he does, he then continues.

"The middle zone was more balanced, with the pulmonary artery pressure greater than the alveolar pressure, which allowed perfusion past the alveoli. And the bottom zone was characterized by pulmonary artery pressure that was much greater than alveolar pressure, allowing easy perfusion. Do you remember that?" Paul

nods. Phaedrus continues. "So Paul, why is it that the top zone is different from the bottom zone?"

"Well ... because of gravity, I guess. The pulmonary artery pressure is greater at the base of the lung."

"Exactly, Paul. Now let me ask you this. How could you make the middle zone look more like the top zone—and as you think about this, remember that there are only two variables in this equation: the pulmonary artery pressure and the pulmonary alveolar pressure."

The attending takes the time to review the causes of deadspace ventilation. This will enable a discussion of the less common occurrences of deadspace due to inadequate pulmonary artery pressure, usually as a consequence of overly aggressive ventilation or right ventricular heart failure with excessive preload reduction.

"Well, I guess either increase the alveolar pressure, or decrease the arterial pressure," says Paul.

"Indeed, exactly. At a later date we'll talk about right ventricular heart failure ... or if this patient ends up being intubated, about the consequences of overly aggressive ventilation. Both of these can decrease the pulmonary arterial pressure to a level that causes deadspace. But for now, let's stay with COPD. As the air is trapped in the alveoli by the floppy bronchioles, what happens to the alveolar pressure?"

"Well, it goes up." Paul pauses, "So the COPD causes deadspace, and that's the cause of the elevated CO_2?"

Phaedrus nods, "Exactly. As the alveolar pressure goes up, the deadspace increases. And that decreases the minute ventilation, and that increases the CO_2." Phaedrus pauses. "And that's the hallmark of COPD, Paul. An elevated CO_2. But let me ask you, does this disease that predominantly affects the terminal bronchioles affect the interstitium between the alveoli and the pulmonary capillaries?"

"Well, no. I guess not."

*"So outside of the effect of elevated CO_2 in the alveoli .... Remember Equation 1?" Paul nods. "We can say that impairing oxygen exchange is **not** the predominant feature of these two diseases. Is that right?"*

"Yeah, that's right."

"Okay, we'll return to that in a second. But let's return to how COPD is different from asthma." At that moment, Stef returns with the first ABG result.

"I found the first ABG," Stef says. "It's from a hour ago ... 7.48/30/60. They just did a stat ABG and they are starting the intravenous steroids and albuterol nebulizer."

"Great work, Stef," Phaedrus replies. "Paul and I were just comparing and contrasting COPD with asthma."

"Oh, I know where this is going," Stef says.

"All right, Stef. Let's see if you remember last week's talk. Talk me through what we expect with an asthma attack. Paul, listen carefully to this as Stef describes the physiology of asthma."

The attending leverages a previous teaching discussion to the intern not only to teach the student but to assess the efficacy of the attending's previous teaching session (How well does the intern now perform with the skill on the basis of his previous teaching?).

"Well, asthma is an inflammatory disease. It starts with the bronchoconstriction ... just like a person who was trying to protect his lungs from noxious fumes. Paul, have you ever had ... "

Phaedrus interrupts. "We've covered that part."

*Paul and Stef both smile. Stef continues, "Okay, so there is an inflammatory response that occurs both at the terminal bronchioles and at the interstitium, and that's how asthma is different from COPD. The inflammation in COPD is usually confined to the terminal bronchioles alone. Asthma is **both** the bronchioles and the interstitium." Paul glances at Phaedrus with a look of understanding. Phaedrus nods in approval. Stef continues. "So the inflammation increases the permeability of the capillaries, and fluid leaks into the interstitium. And by Equation 2, this increase in the 'wall thickness' impairs oxygen exchange."*

Phaedrus steps back in, "Paul, look at the ABG again. What would we expect to happen to the P_{O_2} if the interstitial wall thickness increased as Stef suggested ... assuming this is asthma, of course. Use Equation 2 in your answer."

Paul looks at the ABG, studies it for a second, and then comes to his answer. "Well, if the interstitial wall increased because of the fluid leaking into the interstitium, then the oxygen diffusion would decrease. So the oxygen in the blood would be less."

"And is it?" Phaedrus asks.

"It's decreased." Paul replies. "Exactly what we would expect. But the CO_2 is decreased. Wouldn't we expect that to be increased? This is an obstructive disease, right?"

The attending's leading Socratic method has brought the student to the distinguishing feature of asthma versus COPD. An elevated CO_2 is to be expected in the initial presentation of COPD, but it is a harbinger of critical asthma (due to the patient's fatigue).

"Indeed, Paul. This is an important teaching point. Asthma comes in phases. The first phase is the inflammation in the interstitium, which impairs oxygen diffusion from the alveoli to the blood, just as you noted by way of Equation 2. And then, Paul, this hypoxia drives an increased respiratory drive, which lowers the CO_2. What we might have lost due to the increased deadspace is compensated for by the increase in respiratory rate and tidal volume." Phaedrus pauses. "That's the first phase, but over time, Paul, the patient begins to fatigue. The deep, fast breathing starts to become slower and more shallow, and the result is that you start to see the deadspace take over. No longer does the patient have the ability to compensate for the deadspace with increased tidal volume and respiratory rate. The CO_2 starts to rise."

As if on cue, the respiratory tech approaches the team with a new ABG. "Here's the new ABG."

"Thanks, Janice." Phaedrus studies it. "Have a look at this, Paul."

Paul reads the results, "7.32/50/55." He pauses. "It looks like she is starting to tire out."

"I think you're right, Paul. Is the ICU team here yet?"

"Yeah, they just arrived," says Stef. "They are over there."

"Stef, can you walk this ABG over to them? I think they will want to see this. She is probably going to require intubation, but a trial of noninvasive ventilation might be worth a shot."

Stef walks away, and Phaedrus continues, "Paul, we'll walk through all of this, especially how we could have better managed this as a team. But before we do so, let me ask you, how is asthma different from COPD?"

"Well, I guess it has to do with the inflammation in the interstitium. It seems like asthma starts there with its first phase, inflammation, and then the bronchiolar constriction declares itself next."

"Correct, Paul, and the management follows the pathophysiology. COPD is due to the floppy bronchioles, with exacerbations being due to viral or bacterial infections causing inflammation in the terminal bronchioles. The result is that COPD exacerbations are characterized by wheezing or dyspnea, but the predominant feature of the presentation is due to bronchiolar obstruction, and thus an elevated CO_2 due to the increased deadspace from the trapped air. The treatment for a COPD exacerbation is to dilate the bronchioles with albuterol, decrease the bronchiolar secretions with ipratropium, or inhaled or system steroids. After the first insult is resolved, the attack is more or less over. There is no rebound inflammation with COPD, so we usually prescribe a short dose of oral steroids for the week, with no taper." Phaedrus pauses to highlight the distinction between the two diseases.

"Asthma, on the other hand, is due to spontaneous or overreactive smooth muscle constriction, in addition to inflammation that affects the interstitium between the alveoli and the capillaries. The presentation begins with hypoxia and hyperventilation. Even though airway obstruction is present, the CO_2 will be initially decreased because of the hypoxia-induced hyperventilation. Once the patient starts to tire, however, the respiratory rate and tidal volume can't keep up, and the CO_2 starts to rise. That's a harbinger of very bad things to come, Paul. Once asthma starts, it's very hard to turn it off, and getting early and aggressive steroids started from the beginning is very important."

"Well, they did start the prednisone when she arrived."

"Yes, they did. But they started with a low dose and an oral route. This would have been fine for COPD, but for asthma, it needs to be a higher dose and intravenous. Especially if the asthma attack appears to be severe."

The attending's line of Socratic questioning has accomplished the first two goals: distinguishing asthma from COPD and defining the treatment of asthma. Now the attending circles back to the entry point (precipitants causing bronchoconstriction) to emphasize using this historical information as a clue in the severity of each patient's asthma.

"How do you know if it's going to be severe?" Paul asks.

"Great question. Let's return to our discussion about fumes. When you inhale fumes, you have a bit of bronchiolar constriction, right?"

"Right. And coughing."

"Indeed. Great point. So you know, coughing can be a sign of an 'asthma variant.' But let me ask you. What was her precipitant?"

"Well, nothing. She was sleeping and just awoke with the symptoms."

"Right. So again, I want you to see bronchiole constriction as a spectrum. On the far left is you, having only mild bronchiolar constriction to significant toxins. Toward the right are those who have been dealt the bad deck of cards and have excessive bronchiolar constriction in response to relatively mild irritants, such as perfumes, household allergens, smoke, or automotive exhaust." Phaedrus pauses for effect. "And on the far right of the spectrum is our patient, who has spontaneous bronchiolar constriction to no apparent stimulus at all. Nocturnal asthma, Paul, or patients who give you a history of severe reactions to mild precipitants— as assessed by the number of times that they have been intubated—those are the people about whom we should really worry. As a team, we should have recognized that she was far to the right on the spectrum, and we …"

Paul interrupts. "We should have started the steroids much earlier … and at higher doses."

"Right, Paul. And one other tip to assess the severity of asthma. I want you to do this for me." Phaedrus produces a page out of Mrs. Eggerding's chart. "I want you to take a deep breath, and then I want you to read as much of this out loud as you can without taking a breath. Just keep going as long as you can, but don't take a breath."

Paul begins to read, finishing three or four sentences before his voice begins to shudder and soften. Phaedrus intervenes. "Okay, now don't breathe. Don't breathe." Paul looks at him as Phaedrus continues, "Now read as much of the next sentence as you can,"

Paul continues. "The ... patient ... has been ... seen ..." he says followed by a deep gasping inspiration.

"When you talk, Paul, it is because of your ability to take a deep inspiration, and then slowly regulate your exhalation past the vocal cords. When exhalation is impaired, it is very difficult to talk without speaking in broken, one-word sentences. Isn't it?"

Paul feels the analogy. "Just like I did for that last sentence. That was hard to do ... and frightening."

"And it sounded a lot like Mrs. Eggerding's history, didn't it? Those one-word sentences?"

"Yeah, it sure did."

"So lesson learned, Paul. The best predictors for the severity of an asthma attack are one, the inability to speak full sentences; two, asthma attacks that begin, or have begun in the past, spontaneously, especially nocturnal asthma; and three, a history of severe attacks, as measured by prior hospitalizations or intubations."

"Wow, that's really useful," says Paul.

"One last thing, Paul. Asthma, unlike COPD, is predominantly an inborn trait. Most patients with inborn asthma have their first attack in childhood or early adulthood. In contrast, most patients with COPD have their first attack later in life, after years of bronchiolar damage from the smoke or occupational exposure. If you see asthma in an older patient who has never had it before, I want you to think about endogenous chronic precipitants, namely gastric reflux with acid going into the bronchi, or postnasal drip, with secretions draining into the bronchi."

"So I guess the history of her asthma attacks was more than just past medical history, huh?"

"Yes, you have the point.

Essential Components of Teaching COPD/Asthma

1. Get students to see the difference between COPD and asthma.

2. Ensure that students understand that asthma is an inflammatory, as well as a bronchoconstrictive, disease. This will help them understand the need for early and aggressive steroids in severe cases. It will also disentangle a point of confusion. That is, why would an obstructive disease initially present with a low CO_2, and why would a high CO_2 (otherwise expected for a bronchoconstrictive disease) be such an ominous harbinger?

3. By beginning the talk with "a spectrum of bronchoconstriction," the attending sets the stage for the "range of severity" talk that is critical to understanding asthma, and offsetting a potential risk that awaits the learner. Asthma, like sickle cell anemia, is a disease that frequently "lulls physicians to sleep"—that is, so many mild cases admitted to the hospital that learners may be at risk for interpreting asthma (or sickle cell anemia crises) as "no big deal." But eventually a severe case of asthma does arrive, and if treated like the mild cases (as in this dialogue) will have a bad outcome.

4. Intrinsic causes of asthma should also be addressed in the course of the discussion, especially for older patients (sinus drainage, reflux).

❖ Acid-Base

Purpose

Acid-base may be the most difficult topic an attending will teach. By its nature, it is filled with complexities, made more confusing by words such as "compensation" and "double, triple disorders." It is an opportunity, however, for the attending to turn a complex topic into a simple one, and to simultaneously teach the value of methods and mental discipline.

The attending who teaches acid-base must be prepared for how students will probably approach the problem: 1) They will have resorted to complex nomograms, or 2) they will have memorized formulas, although without understanding the disease they will be misapplying the formulas and introducing even more confusion.

Teaching acid-base requires five essential elements. First, time must be devoted to the discussion. Given the pace of the wards, it is unlikely that the whole topic can be addressed in one sitting. As portrayed in the following dialogues, it is best to block the topic along the following lines: block 1, step 1 and 2 of the method; block 2, respiratory silos; block 3, metabolic acidosis; block 4, metabolic alkalosis. Second, the student must have a method. The dialogues below provide a sample method. Third, here more than any other topic, the attending has to ensure that the student exercises mental discipline in going through the method. Students will try to jump ahead, or jump side to side, and if allowed to do so, this will create the confusion that will unravel the whole effort. Fourth, the attending has to concentrate. One misused word (for example, saying "alkalosis" when you meant "acidosis") can send the student into a tailspin. And finally, this will require a lot of practice on the student's part. The attending must ensure, through practice with multiple sets of numbers (such as arterial blood gas or electrolyte numbers) that a student has mastered the "step" before moving to the next step. Depending on the student, a whole teaching session may have to be devoted to just one task, such as calculating the anion gap or reading the pH/CO_2.

Setting, Cast of Characters, and Abbreviations

This dialogue takes place on the day after a post-call day. The attending, Phaedrus; student, Paul; and intern, Stef, are at a nursing station. The attending is between notes, and takes the time to check in on the student's progress.

The following abbreviations are used in this dialogue: ABG = arterial blood gas; ATPase = adenosine triphosphatase; BUN = blood urea nitrogen; CHF = congestive heart failure; GFR = glomerular filtration rate; JG = juxtaglomerular; MRI = magentic resonance imaging; Pco_2 = partial pressure of carbon dioxide.

Dialogue Part 1: The Entry Steps and the Respiratory Silos

"Hey, Dr. Phaedrus."

"Hello, Paul. What's going on?"

"I'm working on Mr. Robert's care plan."

"Indeed. Did the ABG come back yet?"

"It did, but I'm not sure I can figure this out." Paul looks puzzled as he stares at a nomogram that resembles an AC/DC album cover.

Nomograms are fine, but they do not inspire the student to learn the pathophysiology that underlies the disease. The attending moves the student back to the reasoning approach to diagnosing the acid-base disorder.

"Well," Phaedrus responds, "What do you think is the problem?"

"Respiratory acidosis, I guess."

"Why do you think that?" Phaedrus asks.

"Umm, honestly, because that's what the night-float resident says it was."

"Hmm. She's probably right, but let's make sure. What are the electrolytes and ABG results?"

The student is locked in an anchoring heuristic. The night-float resident may be correct, and the attending acknowledges this lest the student learn the behavior of not considering the opinions of colleagues, but he redirects the student to the importance of confirming the diagnosis on his own.

"The ABG is 7.28/28/88. The bicarb is 18 and the sodium is 135; the potassium is 4.0 and the chloride is 100."

"Do you have a method for approaching acid-base disorders, Paul?"

"Well, I usually just look at this book. But it's kind of hard to interpret. I'm not sure where to start."

"Do you have time to talk through a method?"

The attending shows respect for the student's autonomy and time by asking if this is a good time to talk through the method.

"Sure."

"Okay. But here must be our deal. I'm going to give you a three-step approach, but if you are going to follow this method, you have to promise me that you will always follow these steps in exactly the order I give to you. Will you promise me?"

"I promise."

While creativity is good for most methods, acid-base is the exception. There are too many opportunities for confusion if the method is not followed systematically.

"Okay, Step number 1 ... Look at the pH. Now, I know there are ranges of normal, but for the purposes of this discussion, whenever an acid-base disorder is clinically in play, any pH greater than 7.40 is alkalosis; any pH less than 7.40 is acidosis. Got that?"

"Sure."

"Let's try it out. Step 1. Look at the pH of your patient. Is it less than or greater than 7.40?"

"It's less than 7.40 … so I guess it's respiratory …"

Phaedrus cuts him off. "Exactly in the order I give them to you, Paul. The first step is simply to establish the 'noun.' Is this acidosis or alkalosis?"

"Well, less than 7.40 … so acidosis."

"Great. That's step 1 … you're a third of the way home. Now for step 2. Put your finger over the P_{CO_2} result." Paul follows the instruction. After you have done step 1, always put your finger over the P_{CO_2} result and hypothesize that the disorder is respiratory. Then, knowing that CO_2 in the blood equals acid, ask yourself, 'Self, what would the CO_2 have to be to explain the "noun" that is before me?' In this case, what would the CO_2 have to be to explain the noun of 'acidosis' … again knowing that CO_2 in the blood is equivalent to acid, and knowing that it is the lungs that are responsible for eliminating CO_2 from the body?"

"Well, if it were respiratory … the lungs would not be working properly … that would be the problem. And since CO_2 is equal to acid in the blood … then the CO_2 would have to be elevated to explain the acidosis," Paul says.

"Great. Now, what you're going to do is, you're going to pull back your finger …" Paul begins to move his finger, "Not yet …. you're going to pull back your finger and one of two things will appear. Either the CO_2 will be elevated, that is, greater than 40, in which case you will confirm the hypothesis … or it will be depressed, less than 40, in which case you will reject your hypothesis. You hypothesize respiratory, and since the noun is 'acidosis,' you hypothesize the CO_2 will be elevated. Ready? Go."

Paul pulls back his finger from the CO_2 result. With a strange sense of delight following the suspense, he proudly announces, "It's depressed. I reject my hypothesis!"

"Yes, indeed. And since there are only two acid-base disorders—respiratory and metabolic—if it's not respiratory, it has to be …"

"Metabolic acidosis."

"Well done. Paul. Now you have your first adjective and your noun. Metabolic acidosis. That's the end of step 2."

The method may seem overly regimented, but it is important. The attending is spending extra time on this step to consolidate the lesson that the approach to acid-base disorders must be a disciplined step-by-step method: noun, then adjective, then second adjective. The attending must anticipate that the student's predilection will be to go side-to-side, trying to analyze the mass of data in an acid-base problem in a random sequence.

"Okay, how about compensation?"

"Not yet, Paul. I want to make sure you've learned this first part, so we're going to practice a bit before we go on. I'll give you some numbers, and you go through the step 1 and step 2 method." Phaedrus cups his hand over the paper like a poker player, and writes the following: 7.48/60/60. He immediately puts his finger over everything except the pH. "Okay, step 1 ... talk me through it as you go."

Paul looks for a few seconds and then proceeds. "Okay, well step 1. Find the noun. Is the pH less than or greater than 7.40? It's greater than 7.40, so the noun is alkalosis."

The dialogue to this point is to the "noun." As with all of the acid-base-silo approach, it is very important that the attending be confident that the student has mastered this step before proceeding to the next step. For many learners, this will mean multiple iterations of interpreting the pH and perhaps deferring the instruction of subsequent steps to other teaching sessions.

Phaedrus gives Paul several iterations of interpreting the pH until he is confident that Paul has the first step down. He then proceeds. "Good, now step 2."

"All right. I put my finger over the CO_2 and hypothesize that it is respiratory. Since CO_2 is equivalent to acid in the blood ... if it is respiratory, and it is an alkalosis ... the CO_2 would have to be low ... lower than 40." Phaedrus removes his thumb revealing again the ABG of 7.48/60/60. Paul looks for a second, and then says, "The CO_2 is high. So I reject my hypothesis. It can't be respiratory alkalosis because the CO_2 is elevated ... so it must be metabolic acidosis." Phaedrus spends the next few minutes repeating this same game until he is convinced Paul has it. After a few iterations, Paul asks, "But why do I have to hypothesize that it's respiratory?"

"You don't have to do anything except die, Paul. You always have a choice with every decision in your life, and from that realization comes responsibility. But your choices should always obey principles, and the principle in this case is that respiratory disorders kill

people quickly. The method is to keep you focused on that. Remember the ABCs? Airway, then breathing, and then circulatory."

The risk of the regimented approach, though important for teaching acid-base, is that learners will interpret the method as personal "rules," which are daunting and likely to be broken. Long-term compliance with the method is achieved by redirecting the learner to "principles" that have to be followed, as opposed to arbitrary rules. In this case, the principle is the ABCs.

"I do remember that," Paul says.

"Okay, to keep us focused on that principle, we will always presume it's respiratory until proven otherwise." Phaedrus pauses. "Okay, are you ready for step 3?"

"Absolutely. This is easy."

"It's supposed to be easy, Paul. Like all things in medicine, it's really not that difficult with the proper method." As he speaks, Phaedrus takes out a piece of paper, lays it out widthwise, and draws four cylinders (Figure 7-8). "All right, Paul, based upon

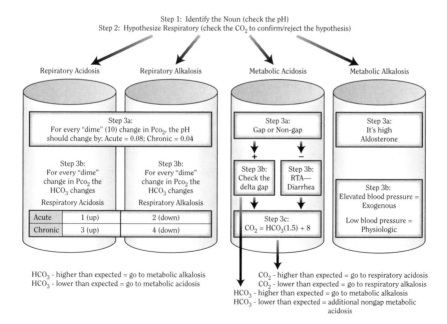

Figure 7-8 The silos of acid-base. Pco_2 = pressure of carbon dioxide; RTA = renal tubular acidosis.

your noun and adjectives, you are going to track into one of these four silos. But here's the gig. Once you enter a silo, you do not leave it until you get to the end of the tube. Will you promise me that you'll follow this method?"

"Sure. But what about mixed disorders and compensation?"

"I don't even want you thinking about that until you get to the end of the silo. At the end of each silo will be a method for determining if there is another disorder at play. But I want you to block that out of your mind until you get to the end of the tube. And at that point, if there is another disorder, then you'll re-enter at the silo at the top of that disorder. It's very important to me, Paul, that you agree to do this. Will you promise me?"

Anticipate that the student will try to jump ahead. He is just following patterns that he has used before: jumping all over the place. The attending has to ensure discipline with the method, or the student will become even more confused. The personal appeal is a good way to communicate the importance of following the method.

"Yes, okay."

"All right then. Which silo do you want to start with?"

"Well, respiratory disorders kill people, so let's go with respiratory acidosis."

"You're learning, Paul. Very good." Phaedrus pauses, then continues. "This is step 3A: respiratory acidosis. The first step is to determine whether this is acute or chronic. The reason for this, Paul, is twofold: First, because if it is acute respiratory acidosis, we need to stop cogitating and intubate the patient so that he can breathe. And second, because we'll need to know this to determine the correct formula for the next step, step 3b. So in front of you, Paul, are some coins."

"I was wondering why you put those there. Can I keep them?"

"Maybe. But tell me, how many dimes are there?"

"There are three."

"Good. And how many pennies in three dimes?"

"30," Paul replies.

Using dimes to equate to every "10 change" of CO_2 makes the content more tangible for the learner.

"Well done. Now let me give you some numbers." Phaedrus writes out, again under a cupped hand: 7.28/70/70, holding his thumb over everything except the pH. "Steps 1 and 2 ... let me hear your think."

"Step 1 ... look at the pH. It's less than 7.40 so it's acidosis ... that's the noun." Paul looks for approval. Phaedrus acknowledges with a head nod. "Step 2, hypothesize that it's respiratory. Since the lungs normally get rid of CO_2, and CO_2 is acid ... then if the hypothesis of respiratory acidosis is correct, the CO_2 should be elevated." Phaedrus removes his thumb from the paper. "I confirm my hypothesis ... it is respiratory."

"Okay, Paul. How many points is the CO_2 over normal?"

"Well, normal is 40 ... so it is 30 points over normal."

"And if each of these points was a penny, how many dimes would you have?"

"Three dimes."

"Well done!" Phaedrus begins to write in the silos (see Figure 7-8). "Okay, here's what you need to know, Paul. As the lungs fail, the CO_2 increases. The body tries to adapt to that by using the kidneys to excrete acid if the lung failure is respiratory acidosis, or excrete bicarbonate if the lung failure is respiratory alkalosis."

"Compensation!"

"Yes, but stop using that word. It will only confuse you. Let me ask you ... if the lungs failed quickly—that is, acutely—would the kidneys have more or less time to compensate for the disorder than if they had failed over a longer period of time—that is, chronically."

"Compensation" is a bad word; it only offers confusion to the student. Failure to compensate is its own disorder, and the focus should be on establishing what the numbers should look like with one disorder; if they are different from that, then there is a second disorder to be addressed (a separate silo).

"Well, if it was quick ... acute ... then less time."

"Right. So since CO_2 equals acid, what would happen to the pH as the CO_2 went up?"

"Well, the acid would go up, so the pH would go down."

"And if this was acute, and the body hadn't had time to adjust, would the pH go down more or less than if it was chronic and the body did have time to adjust?"

"Well, it would go down more if the body didn't have time to adjust."

"That's right. But the question is how much does the pH go down for acute respiratory acidosis versus chronic respiratory acidosis?"

"I have that in my nomogram, let me look."

"Stop, Paul. I want you to know this. The answer is that the pH changes 0.08 points for every 'dime' of CO_2 if it is acute. The change will be less for chronic respiratory acidosis, since the body has time to adapt…. So let's say half as much of a change in the pH, or 0.04 points in the pH for every dime."

"Okay. The pH will change 0.08 points for every dime of CO_2 if it is acute, and 0.04 points for every dime of CO_2 if it is chronic," Paul says.

"Okay. Let me summarize step 3a for you. You are going to count the number of dimes that the CO_2 has gone up. Put your finger over the pH … then you are going to hypothesize that it is acute. If it is acute, then the pH should change by 0.08 points for every 'dime' the CO_2 has changed. Then you are going to pull back your finger and look at the pH and determine whether your hypothesis is correct." Phaedrus puts his thumb over the pH. *"With three dimes of CO_2, how much should the pH change if it was acute versus chronic?"*

"Well, three dimes. I hypothesize that it is acute … so three times 0.08 is 0.24 pH points. So subtracting that from 7.40, it should be 7.16."

"Okay, now look at your numbers. Does your hypothesis that this is acute hold up?"

Paul looks at the pH of 7.28. "No. The 7.28 is higher than what I would expect if it was acute."

"Okay, then, so do you confirm or reject your hypothesis that this is acute?"

"Reject it. It must be chronic respiratory acidosis."

"Do the math again, but subtract 0.04 pH points from the pH for every dime."

"Okay, I get it. If it is chronic, then it should be 0.04 points for every dime. Let's see ... 0.04 times 3 is 0.12. Subtracting 0.12 from 7.40, the answer should be ... hey, it's 7.28, just like our patient has."

"Indeed."

"But what if the formulas don't work perfectly? What if the number falls between what the pH should be for acute and chronic?"

"Well, then, Paul, you assume that it is acute-on-chronic, and I would treat that the same way as you would pure acute respiratory acidosis."

Frequent summaries and reviews are important in this method. Frequent practice with hypothetical numbers is important to ensure that the learner has mastered the approach.

Phaedrus takes some time to give Paul several sets of numbers, starting with the CO_2, and asking him to predict the pH if it was acute versus chronic respiratory acidosis. Finally, he returns to the actual patient's numbers.

"Okay, now for step 3b ... the end of the silo. Remember that we agreed that with acute insults, the kidney wouldn't have time to accommodate as well, so less bicarb would be retained." Phaedrus looks to Paul to assure that he has this point. Paul nods. "Now this part, Paul, you do have to memorize, but I'm going to give you an easy way to remember it. Make a two-by-two table (see Figure 7-8). On the side put 'acute' and 'chronic' in alphabetical order; acute on top and then chronic below. On the top side, put 'acidosis' and 'alkalosis' in alphabetical order; acidosis first and then alkalosis. Now, for every 'dime' of CO_2, the bicarb will change by 1 point for respiratory acidosis. Which direction will it go, Paul? Up or down?"

"Well, if CO_2 is retained, that's more acid. So you would want more bicarb to buffer that acid. So the bicarb should go up."

"Great. Now we haven't gotten into the respiratory alkalosis silo yet, but I'm giving you the numbers for that as well to complete the two-by-two table. You'll see in a minute, the silo for respiratory

alkalosis is the same, just with all of the numbers going in the opposite direction. Again, for every 'dime' of CO_2, the bicarb will change by 1 point for acute respiratory acidosis. But for acute respiratory alkalosis, the bicarb changes by 2 points. For chronic respiratory acidosis, the bicarb changes by 3 points, and for chronic respiratory alkalosis, the bicarb changes by ... any guesses?"

"Four points?"

"Actually a little more than that, 4 to 5, but you get the point. 1, 2, 3, 4. ..." Phaedrus moves his pen as he says the numbers, pointing to each the squares on the two-by-two table. "Look at your numbers again, Paul. Step 1 you said it was acidosis as the noun. Step 2 you hypothesized ... and the hypothesis was correct ... that it was respiratory acidosis. That's the adjective. For step 3a, you hypothesized that it was acute, but we rejected that hypothesis because the pH was too high for that number of dimes, so we called it chronic respiratory acidosis. Now, looking at this two-by-two table, how much should the bicarb go up if it is chronic respiratory acidosis?"

"Well, it should go up 3 points for every dime. So three dimes times three is 9 points. If the normal is 24, then the bicarb should be 33."

"Well done, Paul. Now look at your numbers. Is this what you expected?"

"It's 32," Paul replies.

"That's close enough ... no need to evoke another disorder. But what if the bicarb had been 42. How would you have interpreted that?"

"Compensation disorder?"

"Man, you love that compensation thing. Let's make it simple. Just take the word 'compensation' out of your vocabulary. A failure to compensate is its own disorder. If you looked at a bicarb on a different patient and it was elevated, what would you say?"

The student will try to add on another layer of memorization. The attending takes him back to a previous setting: "If you looked at a bicarb on different patient and it was elevated, what would you say?"

"I guess I would say that the patient had a metabolic alkalosis."

"And if you looked at a bicarb on a different patient and it was too low, what would you say?"

"Metabolic acidosis."

"Correct. So at the end of the silo, if actual bicarb is higher than you expected, then it is a metabolic alkalosis. You enter the metabolic alkalosis silo. If it is lower than expected, then it is a metabolic acidosis, and you enter the metabolic acidosis silo. If it is just what you expected, then you are done. It is one disorder.

"Okay, quickly," Phaedrus says. "Let's traverse the respiratory alkalosis silo and then we'll stop for the day. We can pick up the other two silos later." Paul nods. "The nice part of this method, Paul, is that respiratory alkalosis is a 'two-fer,' meaning the method for the respiratory alkalosis silo is exactly the same as for the respiratory acidosis silo. The only difference is that we expect the pH and the bicarb to go in opposite directions than they did for respiratory acidosis."

Phaedrus takes the time and writes down some new numbers, all of them respiratory alkalosis. When he is confident that Paul has mastered the two methods, he shifts gears to consolidate the approach with clinical management.

"Okay, Paul, one last point. For both respiratory acidosis and respiratory alkalosis, I want you to have a method for diagnosing the cause as much as the disease's presence. So here's the method, Paul. Start at the brainstem, and then follow the nerve all the way to the diaphragm. Once you are at the diaphragm, work anatomically through the lungs: first the chest wall, then the pleural space, then the lungs themselves. So for respiratory acidosis, the inability to breathe sufficiently, starting at the brainstem...?"

There's a risk in teaching acid-base that it becomes its "own entity," separate from clinical utility. After each silo, it is important to relink the skill to the patient.

Paul replies, "Oh ... okay ... a brainstem stroke."

"Fantastic. Or any brainstem disease—the spinal cord is next, which would be amyotrophic lateral sclerosis or multiple sclerosis." Phaedrus proceeds to go through step-by-step with Paul each cause of respiratory acidosis: phrenic nerve damage, damage to the diaphragm, chest wall damage or obesity, pleural

effusions/pneumothorax, COPD, asthma, and sleep apnea. He repeats the same method with respiratory alkalosis.

The use of the terms "bicarb" (instead of "total CO_2") and "CO_2" will send nephrologists into orbit, as will the indiscriminate use of "acidosis" versus "acidemia." But you pick your battles: Being picky on these points will confuse the student up front. After the student has mastered the silos as an approach, further teaching can be given to correct the finer points of these terms.

Dialogue Part 2: The Metabolic Acidosis Silo

"Phaedrus, I was hoping we could go through the approach to metabolic acidosis. You said that when we had time, we would do that."

"Indeed. It does look like we finished rounds a little early, so let's sit down and go through it." The team retires to a conference room, where Phaedrus has access to a whiteboard. "Okay, Paul, review steps 1 and 2 for me—the noun and the adjective." Phaedrus provides a few sets of numbers to ensure that Paul has the first two steps down. On the last set, he chooses numbers that will bring Paul into the metabolic acidosis silo: 7.25/25/90; sodium 135, chloride 100, bicarb 12. "Okay, Paul, go at it ... "

Instruction of each silo should begin with reviewing steps 1 and 2; that is, how the student would find herself at that silo.

"Well ... step 1. I look at the pH to get the noun. In this case it is less than 7.40, so it is acidosis." Paul places his finger over the CO_2 and looks for approbation; Phaedrus obliges. "And then I hypothesize that it is respiratory, because that is what we would want to deal with first. And if it's respiratory ... since CO_2 is acid ... then the CO_2 would have to be high. So I then pull back my finger and check my hypothesis." Paul does just that. "And the CO_2 is not elevated ... so I reject my hypothesis. And since there are only two causes of acid-base disorders, and since it's not respiratory, then it must be metabolic."

"Well done, Paul. Fantastic discipline." Phaedrus pauses. "Okay, that takes us to the metabolic acidosis silo. Paul, the next step in this silo—we'll call it step 3a—is to determine whether the acidosis is a 'gap' or 'nongap' acidosis. But before we get to that, we need to talk about the 'gap' equation for a minute because I want you to understand this, not just memorize it." Phaedrus draws out

the gap equation and continues. "Let me walk through this equation, and Paul, you do need to know this one." Paul nods and writes it down. "The anion gap is the difference between two teams—the 'positive team' and the 'negative team.' In our equation, the positive team comprises the sodiums, and the negative team comprises the chloride and the bicarb. The normal anion gap is 12, which would suggest that there are more positives in the body than negatives." Phaedrus then turns to Stef. "Stef, is that right? Do you actually have more positive ions in your body than you do negative ions?"

The "gap" equation has to be explained before a discussion of this silo begins. Failure to do so will prevent the learner from understanding how adding acid reduces the bicarbonate, and this will prevent understanding the delta gap discussion that will follow.

Stef replies, "Well, I think they are equal."

"Indeed. If the two teams were not equal, you would be polar ... and your magnetic body would gravitate to one of the two poles of the earth." Phaedrus pauses. "Not to say that you don't have a magnetic personality or anything ... you seem like a charming guy." Stef smiles. "But how do we explain this discrepancy between reality and our equation? How do we explain this anion 'gap'? If we have the same number of positive ions as we do negative ions in our body, why is there a gap in the equation?"

Stef replies, "It's just because of the way the equation is set up."

"Right, Stef. It's just because of the way the equation is set up. Paul, do you get that?" Paul nods. Phaedrus continues. "Indeed, there are many ions, both positive and negative, that are not represented on this equation at all." Phaedrus pauses. "There are also other positive ions in the body—for example, potassium, calcium, and, importantly, Paul ..." Phaedrus looks at Paul. "...hydrogen." Phaedrus pauses. "So we have a positive team in the body that comprises sodium, potassium, calcium, and hydrogen. But in our equation, it is only sodium that is representing this team for the 'positive team.' Phaedrus pauses again. "And in the body, we have a negative team that comprises chloride, bicarb, and proteins." Phaedrus pauses once more. "But in our equation, it is only chloride and bicarb that are representing this team for the 'negative team.'"

"Proteins are negatively charged?" Stef asks.

"Indeed, and this is a very important principle for you. Write this down. I want you to see all proteins in the body as 'negatively charged'—all proteins except the antibodies. So for example, albumin is a protein, isn't it?" Paul nods. "So albumin is negatively charged." Paul nods again. "So let's say we could measure albumin as an electrolyte—normally we measure it as its weight, not its charge … but let's say we could measure it as an electrolyte. If you added in albumin to the equation—that is, sodium representing the positive team." Phaedrus pauses. "…minus the negatively charged team of chloride, bicarb, and albumin." Phaedrus pauses again. "What would the gap be then?"

Paul looks for a moment and then responds. "I guess it would be zero."

Not all of the proteins in the body are negatively charged, though most are. Staying with the general rule will help the student conceptualize why there "appears" to be a gap between the cations and the anions. It will also help explain the reason for the cell-shift of potassium as hydrogen ions enter cells to be buffered.

"Exactly, Paul, and that is what explains the discrepancy between what is happening in reality—an equal number of positive and negative ions in the body—and our equation that 'looks like' there are more positives. It is only because we are not adding in the albumin to the equation. If we could, then there would be no gap in our equation at all."

"That makes sense," says Paul.

"Okay, so we've established that the 'gap' is really just an artificial construction. It's only because of the way we have designed our equation, which, so you know, is based upon what electrolytes we can actually measure." Phaedrus pauses. "But let me ask you, Paul, what would happen if I added 10 hydrogen ions to the body. How would the body buffer that acid that we added?"

"Well, the hydrogen ions would be buffered by the bicarb … to convert it to CO_2 so the body could get rid of it."

"Absolutely, Paul. Now look at our equation for the anion gap. As we added 10 hydrogen ions, 10 bicarbonates were removed." Phaedrus pauses. "It's a one-for-one reaction." He pauses again. "What happens to the 'negative team' as 10 bicarbs are removed from the body, Paul?"

"The negative team goes down."

"So what happens to the anion gap?"

"Well, since the negative team went down, the anion gap would go up ... provided the sodium stayed the same."

"Correct, Paul, and you've tapped into a very important point. Sodium really doesn't play in acid-base at all. Remember that sodium disorders—too high, or too low—are actually disorders of water. So if sodium goes up in concentration, it's because we have lost water, which will cause the concentrations of all of the other electrolytes to go up proportionally. So the gap will stay the same in our equation as sodium changes." Phaedrus pauses. "The big point, Paul, is that sodium disorders do not play at all in acid-base."

It is important to establish that sodium does not "play" in this equation, because students will get confused on this point. It is important that they focus on the bicarbonate/chloride component of the equation, since this will enable them to see how adding a hydrogen ion causes a decrease in the bicarbonate, and that (assuming chloride was not also added) links to a proportional increase in the anion gap. In addition, this teaching point will eliminate the confusion that comes with sodium levels that have been "corrected" for hyperglycemia: *"Which do I use in calculating the anion gap, the corrected sodium or the actual sodium?"* The answer is the actual sodium, because although it is diluted by the extra intravascular water inspired by the hyperglycemia, the other electrolytes are proportionally diluted. Sodium disorders are disorders of water.

"Okay, got it. Sodium doesn't play." Paul nods.

Phaedrus continues. "But Paul, we can't just add hydrogen ions. The hydrogen ions come with a corresponding anion. For example, ketoacidosis is the hydrogen ion ... that's the acid part ... plus the ketone ... that's the base part. Lactic acidosis is the hydrogen ion ... that's the acid part ... plus the lactate ... that's the base part." Phaedrus writes 'Ketone- and H+' and 'Lactate- and H+' as he speaks. "So let me ask you, if I added 10 units of ketone plus hydrogen, what would happen to the bicarb?"

"It would go down 10 points."

"And is 'Ketone-' on our equation?"

"No," Paul responds.

"So what would happen to the anion gap if the bicarb went down 10 points, assuming we couldn't add in 'ketone-' because it is not in our equation?"

"Well, the anion gap would go up 10 points," Paul responds.

It is worth the time to go through each and every cause of "gap" acidosis in this fashion. The repetition will eventually show the learner that the nonchloride anion does not appear in the equation, even though the H+ ion does. This is what separates gap acidoses from nongap acidoses (since in nongap acidoses, the chloride ion does play in the equation).

"Great." Phaedrus repeats the same line of questioning with 'Lactate- and H+', then 'Methyl- and H+', and so forth, until he is sure that Paul has the principle. Then he continues, "And what if I added 10 units of 'H+ Cl-' to the body? How much would the bicarb go down?"

"10 units."

"And is chloride in our equation?"

"Actually, yes. So the chloride would go up 10 points," Paul responds.

"Indeed. So if the bicarb went down 10 points, and the chloride went up 10 points, what would happen to the anion gap?" Phaedrus asks.

"It would stay the same."

"But we added 10 hydrogens, right?" Paul nods. "So it would still be an acidosis, would it not?"

"It would be ... hey, is that the nongap acidosis?"

"Exactly, Paul. We are going to talk about nongap acidosis on a different day, but for now, I want you to remember this principle. All nongap acidoses have this in common: the addition of hydrochloric acid."

"Really? When would that ever happen?"

"Well, in broad strokes, Paul, on two occasions: diarrhea and renal tubular acidosis. In diarrhea, you lose 10 bicarbs in the stool, which is the same as gaining 10 hydrogen ions—that's the acidosis part. And then the kidney, in an effort to maintain electroneutrality, holds on to more chlorides to build up the 'negative team,'

*since it can't hold onto bicarbs that are lost in the stool."
Phaedrus pauses. Paul nods in understanding. Phaedrus continues. "In renal tubular acidosis, the kidney can't salvage bicarb.
That's the disorder, and losing 10 bicarbs in the urine is the same
as adding 10 hydrogens." Paul nods again, "So the kidney, without the luxury of holding on to bicarbs, grabs 10 chlorides to
maintain electroneutrality. Same gig as with diarrhea."*

*Paul nods in acceptance again. "That makes sense. So that I have
this right, all nongap acidoses are due to adding hydrochloric
acid. What about the gap acidoses?"*

Even though it will be addressed on a different day, the introduction to
nongap acidosis is important here to distinguish it from gap acidosis.

*"Great question, and the answer is, all anion gap acidoses are due
to adding an acid that comes with any nonchloride anion."*

"Wow, that's easy."

*"Exactly, so to review your steps, Paul. Step 1, you look at the pH
to get the noun. Step 2, you hypothesize respiratory and then look
at the CO_2 to determine whether your hypothesis is correct. This
will give you the adjective. And then you go to the appropriate
silo. And once in the metabolic silo, step 3a is to determine
whether it is gap or nongap acidosis. If it is nongap, then you
know it was hydrochloric acid that was added, either from diarrhea or a renal tubular acidosis. If it is a gap acidosis, then it is a
'nonchloride anion acid' that has been added to the solution."*

*"Wow, this is a lot easier than I've seen before. What's the next
step?"*

*"Well, if it's a gap acidosis, then you go through your mnemonic
of gap acidoses. What do you use, Stef?"*

*Stef has the mnemonic on the tip of his tongue: "Mulet Sack."
Phaedrus laughs as Stef continues, "Methanol, uremia, lactic acidosis, ethylene glycol, toluylene, salicylates, cyanide, ketoacidosis."*

*Phaedrus replies, "You have adapted to being in the South,
haven't you?" Moni laughs. "The next step, Paul, is to sequentially
get the lab tests to measure each of these … for example, a BUN
to assess uremia, a lactate or ketone or salicylate level, et cetera."*

"That's easy," Paul pauses. "But what about the mixed disorders?"

"Good question. Just like we did with the respiratory acidosis and respiratory alkalosis silos, the end of the silo is to determine whether any other disorders are present. And that, Paul, is step 3b … the delta gap." Phaedrus pauses, "But before we get to that, let me ask you this. The normal bicarb is 24 … if I told you that a patient had a bicarb of 10, assuming the lungs are working fine, what would you say he had? Acidosis or alkalosis?"

"Well, since bicarb is base, I would say he had an acidosis."

"Correct. And if he had a bicarb of 32?"

"I'd say he had an alkalosis."

The attending is setting the student up for interpreting the result of what comes next: step 3b. That is, he is simply asking the student, *"If you saw this (a bicarb of 32) what would you say?"*

"Great … So this is step 3b, and it has a very precise mantra, and there are six questions to this mantra. If you are going to do this, Paul, you have to follow the mantra exactly as I lay it out. Can you promise me you will do that? You don't get the mantra until you promise."

"I promise."

"Okay," Phaedrus writes some numbers, "Question 1 on the mantra. If the patient's sodium is 135, the chloride is 100, and the bicarb is 15, what is the anion gap?"

Paul does the mental math. "20 … 135 minus 115 is 20."

"Correct, now for question 2. Assuming that everything was normal before this started … that is, before we added the acid, what WAS his anion gap?"

"Well, before all this started, it should have been normal. So 12."

"Correct, now question 3 on the mantra: How many hydrogen ions would we have to have added to the body to increase the gap from 12 to 20?"

"Eight," Paul replies.

"Right again, Paul. And now question 4 on the mantra: If we added eight hydrogens, how many bicarbonates were lost?"

"Eight," Paul replies.

"You are on a roll, Paul. And now look at the patient's bicarb. What is it?"

"Well, it's 15."

"So question 5 on the mantra: If the patient's bicarb is currently 15, and we recently lost eight bicarbs, what WAS the patient's bicarb before the gap-acidosis started?"

"Well, if it's 15 now, and we recently lost eight, then it had to be 23 before the gap-acidosis started."

"And final question on the mantra, question 6: If you looked at that bicarb of 23, what would you say the patient had, everything else being equal?"

"That's pretty close to normal … so I would say that nothing else is wrong."

"Exactly. You are at the end of the silo, there is one more step, step 3c, which will assess the respiratory function, but we'll come to that in a minute. Do you want to try another one?"

"Sure."

The student has to practice the six steps of the mantra. The attending might find that this block ends here, with the remainder of the time devoted to just going through the six steps. Importantly, each step has a question that focuses on the "reasoning" of the process, diverting the student away from just memorizing the formulas.

Phaedrus writes out the following numbers: "If the patient's sodium is 135, the chloride is 110, and the bicarb is 5, what is the anion gap? That's question 1 on the mantra."

"Well, it's still 20."

"Correct, now for question 2. Assuming that everything was normal before this started …what WAS his anion gap?

"12," Paul replies.

"Right, and question 3 on your mantra: How many hydrogen ions would we have to have added to get from 12 to 20?"

"Eight," Paul replies.

"And question 4 on the mantra: How many bicarbonates were lost if we added eight hydrogens?"

"Eight," Paul replies.

"Now question 4 on the mantra: What WAS the patient's bicarb before the gap-acidosis started?"

"Well, his current bicarb is five, so adding back the eight that were lost, it must have been 13."

"Indeed, Paul, and if you looked at a bicarb of 13—everything else being equal—what would you say?"

"An additional metabolic acidosis?"

"Correct, and since two gap acidosis of four hydrogens each would be the same as one with eight hydrogens—that is, all of our calculations would be the same—we can say the metabolic acidosis you are talking about must be an additional nongap metabolic acidosis." Phaedrus pauses. "Okay, one more time. Now it's your turn to ask the questions. Stef, Paul, I want you to do this one together, but I want to hear you asking the questions in the mantra. Eventually, we have to go our separate ways, and it's important to me that when that day comes, you can run through these questions on your own. But remember, you promised that you would follow the mantra exactly as I laid it out. You ready?" Paul and Stef nod. "Okay, the patient's sodium is 137, the chloride is 95, and the bicarb is 22. Begin."

The important skill is not to be able to answer the questions. The important skills is that learner be able to ask herself the questions. The attending at this point is watching not only for the correct answers but also that the learner is asking the right questions and in the correct order.

"Okay," Paul says, "The first question is what is the anion gap? And it looks like 137 minus 117 is 20. So a gap of 20."

Stef takes the next one. "And the next question is what was the anion gap before this started? Which would be 12."

Paul follows with, "Okay, next, How many hydrogen ions would we have to have added? And that would be 20 minus 12, or eight."

Stef takes the next two questions on the mantra. "And then question 3: How many bicarbonates were lost? And that too would be eight. Question 4 is what WAS the patient's bicarb before the gap-acidosis started? So if it's currently 22, adding in the eight, that would be 30."

Paul concludes, "So if the bicarb was 30, I would say that's elevated, so it must be an additional alkalosis."

"Indeed, Paul." Phaedrus jumps back in. "And since an elevated bicarb is the station of the kidneys, we would say that there is an additional metabolic alkalosis."

"So I would go to the metabolic alkalosis silo?"

The teaching session will probably end here, and probably should, because remaining time in the session should be devoted to copious practice of the mantra. Even if it is not addressed in detail, however, the learner should not leave the teaching session without being told that there is a step 3c: assessing respiratory function in response to the metabolic acidosis.

"I think you have it. So the very last part of the method is this. At the end of the metabolic acidosis silo, after you have done step 3a—gap versus nongap—and step 3b—other metabolic disorder—comes step 3c: Is there an additional respiratory disorder? And this one, Paul, is simple. You simply take Winter's formula, which states that the expected CO_2 should be 1.5 times the bicarb plus eight. So if the bicarb is 15, what would you expect the CO_2 to be?"

"Well 1.5 times 15 would be 22.5 ... adding eight ... it should be 30.5."

"And if the CO_2 was higher than expected .... Let's say it was 40, what would you say? Just think in general ... a CO_2 higher than expected is ... "

"Respiratory acidosis."

"Indeed. And to the respiratory acidosis silo you would go, though there will be no need to do the end part of that silo where you determine if another metabolic disorder is in play ... since you've already been down that silo and you know for sure the answer is yes." Phaedrus pauses. "And what if the CO_2 was less than expected?"

"Well, then I would go to the respiratory alkalosis silo."

"Right-o. Okay, team, we'll pick up on the metabolic alkalosis silo a different time. But tonight, I want you to practice this silo. Draw out numbers and work through it. Moni, perhaps on our next call day when there is some down time, you can feed them some numbers to practice?"

"Happy to do that," replies Moni.

Practice is the key. Learners will master this approach quickly because once it's put in motion, it's pretty straightforward. But unless they practice, they will revert to the nomograms and scattered thinking. Using the resident to use downtime "on-call" is a useful way for learners to practice this skill (and a useful way to consolidate the mantra in the resident).

Dialogue Part 3: The Metabolic Alkalosis Silo

"Hey, Dr. Phaedrus. I have a patient with metabolic alkalosis!"

"Did someone tell you that, Paul?"

"No ... well, yes ... but I followed my steps ... steps 1 and 2 ... and I confirmed it. Do you have time to show me the metabolic alkalosis silo?"

"Okay, let me finish this note." Phaedrus finishes his note, and turns back to Paul. "Okay, Paul. Here's the simple rule ... you ready?" Paul nods. "All metabolic alkalosis is due to increased aldosterone."

"Really?" Paul looks amazed.

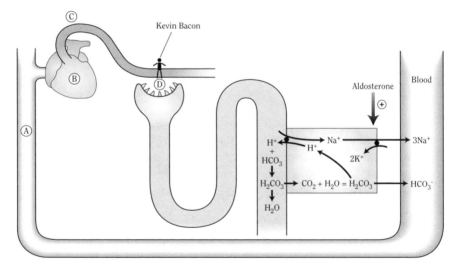

Figure 7-9 The kidney and metabolic alkalosis. A = decreased preload volume returns to the heart; B = decreased preload volume returning to the heart decreases stroke volume; C = decreased stroke volume from the heart decreases cardiac output; D = decreased cardiac output from the heart decreases volume, and thus pressure, at the glomerulus—the glomerular filtration rate decreases.

"Truthfully, there are some super rare causes—like someone eating too many Tums—but for 99% of the cases, it will be high aldo, and that's how I want you to remember it."

The attending is honest in noting that there are some other causes of metabolic alkalosis, but he correctly gives the learner perspective that matches prevalence: Establish early that for all intents and purposes, metabolic alkalosis is equal to increased aldosterone.

"Well, why is that?" Paul says.

Phaedrus draws out the picture of the nephron (Figure 7-9). "Do you remember this?" Paul nods. Phaedrus draws in Kevin Bacon. "Okay, I'm going to talk you through what aldosterone does ... it will seem very detailed at first, but it's the big picture that I'm after, and after you see these details, it will firmly establish that big picture. But first, Paul, what did your patient come in with?"

"Well, he's been here awhile. It's Mr. Lawrence ... you know, our gentleman with congestive heart failure. We've been diuresing him."

"I can see that," says Phaedrus, noting that the bicarb is now 40. "Okay, he came in with CHF, right?" Paul nods. "And we started furosemide, which you call Lasix." Paul nods again, feeling Phaedrus's nudge against trade names. "And the furosemide blocked sodium reabsorption, which caused him to urinate lots of sodium and water. Okay, Paul, talk me through what happened next. Starting with the preload." Phaedrus points to point A in Figure 7-9.

Redirecting learners to see "diuresis" as "preload reduction" and "fluids" as "preload augmentation" will prevent them from doing something silly later on: "Preload reduction" simultaneous with "preload augmentation" will appear as an obvious mistake to them. For some reason, "diuresis" with "fluids" is a less apparent mistake to novice physicians.

"Well, it reduced his preload. That was our goal, and that reduced the volume in his left ventricle, which decreased the pressure in the pulmonary veins that was pushing fluid into his lungs. So his symptoms of dyspnea are much better."

"Indeed, just as we planned. But what happened to his stroke volume?" asks Phaedrus, as he points to point B in Figure 7-9.

"Well, that went down as we expected, as did his cardiac output. His pressure dropped a bit but it's stabilized. His only symptom now is the dizziness, which we are getting an MRI for."

"Oy veyh," says Phaedrus. "All right, well, maybe it is good that we are talking through this right now. Tell me, Paul, what happened to his perfusion of his brain, I mean his kidneys, when the preload, the stroke volume, the cardiac output, and eventually the mean arterial PERFUSION pressure went down?" Phaedrus emphasizes perfusion, making the "brain/kidney" slip on purpose.

"Well, it went down.... Hey, do you think his dizziness is due to not perfusing his brain?"

"In a word, yes. We'll cancel the MRI in a moment, but for now, let's continue with the metabolic alkalosis. As the perfusion to Kevin Bacon here went down, what happened to the GFR?" Phaedrus points to point D in Figure 7-9.

On the basis of the student's responses, it is apparent that the attending has been through this cycle before, but it is a good reiteration. The ultimate treatment for metabolic alkalosis, assuming it is physiologic, is more preload (fluids). Linking the problem to the physiology will enable the learner to link the problem to its solution.

"It went down," Paul answers.

*"Good, and what happened to the **total** sodium delivery to the JG apparatus?"*

"It went down," Paul replies.

"Good, and based on what you know, what happened to the renin level?"

"Well, I'm sure it went up ... which would have increased the angiotensin and eventually the aldosterone," says Paul.

"Great, and remember, that's the body's way of trying to get more sodium, and thus water, back into the body to offset the low preload that started all of this." Paul nods. "But let's look at what aldosterone does." Phaedrus points to the cell in Figure 7-9. "Remember that aldosterone is a steroid, so it will go to the nucleus to increase transcription of some DNA/RNA—in this case, the transcription of the sodium-potassium ATPase pumps." Phaedrus looks to Paul to see if he is following. Sure that he is, Phaedrus continues. "As these pumps work, what happens to the amount of

sodium that is being pumped into the body from these cells?" Phaedrus points to the enlarged tubular cell to the right of Figure 7-9.

"It should be increased," Paul replies.

"Right, and what would happen to the sodium in the cells?"

"It will be decreased."

"Correct, Paul. And this creates a 'sodium sink' whereby sodium from the urine flows into the cells through a 'turnstile' that kicks out hydrogen into the urine. It's like a revolving door." Phaedrus pauses as he points to the sodium/hydrogen exchange channel on the luminal side of the cell. "Do you see how the sodium flowing into the cell, down its concentration gradient, is exchanging a hydrogen ion into the urine?"

"I see that," Paul replies.

"Okay. So the hydrogen is going to find bicarb that has been filtered from the body into the urine, and for a moment, it will combine to form H_2CO_3. But you know that this is very unstable, and the result will be the generation of CO_2 and H_2O. The H-2-O ... " Phaedrus says in his best Adam-Sandler-in-Waterboy voice, "will continue out as urine. The CO_2, on the other hand, being the 'Patrick Swayze of Ghost,' will walk right through these lipid bylayers of the cells and enter the tubular cells." Phaedrus pauses. Paul is enjoying the references, but he appears to be following this explanation. Phaedrus continues, "Okay, once in the cells, the CO_2 joins with water to make H_2CO_3, which then degrades to make bicarb ... HCO_3, and a free hydrogen, which is recycled to go back to that sodium-hydrogen revolving door we talked about. Are you following all of this, Paul?"

"Sure. I remember this from physiology ... but how does this cause alkalosis?"

"Good question, and here's the answer. The increased concentration of bicarb in the tubular cells pushes the HCO_3 into the body, and there you go ... metabolic alkalosis."

"Wow. So what's my approach in the metabolic alkalosis silo?"

"Real simple, Paul. First, say to yourself, What is the cause of the increased aldosterone? Is it physiologic, that is, an appropriate response in which the kidney is trying to increase preload to offset *the inadequate perfusion pressure? Or is it nonphysiologic, that is, additional aldosterone that is being produced or ingested?"*

"How do I determine that?" Paul asks.

"You can figure this one out. What would you look for to determine if the patient had inadequate perfusion pressure ... go back to Equations 4, 5, and 6."

"Well, their blood pressure would be low."

"Right. And on the other side ... let's say someone had a tumor that was producing aldosterone—which is rare, by the way—what would their preload be?"

"Well, with lots of aldo, there would be lots of salt and water reabsorption, so their preload would be very high."

"And their stroke volume?" asks Phaedrus.

"It would be high as well ..." Paul is following the methods as habit. It makes Phaedrus feel good. "So the cardiac output would be high, and the blood pressure would be high." Paul pauses. "So if it's extra aldosterone, the blood pressure will be high, and if it's physiologic, that is, in response to a low perfusion pressure, the blood pressure will be low."

"You got it, Paul. One more point ... I told you that the 'nonphysiologic' causes of high aldo were rarely due to a tumor. But let me ask you, can you think of any names that rhyme with aldost-ERONE?"

"Well, prednisone ... and cortisone ... and ..."

Phaedrus steps back in. Paul has it. "Have you ever seen a patient who has been on long-term prednisone ... or seen those pictures of patients who have Cushing syndrome?"

"Yeah, I've seen pictures," replies Paul.

"They had lots of swelling, didn't they? Almost like they were absorbing lots and lots of salt and water." Paul nods. "What you can't get from the photos is that they are hypertensive. Think through that for me. Tell me later why that might be, and what you think their bicarb might be." Paul is about to give the answer, but Phaedrus wants him to wait. He continues. "And Paul, it might be worth dialing down our diuresis of Mr. Lawrence."

Essential Components of Teaching Acid-Base

1. Teaching acid-base requires a disciplined approach. The attending should recognize the learner's predisposition to move horizontally, jumping from one part of the assessment (such as respiratory acidosis) to another (such as metabolic alkalosis) and then back again. Eventually the learner becomes confused, trying to use formulas to assess compensation for another compensation.

2. By starting with steps 1 and 2, the attending can focus the student on the primary disorder.

3. The next step is to get the student into one of the silos, which will prevent his jumping around the algorithm. There are really only two silo methods to learn: the respiratory acidosis/alkalosis method and the metabolic acidosis method. Metabolic alkalosis is straightforward in most cases (that is, finding the cause of the increased aldosterone).

4. The respiratory silo method should emphasize acute versus chronic assessment first because this will direct the student to the acuity of the disorder (with very acute disorders, the goal is for the learner to cease cogitation and begin immediate treatment of the patient) and enable interpreting the bicarbonate change (Does the learner need to address another problem and enter another silo?).

5. The critical component to teaching the metabolic acidosis silo is that the learner understand what defines the anion gap. With this understanding, she will be able to see that nongap acidoses are due to a loss of bicarbonate with a gain of chloride: RTAs and diarrhea. Gap acidoses are due to a loss of bicarbonate (because of an added H+), with a nonchloride anion.

6. The metabolic acidosis silo should end with a discussion of the "gap-gap" (addressed by asking what the bicarbonate was before the acidosis occurred and then using Winter's formula (Is the P_{CO_2} appropriate for this level of acidosis?), to determine whether the learner needs to enter another silo for a second or third disorder.

❖ Chest Pain

Purpose

Chest pain is perhaps the most common of admitting diagnoses to the inpatient ward. The risk to the learner is that she comes to see chest pain as merely a "rule out myocardial infarction" routine, governed by a protocol that does not integrate clinical reasoning. This dialogue does not address the intricacies of managing chest pain (which is beyond the scope of this book), but it does illustrate an essential teaching point for the attending: Learners have to have a method that enables them to consider the nonmyocardial causes of chest pain.

Setting, Cast of Characters, and Abbreviations

The team is on-call. Phaedrus, the attending, is conducting attending rounds when the team gets a call from the emergency department for a new admission. With him are Paul, the student; Stef, the intern; and Moni, the resident.

The following abbreviations are used in this dialogue: ABCs = airway, breathing, circulation; CT = computed tomography; EKG = electrocardiogram; ER = emergency room; GFR = glomerular filtration rate; ICU = intensive care unit; ID = Infectious Diseases; MRI = magnetic resonance imaging.

Dialogue

"Dr. Phaedrus, we just received a page from the ER. They have an admission for us to see. Should we continue rounds or go see him?" asks Stef.

"We'll, it looks like we have four patients remaining. Is that correct?"

"Yes, I think that's right."

"Let me ask you. Are any of these four patients going home today, critically ill, or needing rate-limiting tests?"

The attending capitalizes on the opportunity to teach the team prioritization by pointing to the "three Ds:" disability, diagnostics, and discharge.

"We've already rounded on those going home today. All four are stable … I don't think any of the four are at risk for dying or going to the unit. What's a rate-limiting test?" asks Stef.

"Let me put it another way. Is anyone in need of a test or procedure that takes a long time to complete, and that will yield infor-

mation that will change our management later today. For example, a CT, MRI, or a consultation?"

"Actually, yes. We need ID to see Mr. Saint … you'll remember he's the man with HIV and cryptomeningitis. I think he might be able to go home, but ID wanted to see him before we discharged him. And Neurology wanted an MRI on Ms. Spangle, our 35-year-old woman with multiple sclerosis, before they saw her," says Stef.

"Great. Let's do this. Go write the orders for the MRI and give ID a call. I'll head to the ER with Paul, and I'll meet you there. We can round on the remaining four patients after we see this admission. If we need to review the MRI, we can do it at that time."

It is far enough into the rotation that the attending elects to correlate his surrogate assessments of the student's clinical reasoning (the admission note and oral case presentations) with the gold standard (actually watching the student conduct the history and exam).

"So, Paul, let's go see Mr. Flanders, and I want you to take the history."

"Uh, okay." Paul begins to dig in his lab coat to find a laminated, fourfold card with questions to ask. Phaedrus recognizes the move.

"But here's what I want you to do. Put that card away. I just want you to go in there with me, and find out the chief complaint. Then I want you to ask each of the questions on the FAR COLDER mnemonic: the frequency, associated symptoms, radiation, chronology, onset, location, duration, exacerbating and relieving positions. Can you do that?"

"Okay. FAR COLDER … I remember that."

"All right, that's all I want you to do. Then we are going to leave the room and talk about a differential diagnosis based upon what information you garnered from the FAR COLDER. Then we'll go back in together to ask some more questions based upon your differential diagnosis."

Phaedrus and Paul enter the room. Paul performs the first part of the history, using the 'FAR COLDER' approach, and then both exit the room. At this time, Stef and Moni arrive at the ER.

"Okay, Paul, what is your method for approaching chest pain?"

"I don't really have one."

Stef interjects, "We usually just use the chest pain protocol. It seems to work."

There is nothing wrong with protocols, but implicit in their use is that the physician has enough clinical experience to know when to exit the protocol because of circumstances unique to the patient. Most students and residents do not have that experience, and they often rely on protocols because they are an easier (though mindless) way to treat patients without having to invest intellectual energy in reasoning through the diagnosis and treatment. The attending wisely redirects the team away from the protocol so that they learn an approach to chest pain.

"Hmmm ... 'seems' might be the operative word. Let's talk through a method together and then you can decide. In doing so, I'm going to try to convince you why blindly following these protocols is not necessarily the best thing. Has the ER ordered a posteroanterior chest film on this patient?"

"Yes, though I thought you didn't want us to jump to diagnostic tests before doing the history and exam," Stef notes.

Many tests can be used as springboards in organizing the learner's approach to a disease: Radiographs, MRIs, and echocardiograms are examples. When the attending elects to use a test as a way of illustrating the method for approaching the disease, he should clearly note that he is using it for that purpose and not for actually reading the test (which would be a violation of the "history first, then tests" standard).

"Correct, you are, Stef. I just want to use it for illustration purposes."

"Okay, it's over here." The team walks to the computer screen where the lateral chest radiograph was uploaded. Phaedrus stands for a second, and then walks over to the nurse.

"Are you taking care of Mr. Flanders?"

"I am," replies the nurse.

"Well, thank you for doing that. I wonder if we can't get a STAT CT ordered for him. Can you take care of that for us?"

"STAT CT. Okay, I'll put it in right now. Is it really STAT?"

"Yes. It's pretty important." Phaedrus returns to the team. Moni looks at Phaedrus. "We'll get to it in a minute." Phaedrus redirects

his attention at the screen. "Okay, Paul. Look at the film. Now, what I want you to imagine is an arrow going through the body, front to back. As the arrow passes each layer of tissue, I want you to think of a cause of chest pain. Are you ready?"

The student's predisposition, made worse as training proceeds, is to jump to myocardial infarction for all presentations of chest pain. The method is designed to prompt the learner to at least consider alternative causes before entering the "chest pain protocol."

"Umm, yeah. Okay."

"You look nervous. Do arrows make you nervous?"

"Yes … I mean … no, not arrows. It's just I haven't read about chest pain yet."

"All right. It's important to me that we get you to a point where you are not nervous. So here's what we are going to do. First, what you read about will flesh out the details you'll need to be a great physician. But I never want you to feel that you have to have read everything about a topic before you practice it. The methods you learn here on the wards are meant to give you an approach to the problem, and I want the approach to guide your reading. Second, I want you to visualize using the method even as you learn it. This will help you master the method in the setting of true stress, such that when the day comes when you are all alone, the method will flow from you with equanimitas … keeping your emotions in check, allowing rational and methodical thought. That's my vision for you, Paul. It will take some time to get you there, but I can if you will, because I'm here to help you. Are you down with that?"

"Sure."

"Okay, here we go. I want you to imagine yourself in the ER … in that third trauma room over there." Phaedrus points to the room down the hall. "Can you see yourself there?"

It doesn't count if the learner can't some day use it. The attending's question places the student in the actual clinical setting, using the skill, thereby raising the level of the emotion in the vision to the same level the student will someday experience. If the student can perform in the vision, at that level of emotion, and still maintain control, the attending can be assured that performance will be preserved.

"Yeah. That's where they take the patients with chest pain."

"That's right, the one with all of the monitors. Can you see yourself there? Three years from now, you are the physician on call, and there is the patient ... A 60-year-old man lying on the table with his shirt unbuttoned. The nurses circling around him, with monitors already hooked up. You're the doctor now, Paul. What are you going to do?"

"Umm, call 911 I guess."

"Well, good choice ... except that you are 911." Phaedrus laughs. "Okay, here is what you are going to do. You are going to walk into the room and ensure that he is breathing and he has a pulse. The ABCs. Then you are going to take the first part of the history. The FAR COLDER ... just like we just did. Can you see yourself doing that?"

"Sure, that's not so hard." Paul's anxiety begins to subside.

"All right. Then you are going to walk over to this computer, and you are going to look at the lateral chest x-ray while the nurses get the EKG."

"Okay, I can see myself doing that."

"Great. So now ... imagine that arrow hitting the chest. What is the first layer of the body as the arrow passes?"

"The skin and muscles."

"Indeed. Stef, can you think of a cause of chest pain that originates from the skin and muscles?" asks Phaedrus.

"Herpes zoster ... shingles for the skin. For the muscles, I would guess costochondritis."

Instead of merely listing the diagnoses and giving the details, the attending is letting the learners build the differential. This is much more powerful for long-term retention because they will already have had one repetition in building the differential. The attending merely adds in the details and corrects their omissions.

"Don't guess, Stef, you're right. Now let me give you some things to ask about and look for when you go back into the room once the differential diagnosis has been constructed. Remember that with shingles, sometimes the pain can precede the rash. The pain will be sharp and constant, limited to one or two dermatomes.

Shingles is rare in young people, but a reasonable diagnosis in the immunocompromised or the elderly. If it's muscle pain, the pain will worsen with movement or pressure on the chest, but don't put too much stock in that. Many causes of chest pain will worsen with pressure applied to the chest. Okay, Paul, what tissue layer is next?"

The way in which information is presented to learners is the way that they will most easily recall it. The attending is giving the learners the questions they should be thinking about for each diagnosis by linking the characteristics of each diagnosis as it is presented. This will make it easier for them to recall what questions should be asked, and what should be looked for on exam, when the learners later evoke this method for a different patient.

"The bones," Paul replies.

"Stef, causes?" asks Phaedrus.

"Well, rib fractures, or metastatic lesions to the bone."

"Good. And questions about trauma to the chest or symptoms of cancer might be useful. Again, metastatic cancer is a higher probability as patients age, especially those who have not had regular age-appropriate cancer screening. Something worth asking about … Paul, what's next?"

"The pleural lining."

"Well done, Paul. I thought you would skip past that and go to the lungs. Moni, your turn, causes?"

"Well, pleuritis from, say, lupus … or just an empyema or pneumonia that is peripheral."

"Great. For all of these, the pain will be worse with inspiration. For pneumonia or empyema, you might also get a history of cough with sputum production or fever. Again, some things to ask about to change your pretest probabilities. What's next, Paul?"

"The lungs."

Stef jumps back in, "So that would be pneumonia, pulmonary embolism, or alveolar hemorrhage. I would ask the same questions as above, I guess, but also add some questions about stasis, hypercoagulable conditions, and leg swelling."

"Now we're cooking with gas. Well done, Stef." Phaedrus points to the pericardium. "Can you think of any causes of inflammation of the pericardium?"

"Pericarditis and myocarditis."

"Indeed. I'll give you the full list of pericarditis diseases later, but for now remember that any disease that traverses the chest lymphatics has a shot of dropping off into the pericardium. So ... lung cancer, lymphoma, breast cancer, sarcoid, tuberculosis, viruses, and finally, serositis, like you might see with lupus or with renal failure. Now, Paul, what's next?"

"Acute coronary syndrome."

"Good, but what do you mean by acute coronary syndrome?"

"I don't know. I guess that means a heart attack."

The downside to the apprenticeship model is that learners may merely mimic their superiors without fully understanding what a word means. If this is in doubt, the attending should inquire of the student exactly what he means by the term.

"Well, that's right, Paul, but say what you mean, and mean what you say. Myocardial infarction, unstable angina, and stable angina are good words to describe inadequate oxygen to the heart muscle. Myocardial infarction means that there has been actual damage to the muscle; unstable angina implies that the chest pain is due to thrombus in a coronary artery, and angina implies that the chest pain is due to a coronary artery stenosis, but not necessarily with an unstable plaque and/or thrombus. The distinction is important, since if it is myocardial infarction, we need to be thinking about immediately moving the patient to the cath lab for immediate intervention. If it is unstable angina, then we need to be thinking about anticoagulation. Regular angina is secondary to a fixed plaque and usually increased myocardial work ... like you might see with tachycardia of any cause, exercise or hypertensive crisis."

"The EKG would be good for all three." Paul interjects.

"Now you're getting it. You're letting your method drive your tests, not the other way around. I'm sure we'll be talking much more about these later, but let's stay focused on finishing our method. What's the tissue behind the heart?"

"Well, there's the esophagus and the aorta." Paul points to the screen.

"Moni? What are the causes?"

"I would think about esophagitis, gastroesophageal reflux disease, esophageal rupture ... and then an aneurysm."

"Perfect. How would you diagnose an aneurysm?"

"Well, there would be an enlarged mass behind the heart ... " Moni stops in midsentence.

"Wow, that aorta looks kind of big, huh?" Paul says, pointing to the screen. *"So that's why you ordered the STAT CT."*

"Yes ... congratulations, Paul." Phaedrus pats Paul on the shoulder. *"You've just diagnosed your first dissecting aneurysm."* Phaedrus pauses. *"We'll finish the history after the CT comes back."* Phaedrus begins to walk away.

"And Paul ... "

"Yes, Dr. Phaedrus."

"Don't ever forget this feeling. It's what is almost always on the other side of a really good method."

"I won't. I promise you, I won't."

Essential Components of Teaching Chest Pain
1. The attending should empower the resident with a method that enables considering each of the diagnoses that could cause chest pain.
2. Once the method is established, the learner should be trained to ask questions and order diagnostic tests that would increase or decrease the probability of each of the diagnoses being considered. This will move the student away from defaulting to the myocardial infarction protocol.
3. Once a diagnosis has been established, the attending can return the learner to using the management protocol appropriate for that diagnosis.

❖ Antibiotics

Purpose

The use of antibiotics is one of the most common decisions on the inpatient wards. Unfortunately, the complexity of this decision frequently causes learners to default to an inappropriate and thoughtless default decision. The number of antibiotic choices and combinations, and the number of indications (types of infections), frequently results in learners defaulting to "broad-spectrum antibiotics," with some learners not even knowing what those three words mean.

This dialogue is meant to provide an approach to empirical antibiotic use, and to provide the learner with the general rules that define initial antibiotic decision-making. A discussion of antibiotic use for each infection is beyond the scope of this book, and addressing all of the possible exceptions to the general rules is also not possible to integrate into one teaching script. This dialogue, however, operates under the principle that "perfection is sometimes the enemy of the good," and that failing to provide learners with a method of general rules can lead to the adverse consequences of prescribing excessive antibiotics or prescribing with no rational basis for their decision.

Before proceeding with this method, the attending physician should make it clear that this is a method designed to 1) establish some general rules as to what specific antibiotics can and cannot do, 2) explain that there are many exceptions to the rules, 3) show that by understanding the rules, the learner will be in a better position to understand and assimilate the exceptions, 4) explain that the method is for empirical choices only (and that cultures and sensitivities, when available, should guide subsequent antibiotic selection), and 5) reinforce that the learner will still be accountable for knowing which types of bacteria affect different parts of the body (for example, determining what level of coverage is required for the pneumonia vs. cholecystitis). But the overall message of the method is this: There should be a reason for why antibiotics are chosen, and the choice should not be a blind default to the most potent antibiotic available.

Setting, Cast of Characters, and Abbreviations

The team is on call. The attending, Phaedrus, has touched based with the team at the conclusion of his solo afternoon rounds, during which he has completed his billing, coding, and second visits for the day. The discussion begins with Paul, the medical student, who is later joined by Moni, the resident, and Stef, the intern.

The following abbreviations are used in this dialogue: MRSA = methicillin-resistant *Staphylococcus aureus*; PCN = penicillin; TMP-SMX = trimetho-prim–sulfamethoxazole; VRE = vancomycin-resistant enterococci. The following brand names are also used, followed by the generic names: Augmentin = amoxicillin–clavulanate; Timentin = ticarcillin–clavulanate; Unasyn = ampicillin–sulbactam; Zosyn = piperacillin–tazobactam.

Dialogue

"Paul, what are you up to?"

"Well, I have a patient, but I'm not sure I'm ready to present him yet."

"That's okay, tell me what you are doing now," says Phaedrus.

"Well, we have a 42-year-old man who presented with a fever. We have a bunch of tests pending. I'm just trying to decide what types of antibiotics to start."

"Sounds good. Maybe we could do this part together," Phaedrus says.

"That would be great, since I have no idea which of these drugs I should choose," replies Paul.

"Well, what are you thinking of thus far?"

"I guess I want something with broad coverage," Paul replies.

"What does 'broad coverage' mean, Paul?"

"Uh … I don't really know. It's just what everyone says."

"Indeed. Who would opt for razor-narrow coverage? Well, tell me what you are thinking about starting."

"I'm thinking ciprofloxacin, piperacillin-tazobactam, and imipenem."

"Good God! Sounds like he might die, huh?"

"Really?" Paul looks alarmed.

"No, not really. I'm just being dramatic. Those are some pretty big guns for a patient like this, unless of course he really is that sick. Are you sure you need all of those?"

"Broad coverage," like "acute coronary syndrome," is one of those terms that learners will have adopted from their superiors, but may not have understood what it means. Similar to blindly following an acute coronary syndrome protocol, novice physicians may evoke multiple antibiotics as an easy way of "not missing anything" without applying the appropriate thought to what is required for a particular patient.

"No, I'm not sure at all."

"Well, tell me how you came to select those drugs." Phaedrus says.

"Well, last month that's what I saw in the ICU. I guess that was wrong, huh?"

"No, not necessarily wrong for the patient you had in the ICU. But remember that each patient's needs are unique; what was done last is not necessarily best for the patient that comes next. Every patient is different, Paul, and I want you to have a method that allows you to adapt to each unique patient."

Disparaging past teaching, teachers, or lessons, even if they were wrong, is daunting to learners because it inspires the internal dialogue, *"Wow, I wasted my time in the past. I wonder if what I am learning here might also someday be wrong. I don't want to waste more time."* This sentiment is the beginning of the learner's mentally checking out. The attending here validates the correct part of previous teaching, and then adds to it.

"Well, what's wrong with using a lot of antibiotics? It won't hurt him."

"Let me give you a method for using empiric antibiotics while you are waiting for the cultures to come back. And at the end of it, I'll swing back to your question and try to make the case that using too many drugs might actually hurt him." Phaedrus takes out a sheet of paper and lays it down lengthwise. "Paul, have a look at this sheet of paper. Now imagine that this is a wall. And your task is to paint over blemishes in the wall as they appear. Let's say a scratch in the paint occurs over on the far left side of the wall." Phaedrus draws a small asterisk to the left of the page. "Are you going to paint the whole wall just to cover that one spot?"

"Well, no, of course not. I would just paint that spot."

"Right. And let's say that spot was ... oh, say, 2 feet off the ground. Are you going to bring in a ladder to paint that spot, such that you stand on the bottom rung and have to reach down and around the ladder to paint the spot?"

"No, of course not. I'd just stand on the floor and paint it."

"Good. But let's say the spot was high up on the right side of the wall. What would you do then?"

"Well, I would then bring in the ladder to reach it."

"Right, and where would you position the ladder? Far to the left, or far to the right?"

"Well, far to the right, of course."

"Indeed. And if there were multiple dings we needed to paint over, then we would probably have to have more paint ... maybe a couple of quarts ... something that would cover the whole wall. Right?" Phaedrus asks.

"That sounds right," Paul replies.

The attending takes the student through a brief Socratic dialogue to emphasize the rationale of a response that is proportional to the need. The painting metaphor works well because the natural synchronization to the concept of "coverage" will be easy. The ladder, too, works as a good metaphor, since climbing up the ladder can actually impair the painter's ability to reach spots lower down on the wall, and certainly impairs his ability to reach spots on the other side (left to right) of the wall. The attending is anticipating that the student is approaching antibiotics the way many learners do—the false belief that escalating to higher-level antibiotics is without consequence. In reality, there is usually a price to pay: Escalating to higher-level antibiotics may sacrifice some coverage that was provided by lower-level antibiotics (being at the top of the ladder makes reaching down to the bottom of the wall more difficult).

"Okay, Paul," Phaedrus continues, "If we are going to paint this wall, we are going to need to know which parts of the wall need to be painted. Am I right?"

"Yes, that seems reasonable."

"And that's where it isn't so easy, because in medicine we don't always know where we need 'coverage.'" Paul suddenly makes the link between "holes in the wall" and "holes in antibiotic coverage." Phaedrus continues. "But often times, Paul, we can figure it out. And when we can't figure out where the 'hole' is in coverage, then we will be forced to paint the whole wall. That is what you referred to earlier as 'broad coverage.'"

Paul smiles. "I think I see where you are going. When we know that we only need coverage in a specific part of the wall, then we

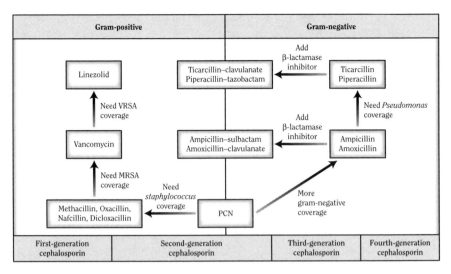

Figure 7-10 The antibiotic ladder. A note about cephalosporins: First-generation have gram-positive coverage, including *Staphylococcus* species; second-generation cover gram-positive organisms, *Haemophilus* organisms, *Moraxella* species, and *Streptococcus pneumoniae*; third-generation cover gram-negative organisms; fourth-generation (cefepime) should be reserved for neutropenic fever. PCN = penicillin; MRSA = methicillin-resistant *Staphylococcus aureus*; VRSA = vancomycin-resistant *S. aureus*.

only paint that part of the wall.... That is, we only use the antibiotics need to cover that whole."

"Exactly, Paul. The method that I am going to give you is for empiric antibiotic selection ... when you don't fully know which specific bacteria are present. Once the culture comes back with the species and sensitivities, we'll use that to guide our antibiotic choices. But until then, we still do need a method of selecting antibiotics, because we can't afford to paint the whole wall every time there is a ding. We'll run out of paint."

"So how do we know what is the best choice?" Paul asks.

"Well, to use our analogy, we won't know exactly where the ding in the paint is, but we can guess as to its general area. For example, if a patient has a skin infection, it is most likely strep or staph. Am I right?"

"Sure."

As he speaks, Phaedrus draws the spectrum of gram positive to gram negative across the top of the sheet (Figure 7-10). "So in *that case, we would choose an antibiotic that was good for that part of the wall." Phaedrus points to the "gram positive" title at the top left of the page. "And if it was a reasonably simple infection—that is, we had no concerns for resistance or the severity of the infection—then we stay pretty close to the base of the wall." Phaedrus points to the left lower quadrant of the page.*

"That sounds reasonable. But which drugs go where?"

"And that, Paul, is your antibiotic ladder. So here's the gig. The default antibiotic is penicillin. You always use penicillin unless you have a reason to use something else. This will cover the middle part of the wall toward the base." Phaedrus writes "PCN" at the base of the diagram.

The goal of the attending is not to get the learner to use penicillin. He is starting with penicillin as the base default, knowing that there are several reasons that penicillin is inadequate. But by starting there, he will entice the learner to argue against it, and in doing so, he will prompt the learner to ask the questions that he (the attending) wants the learner to ask later on: "What is present that penicillin will not cover?" The answer to that question will guide the learner to his antibiotic selection. The method stimulates reason ("What is the reason to move up the ladder?") and not a cookbook with which to choose antibiotics.

"Really? Why? I haven't seen people use penicillin. Seems old-fashioned."

"Well, there are several reasons, First, penicillin is 'cidal' in vivo, and the quick kill of the bacteria is what we're after. The longer you let bacteria live, the greater the exponential increase in the bacterial, and antigenic, load. Second, can you think of the last time you saw penicillin toxicity?"

"Umm, no," Paul replies.

"That's because it doesn't exist. It is a salt, hence the 'PCN-' when written in shorthand. And it is purely excreted by the kidneys. That means you only have to adjust the dose based on the GFR, and there is very little to worry about with respect to hepatotoxicity or drug-drug interactions for drugs cleared by the liver. And you'll appreciate that freedom, Paul, especially for patients with other medication and multisystem disease. The final reason is that it is safe in pregnancy, and many of your patients might not know that they are pregnant at the time that you give the antibi-

otic. But the biggest reason to start with penicillin, Paul, is ... Do you have a guess?"

"No."

"Because why use a drug that comes in 200-, 300-, or 400-mg doses when you could use a drug that comes in 1.5 MILLION units?" Phaedrus notes with a smile as he placed his pinkie finger to his lower lip, imitating his best Dr. Evil from the Austin Powers *movies.*

Paul laughs, "Okay, I see your point."

"Seriously, Paul, penicillins are a good class of drug, and I want that to be your default. It will keep you grounded without going crazy on the higher-end drugs that we need to reserve for really serious infections. But should you need to cover a part of the wall that penicillin doesn't cover, then we will need to move up the ladder to a higher-level drug that does provide that coverage." As he speaks, Phaedrus draws four blocks at the base of the diagram. "If we are going to use a ladder, Paul, we'll need a good foundation. So at the base are four blocks that will be the foundation for our 'antibiotic ladder.'"

"Okay, sounds good," Paul replies.

Phaedrus continues, "There are more sophisticated drugs than penicillin as you climb the ladder. But here's the rule I want you to follow: You only move up the ladder if there is a reason to do so. So, let me ask you, are there any bugs that regular penicillin would not cover?"

The attending's goal in this session is not to tell the student what to use when but to teach the student that there should be a reason why he selects the antibiotic he chooses.

"Sure. How about staph?"

"Correct you are. Can you think of a drug that rhymes with '-illin' that would cover staph?"

Paul smiles. "Okay, how about methicillin."

"Yes." Phaedrus filled in the left part of the graph as he speaks. "We'll move up the latter to the 'M-N-Os' to reach the left middle part of the wall. Do you remember that from the alphabet song ... 'M-N-O?" Paul nods. "Okay, methicillin, nafcillin, and oxacillin.

*These are all more or less the same drug, designed to make a peni-
cillin moiety effective against staph. But before we move forward,
Paul, what happened to our gram-negative coverage ... that is,
our ability to paint the right side of the wall, as we moved up the
ladder to the M-N-Os? Look at the spectrum of gram-positive to
gram-negative at the top of the diagram."*

"It looks like we lost some gram-negative coverage."

*"Exactly. The principle of choosing antibiotics is not the same as
choosing a stereo. If you buy a higher-priced stereo, you generally
keep the features of the lower-priced models and then add some.
In choosing a "higher-level" antibiotic, you gain some features—
in this case, staph coverage, but you may lose some features as
well—in this case, some gram-negative coverage. So lesson
learned. But back to our diagram, is there anything that methicillin wouldn't cover?"*

Novice physicians will miss this point, entering the antibiotic world
thinking that escalation to "higher-level" antibiotics guarantees that what
was covered by "lower-level" antibiotics will be preserved. The "antibiotic
ladder" method is used to illustrate what is lost as the student escalates to
higher-level antibiotics.

*"Well, some staph is methicillin resistant ... that's MRSA," Paul
replies.*

*"Indeed, and remember that part of your history will be in trying
to determine who might have MRSA. We'll come back to that."
Phaedrus pauses. "But remember, we said that simple infections
were those at the base of the wall. But you're saying, 'Wow, this
could be a resistant infection.' So that being the case, we need to
provide coverage for the top of the wall. So up the ladder we go.
What drug would 'vanquish' penicillin-resistant staph?"*

"Umm, vancomycin?" Paul says with a smile.

*"Spot on correct. But look again, Paul. What happened to our
gram-negative coverage—that is, our ability to paint the right
side of the wall—as we went to vancomycin?"*

"It's substantially less—in fact, it looks like not at all."

*"Substantially right! Well done. Just remember that to move up
the ladder, we have to have a good reason to do so, and it will be
your history and pretest probabilities as to which infection you*

think might be present that will drive that. But as you do so, move up judiciously ... as you are likely to lose some coverage as you do so." Phaedrus pauses for effect. "Okay, let me take you back to penicillin. Is there anything else that penicillin would not cover?"

"Well, it looks like most gram-negative bugs."

"Most is right. It might have some coverage for weak gram-negatives, in the mouth, for example, but if you ever need true gram-negative coverage, you'll need something more than regular penicillin. Can you think of a drug that rhymes with '-illin' that would cover gram-negative bugs?"

"Ampicillin?"

"Say it with pride, Paul. Absolutely right. And add on amoxicillin, since these are the same drug. Ampicillin comes intravenously; amoxicillin comes orally. Both are designed to extend the coverage of penicillin to give greater gram-negative coverage. Once again, Paul, what happened to the gram-positive coverage ... that is, our ability to paint the left side of the wall?"

"It's less."

"Indeed. Ampicillin and amoxicillin will still give you some gram-positive coverage, especially for strep, though not for staph. You will, however, find some occasions where regular penicillin is actually a better drug for strep ... especially strep cellulitis." Phaedrus pauses. "Now, is there anything that amoxicillin and ampicillin wouldn't cover? Because if there is, we have to move up the ladder once again."

"Hmmm .... Oh, pseudomonas."

Phaedrus extends a handshake. "Well done. If we need pseudomonas coverage, we'll need to go up the ladder to piperacillin or ticarcillin. These are more or less the same drug, both intravenous only, and both designed to extend coverage to pick up pseudomonas."

"But what if I need both gram-positive and gram-negative coverage? What if I need to paint the whole wall?"

Phaedrus nods. "Well, the first step is to always ask yourself that very question. 'Do I really need both gram-positive and gram-negative coverage?' If the answer is no, then tailor your therapy according to which part of the wall you need to cover ... use the ladder if you must. If the answer is yes, then, well ... we're probably going to need more paint."

Paul smiles.

"But we do have some options." Phaedrus continues, "Let me ask you this. How does staph develop resistance to penicillins and the other beta-lactams? Not MRSA .... Just the regular staph."

"By a beta-lactamase ... oh, we could add a beta-lactamase inhibitor."

"Indeed we could. And if you add a beta-lactamase inhibitor to ampicillin, you get Unasyn. If you do the same with amoxicillin, you get Augmentin. We could also do the same with piperacillin ... it becomes Zosyn, and to ticarcillin ... it becomes Timentin." Phaedrus draws in the arrows on the diagram. "Do you see how we've extended the gram-positive coverage by adding the beta-lactamase inhibitors?"

"Can we add something to methicillin to make MRSA susceptible to it?"

"Unfortunately, no. MRSA resistance is due to a different mechanism ... so the beta-lactamase inhibitors won't work."

The student in this dialogue is asking all of the correct questions. Should a student not ask these questions, however, it is important for the attending to point out that extending an antibiotic's coverage with beta-lactamase inhibitors is good only for the bacteria that have developed resistance to the standard drug by way of a beta-lactamase.

"Okay, well, how about adding something to methicillin to make it cover gram-negatives?"

"Unfortunately, that's not an option. You have to choose to go up the right side of the ladder if you want gram-negative coverage." Phaedrus pauses. "Oh, one important point, Paul. With respect to Zosyn and Timentin ... adding the beta-lactamase inhibitor only confers greater gram-positive coverage. It will not make pseudomonas that is resistant to piperacillin or ticarcillin susceptible to these drugs."

"But what if you do have pseudomonas that is resistant to these drugs?"

"Well, three thoughts. First, this is not a position you want to be in—pseudomonas is a very lethal bug, and you would like to have all available options to treat it. Second, to answer your very first question——this is how you can hurt your patient by using several broad-spectrum drugs when they aren't needed. Antibiotic resistance is a public health problem, but it can also develop in your individual patient over the course of weeks to months. The ladder shows you to use these "top of the ladder" drugs sparingly, such that when you do need them, there is a greater chance that the bug will not have already seen them. And third, specific to your last question—there is the top-top of the ladder ... the imipenems and the quinolones. And that is a fine time to use those."

Evoking public health concerns of "antibiotic resistance" is not an effective strategy in deterring indiscriminant antibiotic use. In the moment, the physician will default to the person in front of him in needlessly expanding coverage. When the issue is made personal to the patient (too many antibiotics will lead to resistance in *this* patient), the message is more compelling.

"Hmmm." Paul looks at his treatment plan, clearly with an eye on changing it. "But what about the boxes at the bottom of the ladder? The foundation?"

Phaedrus writes in "First," "Second," "Third," and "Fourth."

"Oh, the cephalosporins."

"Indeed. Note as the generations increase from left to right, the gram-positive coverage decreases and the gram-negative coverage increases. I'll be honest in telling you that it is more like a ring than it is a line ... the fourth-generation cephalosporins, cefepime, actually have pretty good gram-positive coverage. But it is important to me, Paul, that you save that drug. That's what I use for neutropenic fever, and for these patients with very little immune function left, I really need this drug to work. If you use it indiscriminately, the probability of resistance goes up. Will you promise me that, Paul?"

"I promise .... So what about the quinolones, I see those used a lot."

"Yeah, a lot more than they should be used. Here's the reason, and I want you to know this so you don't interpret my message as merely a bias or personal preference. There are two bugs that you

don't want to meet: VRE and Pseudomonas. And let me take you through the history of both; I think you will understand why the ladder exists the way that it does." Phaedrus pauses.

The rationale of the "antibiotic ladder" is to direct novice physicians to appropriate antibiotics, but it also exists to prevent antibiotic complications. These complications will be far from novice physicians' minds unless the method alerts them to them.

"Let's start with vancomycin-resistant enterococcus. Where do you suppose "ENTEROcoccus" lives, Paul?"

Paul smiles. "In the gut?"

"Indeed ... in the 'entero' ... the bowel. What else lives in the bowels?"

"Gram-negative rods."

"Indeed ... hence they are called the 'enterics.' Now, enterococcus is more or less resistant to two classes of antibiotics: the cephalosporins and the quinolones. For enterococcus to develop resistance, it has to undergo a mutation. And for every 10 to the 16th division, a meaningful mutation occurs. So how could you get enterococcus to undergo 10 to the 16th divisions? Keep in mind, it is living in the bowel, competing for space and food with the enterics."

"Well, it would have to divide unchecked ... if you got rid of the enterics, it could really grow."

"Indeed. And if you were 'Dr. Evil,' which drug would you choose to get rid of the enterics, while not also killing the enterococcus?"

"I guess I would choose ... oh ... the quinolones ... or the third-generation cephalosporins. Both have great gram-negative coverage, but as you said, no enterococcus coverage."

"Nice work, Paul. Exactly the way I want you to see it. Quinolones do have their place, but for some targeted indications. They do have pseudomonas coverage, and I'll come to that in a second. They are also great at deep tissue penetration, like into the bones or deep muscles or low-perfusion organs. Things like osteomyelitis or prostatitis are good indications for quinolones. But the important point is this. Indiscriminate use of quinolones or third-generation cephalosporins ... leads to 'sterilization of the enterics in the gut,' leaving enterococcus to grow unchecked ... because it is resistant to these drugs ... eventually finding its way

to the 10 to the 16th divisions necessary to develop a vancomycin-resistant mutation."

"Well, what about pseudomonas? You said it was the other one."

"Indeed. And my reading assignment for you, Paul, is to learn about pseudomonas, and who gets it. I want you to have a good sense of which patients are at risk for the infection ... that is, I want you to be able to accurately assess a pretest probability for pseudomonas. This is key, because what we don't want to do, as I said earlier, is expose pseudomonas to all of our antipseudomonal drugs by indiscriminate prescribing, such that when we actually need the coverage, the coverage doesn't work. There are four classes of drugs that are good for pseudomonas coverage: the top-of-the-ladder beta-lactams (that is, piperacillin, ticarcillin, ceftazidime), the quinolones, the 'penems' (carbapenem, imipenem), and gentamycin, tobramycin." Phaedrus pauses as Paul writes this down.

"The thing is, Paul, people with pseudomonas—and you'll find this in your reading—are usually pretty sick and debilitated. The common patients at risk are the elderly, those that have been in a health care setting for a long time, patients with burns, and those with cystic fibrosis. The upshot is that multisystem disease is not a rare event for them, which means you may lose the luxury of using one of the four classes of drugs: gentamycin or tobramycin. In these patients, pseudomonas can also be very aggressive, and it is often worth having double coverage. But you can see how losing one of these classes because of renal failure, and losing another class due to resistance, can really put you in a pinch when it comes to choosing a regimen that will work."

The attending spends extra time on pseudomonas, and assigns reading to that end as well. Novice physicians are prone to escalating to pseudomonas coverage without fully knowing who might be at risk for pseudomonas. It is fear that drives the practice.

"I can see that." Paul pauses for thought. "How about anaerobes? I hear that discussed a lot."

"Good question, Paul." Phaedrus extends the now-familiar hand-shake. "There are two types of anaerobes. Those that are B. frag, and those that are not. B. frag is an intraabdominal or pelvic organism, which is why you probably heard your surgery instructors refer to infections 'above the diaphragm' versus those 'below

the diaphragm.' When they say the latter, they are talking about covering B frag. B frag *needs its own coverage ... namely, metronidazole. Non-*B frag *is usually covered by the penicillins. It's the reason that prophylaxis against endocarditis in those having mouth surgery is penicillin."*

"Hmm. Makes sense. How about sulfas? You mentioned those."

"Sulfa drugs such as TMP/SMX are actually really good drugs. Think of them as 'primer paint.' Inexpensively, we can more or less paint the whole wall!" Paul smiles as Phaedrus continues. *"They provide good coverage for all of the gram-positive bugs, including some MRSA, and really good gram-negative coverage, with the exception of pseudomonas. They are also really cheap, and as I said before, they have great tissue penetration."*

"Why don't we use those more?"

"A really good question, Paul. We probably should. The downside to sulfas is that they can cause a rash, and in rare cases, Stevens-Johnson–like drug reactions. Probably not as safe as penicillins, but still a very good drug. Read about it." Phaedrus looks at his pager. *"Okay, I have to go. But five last principles to tell you, Paul. First, I want to remind you that this is for empiric treatment only. It is still upon you to make sure that you obtain the appropriate cultures, and once you have the bug identified, treat according to its resistance pattern. And if the patient is very sick, then all bets are off. Expand your coverage to address all causes. Second, you are going to have to spend some time with the textbooks learning about what types of bugs typically affect what parts of the body. For example, what bugs typically cause pneumonia versus head and neck infections versus meningitis. You have to know this to walk up the ladder and choose the appropriate drugs. Read about that. As the rotation goes on, we'll talk more about each location of infection.*

"Third, remember that each patient is unique. You'll have to consider all of the patient's history in choosing the right antibiotics ... his allergies, his past infections, the age of the patient, et cetera. Fourth, there are many exceptions to the guidelines I just gave you. Know that I know that. But for you at this stage, I want you to know the general principles first. That way you'll at least have a framework upon which you can learn the exceptions. If we did it the other way around, you would be lost inside that Sanford

Guide *forever. And finally, remember that not every fever is due to an infection. Wise of you to think of infection first, but remember to think about drug fever and other causes, especially if the fever doesn't get better as you do the treatment. I'll share a method with you on fevers later. Okay, Paul, this is 7 East calling. I need to get to that family conference. I'll catch up with you later."*

Essential Components of Teaching Antibiotics

1. Expect that learners will be sufficiently daunted at the prospect of using antibiotics that they will either mimic what they have last seen done or default to overly aggressive "broad-spectrum" antibiotics.

2. Establishing a spectrum of coverage (gram positive to gram negative on the horizontal axis, and simple to severe on the vertical axis) will at least provide the "skeleton of rules" on which the student can start hanging specific exceptions to the rules.

3. It is important to emphasize that drug resistance can have real-time consequences for individual patients and that judicious use of antibiotics has a rationale that is more than just public health.

Index